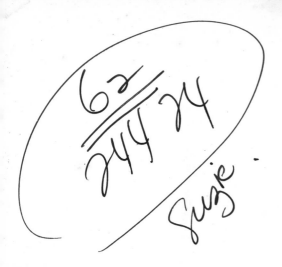

6$\frac{2}{}$
$\frac{244}{}$ 24
Susie -

The
Face and
Body
Book

Suzanne Patricia Niko Archer
69 Eastcombe Ave,
Charlton,
London SE7 7JS.

The Face and Body Book

General Editor
Miriam Stoppard

Pan Books
London and Sydney

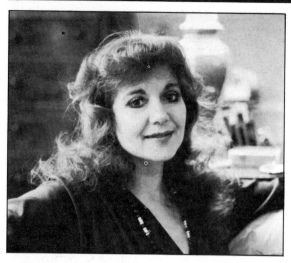

General Editor
Miriam Stoppard MD, MRCP

After qualifying at Kings College, University of Durham, Miriam Stoppard practised as a doctor for eight years, specializing for some time in dermatology. In 1968 she entered the pharmaceutical industry, becoming Managing Director of a pharmaceutical company. She has made numerous appearances on television and radio and has written many articles for newspapers and magazines.

Her first book, *Miriam Stoppard's Book of Babycare*, published in 1977, achieved a remarkable balance of hard fact, sound commonsense, medical insight and lively, expert opinion. It was followed in 1980 by a practical guide to everyday healthcare, entitled *Miriam Stoppard's Healthcare*.

Dr Stoppard is married to playwright Tom Stoppard and has two sons and two stepsons.
● *Chapter I, (except pp. 34–47), Sleep, Chapter IV*

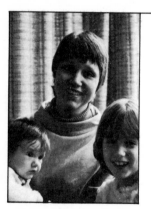

Barbara Dale is a specialist in ante- and post-natal exercises with the National Childbirth Trust. She also runs a body workshop in London. She is co-author with Laura Mitchell of *Simple Movement*.
● *Ante- and Post-natal Exercises*

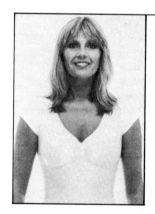

Helene Johnson worked as assistant to Gilda Marx at *Body Design by Gilda* exercise studio in Los Angeles. Among the pupils were Jane Fonda and Barbra Streisand. Mrs Johnson now runs exercise courses in England.
● *Indoor Exercises*

First published 1980 by Frances Lincoln Publishers Ltd
This edition published 1981 by Pan Books Ltd,
Cavaye Place, London SW10 9PG

© Frances Lincoln Publishers Ltd 1980
ISBN 0 330 26565 2

Printed and bound in Great Britain by
Morrison & Gibb Ltd, London and Edinburgh

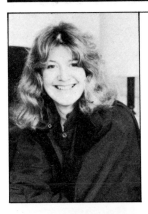

Anne Lambert is a freelance writer and has written features and articles on beauty care and make-up for many women's magazines.
● *Make-up, Manicure, Alexander Principle*

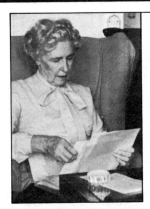

Laura Mitchell MCSP, dip TP has taught physiotherapy and living anatomy for many years. Her method of physiological relaxation is described in her first book *Simple Relaxation*. She is co-author with Barbara Dale of *Simple Movement*.
● *Posture, Massage, Relaxation*

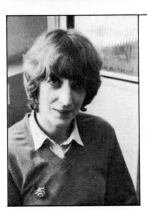

Laura Pank, author of *Women's Words*, has written for many women's magazines, including *Harpers & Queen, Family Circle* and *Cosmopolitan*. She is a keen squash player and skier.
● *A-Z of Exercise, Exercise (pp. 128–129), Exercise Machines and Equipment*

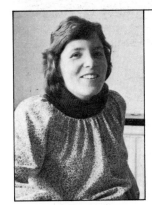

Sally Parsonage BSc, PhD studied nutrition at London University under Professor Yudkin. She has acted as consultant for leading food manufacturers and slimming magazines and has published many articles and research papers on obesity and slimming.
● *Diet and Nutrition*

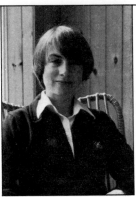

Caroline Richards, beauty editor of *19*, has written on beauty and slimming for many women's magazines, including *Woman's Own* and *Slimmer*. She was Features and Research Editor for *The 1980 Hair Book*.
● *Hair (pp. 34–47)*

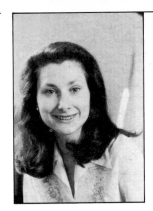

Maxine Tobias is a pupil of B.K.S. Iyengar and has taught the Iyengar method of yoga for many years. She contributed to the yoga section of *The Sunday Times Book of Body Maintenance*.
● *Yoga*

Managing Editor: Daphne Wood
Art Director: Sally Smallwood

Assistant Editor: Clare Meek
Sub-Editor: Kathryn Cave
Designers: Caroline Hillier, Roger Walton, Piers Evelegh
Editorial Secretary: Antonia Demetriadi

Illustrators: Giovanni Caselli, Howard Pemberton, Kathy Wyatt
Photographers: Fausto Dorelli, Chris Harvey
Photographic/Make-up Coordinator: Anne-Marie Mackay

The Publishers would like to thank the following for their help, advice and demonstrations for the Make-up chapter:

Janine Roxborough Bunce and Peter Camburn of **Elizabeth Arden Salon** for Lip Make-up

Eileen Dawson, Eve Gardner and Sue Morris of **Max Factor** for Foundation, Powder, The Art of Camouflage and The Older Face

Vivienne Tomei and Martin Aston of **Revlon** for Eye Make-up

Dennise Choa and Pat Davis of **Helena Rubinstein** for Contour Colour

Natural Good Looks

8   *Exploding the Myths*

10   **Skin**
12   Structure and Function
16   Looking After the Skin
18   Sun and the Skin
20   Facial Skin Care
23   Cleansing and Toning
24   Moisturizing
25   Facial Treatments
26   A-Z of Skin Problems

30   **Hair**
31   Growth, Texture and Colour
34   Equipment and Accessories
36   The Cut and the Style
37   Shampooing
38   Conditioning
39   Blow Drying
40   Setting and Styling
42   Classic Styles
44   Perming and Colouring
46   Body Hair

48   **Eyes**
49   How the Eyes Work
50   Eye Care

52   **Ears, Nose and Mouth**
53   The Interconnecting System

56   Teeth and Gums
58   Mouth Care

60   **Neck and Throat**

62   **Shoulders and Back**
64   Back Care

66   **Hips, Pelvis and Bottom**
67   Structure, Size and Shape

70   **Breasts**
72   Structure, Function and Care
74   Breast Self-examination

76   **Abdomen and Waist**
77   The Effects of Pregnancy

80   **Arms and Hands**
81   Care of the Arms and Hands
82   Nails : Growth and Care
84   Manicure

86   **Legs and Feet**
88   Legs : Structure and Shape
90   Care of the Legs and Feet
93   Pedicure

Make-up

180   *A Facial Statement*

182   Equipment and Accessories
184   Foundation
186   Powder
187   Contour Colour
192   Eyes

200   Lips
202   Party Tricks
205   The Art of Camouflage
208   The Older Face

The Essentials

94 *A Coordinated Approach*

96 **Diet and Nutrition**
98 Proteins, Carbohydrates and Fats
100 Fibre, Minerals and Vitamins
104 A Well-balanced Diet
106 Eating Habits
108 Food Problems and Problem Foods
110 Healthfoods, Wholefoods and Vegetarianism
112 A Rational Approach to Slimming
118 Calorie Controlled Diet
119 Low Carbohydrate Diet
120 Calories and Carbohydrate Units
122 Protein and Fat in Slimming Diets
124 Crash Diets and Fasting
126 Eating to Gain Weight

128 **Exercise**
130 Posture
132 The Alexander Principle

134 Daily Minimum Exercise Programme
136 Abdomen and Waist
138 Bottom, Hips and Thighs
140 Back
142 Breasts, Arms and Hands
144 Legs and Feet
146 Face, Neck and Shoulders
147 Ante- and Post-natal Exercises
150 A-Z of Exercise
162 Yoga
166 Exercise Machines and Equipment

168 **Relaxation**
170 Physiological Relaxation
172 Massage
176 Facial Massage

178 **Sleep**

Professional Treatments

210 *Improving on Nature*

212 The Range of Possibilities

213 **Skin Treatments**

216 **Cosmetic Surgery**
220 Facial Surgery
225 Body Surgery

230 **Cosmetic Dentistry**

232 **A-Z of Alternative Medicine**

238 **Health Clinics**

242 **Beauty Clinics**

248 **Psychotherapy**

252 Index
256 Acknowledgments

Exploding the Myths

Many women are discouraged from looking after their bodies by the confusing wealth of conflicting lore on beauty care. But the myth that a beautiful face and figure require the investment of more time and money than the average woman can afford can be exploded with an understanding of the body's real needs and how to meet them.

Natural

The first principle of caring for the body and for promoting natural good looks is to understand how the body works. Although it is easy to assume familiarity with the way it functions, there are many common fictions and misunderstandings that bedevil the subject. Only with a true appreciation of the facts and fallacies is it possible to avoid wasting time and money on routines that can be of no benefit and to concentrate on those that are essential for well-being and vitality. An educated approach to common health and beauty problems and their causes and cures helps to minimize their impact. This chapter aims to provide an honest appraisal of beauty care equipment and routines, so allowing the reader to make an informed choice that suits her individual needs.

Good Looks

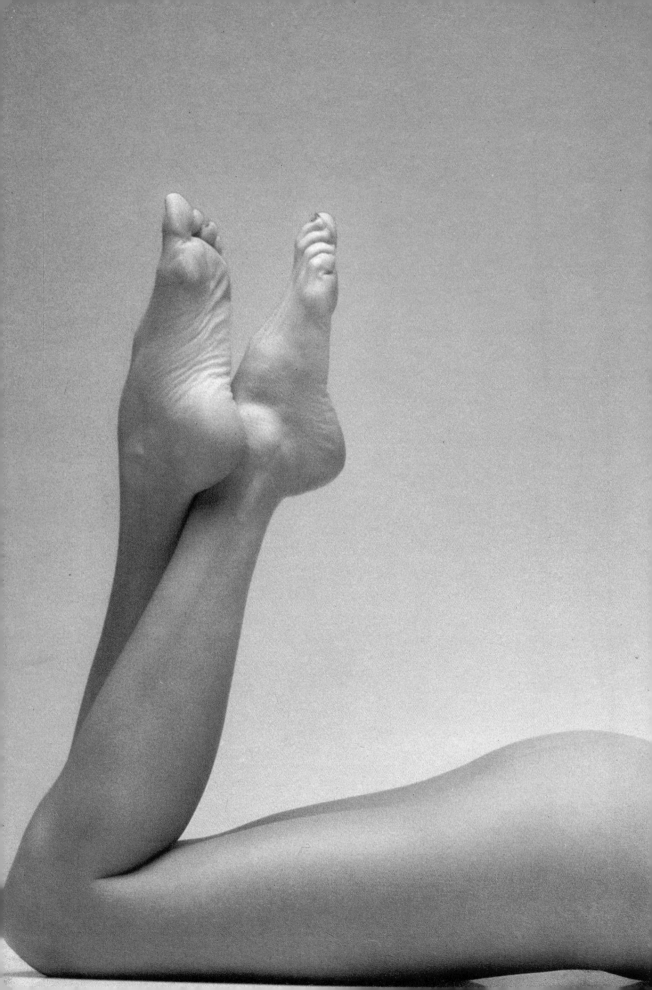

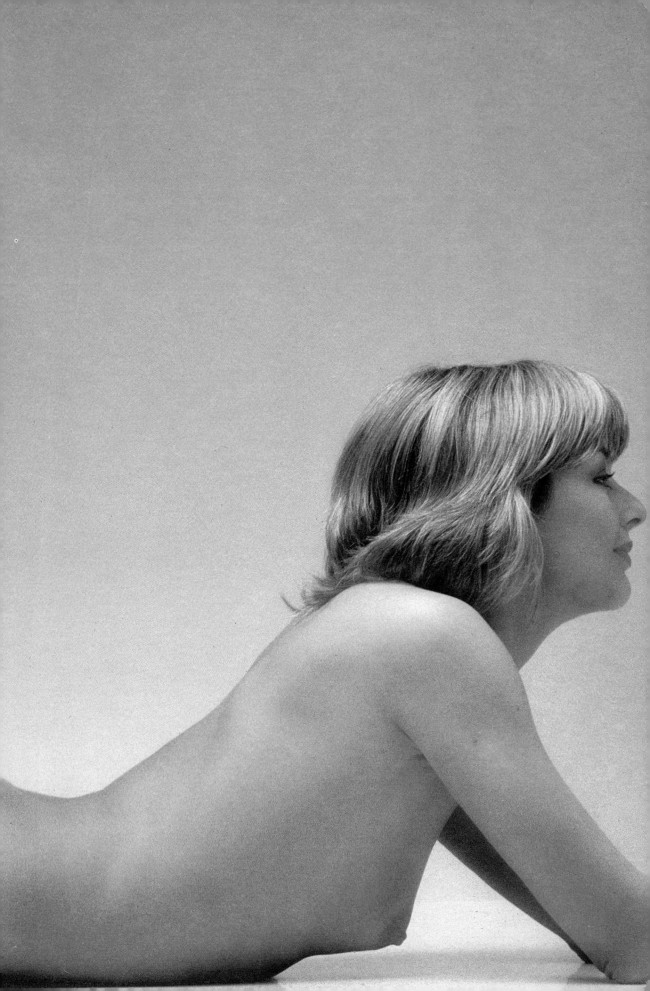

Skin

The skin is the largest organ in the body and one of the most accessible – you can see it and feel it, which can hardly be said of the liver, for example. It is also one of the most interesting organs: it grows from within outwards and is constantly replacing itself; it is involved in some of the most crucial functions of the body; and it is extremely efficient at performing its special tasks.

The skin's four layers

It is useful to think of the skin as composed of four layers: the outer, horny layer of dead cells, then the living, growing epidermis, the dermis immediately beneath that and finally the layer of subcutaneous fat, which varies in thickness in different parts of the body.

Within the epidermis lies the skin's only layer of living, dividing cells. This is called the basal cell layer and it marks the division between the epidermis and dermis. Cells from the basal cell layer bud off, grow, mature, age and ultimately die, moving upwards as they do so through the epidermis to the outer layer of skin. The upper layers of the epidermis are accordingly made up of rather shapeless skeletons of cells, without any cell contents, while the outer, horny layer of skin is just piled up keratin – which is what remains when skin cells have died.

The most obvious function of the epidermis is simply the continual replacement of the outer horny layer, which in its strength and resistance to chemical attack forms a kind of armour plating for the skin. The thickness of the horny layer varies in different parts of the body and is greatest in the areas subjected to most wear and tear, such as the soles of the feet, and, to a lesser extent, the hands. The horny layer of keratin is almost impervious to onslaught from harmful substances, does a lot to prevent moisture evaporating from the skin and also has some anti-bacterial properties.

The epidermis has another, crucially important, function. Research in the early 1960s revealed that in the zone between the dead and the living cells of the epidermis lies a 'membrane' that constitutes the skin's true barrier against penetration. The two surfaces of this barrier between them prevent substances outside the skin getting through to the inner layers and substances on the inside (particularly water) from getting out. So the epidermis shares with the horny layer of skin the work of keeping the skin hydrated.

Within the next layer of skin, the dermis, are the supporting girders of the skin, composed of elastic tissue known as collagen. Through this framework runs a network of nerves, nerve

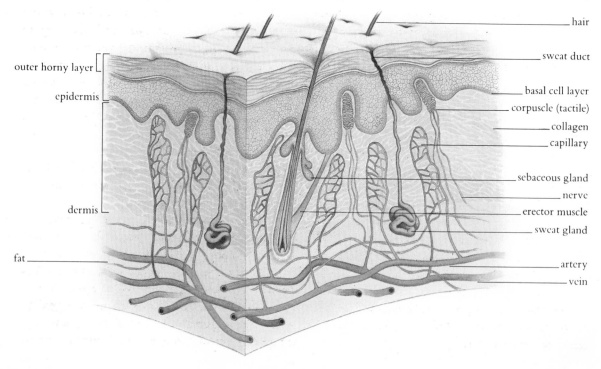

outer horny layer
epidermis
dermis
fat

hair
sweat duct
basal cell layer
corpuscle (tactile)
collagen
capillary
sebaceous gland
nerve
erector muscle
sweat gland
artery
vein

endings and blood vessels (see left). In young healthy skin, collagen is arranged in parallel bundles that lie alongside each other and have the ability to stretch and then resume their original shape. They give young skin its suppleness, smoothness and plumpness. As we get older, the integrity of the collagen bundles is lost, the fibres split, the bundles break up and the parallel arrangement disintegrates. The architecture of the skin crumbles; it sags, wrinkles and becomes thin. These signs of age cannot be prevented and can be removed only by cosmetic surgery, skin peeling or dermabrasion (see pages 213–224). The predisposition to develop them is hereditary so if your parents look young for their age in later life, you have a good chance of doing so too.

Beneath the dermis lies a layer of subcutaneous fat, the main function of which is to provide insulation. Women have more subcutaneous fat than men, concentrated mainly in areas such as the breasts, thighs and bottom. This extra insulation enables us to float better in water and to survive exposure for longer than men.

Blood supply

The skin's extremely rich blood supply is channelled mainly through tiny blood vessels called capillaries. If all the capillaries in the skin were to expand at the same time, they could absorb more than a third of all the blood circulating in the body. This is why we sometimes feel giddy after a hot bath: so much blood has been drawn into the capillaries as part of the process of temperature control (see below) that not enough is reaching the brain. A hard knock or blow can damage the capillaries, causing a bruise. The time this takes to disappear depends on the speed with which the pigments in the blood can be broken down and absorbed; as this happens the bruise gradually changes colour (from purple to brown to yellow) and ultimately vanishes. No medicament applied to the skin will accelerate this.

The strength of the capillaries and their closeness to the skin's surface vary widely from person to person. Some people bruise especially easily; some have capillaries very close to the skin's surface, giving them a rosy-cheeked look in youth and a tendency to develop broken or bluish veins as they get older.

If the skin is injured (cut or torn), the edges of the wound will heal with a bridge of scar tissue. This is a primitive structure – thinner, more stretchy and less even than normal skin. As all healing is accompanied by an increase in blood supply to the site of the injury, a new scar appears pinkish. This colour fades when healing is complete and the extra blood capillaries wither away. The tendency to scar is as variable as bruising: some people get such large, protruding scars that special treatment may be needed, while other people's cuts may heal leaving scarcely a mark behind them.

Nerves

The number of nerves and nerve endings in an area of skin depends on its situation. The most sensitive parts of the body – including the fingertips, face, breasts and genital area – have so many sensitive nerve endings that it is impossible to prick a pin anywhere into them without it being felt. On the back, by contrast, nerve endings are fairly sparse and there may be as much as 4 cm ($1\frac{1}{2}$ in) between painful pin pricks. Most of the traditionally erogenous zones of the body (lips, breasts, genitals and so on) are well supplied with nerve endings – but almost any area of skin will function as an erogenous zone if it is stimulated by touch in favourable circumstances.

The nerve endings are of different types according to their function and look quite different from each other under the microscope. They are very highly specialized: some pick up only pain, others only hot sensations, others cold sensations and there are still others that are sensitive only to the sensation of touch.

The skin's appendages

Distinct from the skin itself but closely related to it in position and function are the sweat glands, hair follicles, sebaceous glands and nails.

The sweat glands fall into two categories. The apocrine glands (found under the arms and around the pubic area and the nipples) begin to function at puberty, when the level of hormones circulating in the body rises. These glands secrete sweat that is said to act as a chemical signal to attract the opposite sex. The eccrine glands are found all over the body and their production of sweat is under nervous control. We sweat when too hot, to lower the body temperature, and we sweat as a nervous reaction when anxious (some biofeedback devices – see page 233 – can monitor stress by detecting minute changes in sweat secretion). Emotional eccrine sweating takes place mainly on the palms of the hands, the soles of the feet, the forehead and under the arms.

Sweat itself has no distinctive smell. The odour that we associate with it is the result of bacterial action. Bacteria are always present on the skin's surface and they are particularly active in areas where sweat is trapped by clothing because they like warm, damp surroundings. A deodorant works by diminishing the bacteria/sweat reaction, but does nothing to reduce the amount of sweat the body secretes. Anti-perspirants, most of which are related to astringents, work along different lines. They dehydrate the upper layers of the skin, including the sweat glands, so that less sweat is produced. No product will stop sweat secretion completely and in general aerosols are less effective than a roll-on anti-perspirant. Some anti-perspirants contain a deodorizer as well. Neither type of product should be used on sore, inflamed or broken skin.

Vaginal deodorant sprays should be used with the greatest caution, if at all, as they cause irritation and allergic reactions in some women. There should be no need to use these products, however, if normal hygiene is maintained: if unusual odour or discharge persist, consult a doctor rather than masking the symptoms with a deodorant.

The hair follicle is a growing, living root with a nerve supply and a blood supply for nourishment. It is because of the nerve supply, which is sensitive to distortion, that it hurts to have our hair pulled. The only visible part of the hair, the hair shaft, is entirely dead and in this and many other respects is closely akin to the plate of the nail. (Hair and nails are dealt with in more detail on pages 31–33 and 82–83.)

The sebaceous gland opens on to and is an appendage of the hair follicle. Sebaceous glands secrete sebum, usually under the stimulation of the male hormone androgen. (Women have androgens as well as men, although of a slightly different type. They are responsible not only for

the secretion of sebum but also for part of our sex drive and for some of our rather aggressive qualities such as ambitiousness.)

Sebum is a fatty substance composed of more than 40 acids and alcohols. It flows from the gland into the hair follicle, where it lubricates the hair. It then spills out over the skin, producing an oily, slightly acid film (called the skin's acid mantle) over most of the skin's surface. The acidity is essential to the skin's health and integrity, mainly because it is an antiseptic and resists bacterial invasion. Sebum also acts as a barrier, preventing the penetration of poisonous substances from outside. The most important function of sebum, however, in the age of central heating, is probably to prevent loss of moisture from the skin. This accounts for the attempts of cosmetic manufacturers – unsuccessful so far – to work out a formula for an exact artificial imitation of sebum for use in moisturizing creams and lotions.

In some people the sebaceous glands are very sensitive to the androgen levels that control sebum secretion. The cells at the mouth of the sebaceous gland increase in number and size, so that they block off the exit from the gland. Upon exposure to the air, the cells at the mouth of the gland undergo a chemical reaction and blacken. The blackhead formed in this way has therefore not the remotest connection with a dirty skin, nor with too rich a diet. Build-up of sebum behind this blockage may eventually cause the gland to burst, liberating sebum into the lower levels of the skin. In this situation it acts as an irritant and results in the formation of an acne pimple. If infected, this pimple will turn into a pustule and, if this is squeezed, the end product is a large hard purplish spot. (For treatment of acne see page 26 and of acne scars pages 213–215.)

Skin colour

The colour of skin depends on how much melanin it has. Melanin in granule form is contained in special cells (melanocytes) found at intervals between the cells of the basal layer. Everyone, no matter what their skin colour, is born with the same number of melanocytes. What varies is their ability to produce melanin: pale-skinned people produce very little, dark-skinned people more, and black-skinned people a great deal. Those with a coloured skin may have as many as three or four different tones on the face: the forehead often looks lighter than the cheeks and chin, and the eye area and lips tend to be much darker. This uneven pigmentation cannot be treated with special creams, but can be camouflaged or evened out with foundation (see pages 184–185).

The function of the melanin is to act as a natural sunscreen. It filters off the harmful wavelengths of sunlight so that they cannot penetrate into and damage the deeper layers of skin. When the skin is exposed to sunlight, the melanocytes are stimulated to produce more melanin to screen off the ultra-violet radiation efficiently. As a result, the skin changes colour. Tanning is therefore the outcome of deliberately injuring the skin.

The skin's growth cycle

The skin does not grow continuously. Cells are budded off from the basal cell layer within the epidermis at two periods each day. One growth spurt comes in the early hours of the morning and a lesser one early in the afternoon – these are the times when the levels of cortisol, the life-giving hormone, are relatively low in the body for most people. Consequently, the best (if not always the most convenient) times to attend to the skin are first thing in the morning and just after lunch, while it is growing and nature is, as it were, working with you. Those of us who do not always go through elaborate cleansing routines each evening may be comforted to know that there is little to be gained from cleansing and massaging the skin while it is resting.

What the skin does

The most important of the skin's functions are:
1 To control the temperature of the body.
2 To eliminate waste.
3 To form a barrier and an outer covering for the body.
4 To produce vitamin D.

Temperature control is achieved by a variety of methods. First, the skin can act in much the same way as a car's radiator does and cool the blood by exposing it to a lower surrounding temperature than the internal temperature within the body. To do this the capillaries in the skin expand and fill with blood. The blood cooled in the skin is then circulated throughout the body, with a cooling effect. This mechanism comes into play when we get hot and the opposite happens – the capillaries contract – when we get cold. This explains why we tend to look red and flushed when we are hot, pale when cold.

The hairs on the skin also help to regulate body temperature. When we feel cold, a muscle in the hair follicle pulls it upright; if this happens all over the body, a layer of air is trapped near the skin. This acts rather like a cellular blanket, to insulate and slow down heat loss when the body is cold. When the body is hot, the hairs lie flat and no insulating layer of air is trapped, enabling us to cool off.

The sweat glands have the job of eliminating some of the cell's waste products from the body as sweat. They get rid of water and also unwanted salts, drugs and certain minerals. This particular function of the sweat glands is interdependent with the excretory role of the lungs and kidneys.

Because of the skin's effectiveness as a barrier, only substances of sufficiently small molecular size to enter it through a sweat gland or sebaceous gland can penetrate. There is therefore no route by which collagen molecules or female hormones (much advertised constituents of many skin creams) can penetrate the deep layers of the skin; they penetrate the outer horny layer of the epidermis only very slowly.

The skin is also an exceptionally elastic covering: it stretches to accommodate the body's movements, particularly over a joint such as the knee, which is continually in use, and contracts back to its original shape without falling into redundant folds of skin.

The final function of the skin is to assist in the manufacture of vitamin D, which our bodies need for strong bones. An inactive precursor of vitamin D is present in the skin. When the body is exposed to sunlight, the precursor is converted chemically into the active vitamin, absorbed into the system and transported by the blood to wherever it is needed. There is no need to sunbathe to facilitate this chemical conversion: exposure to daylight is sufficient and even then not all the skin need be exposed. There is no medical justification for sunbathing (for the harmful effects of the sun on the skin, see pages 18–19).

Looking After the Skin

As the body's first line of defence, the skin is obviously worth looking after. Luckily health, comfort and beauty all dictate much the same so far as skin care is concerned. Setting aside for the moment the skin's arch-enemy, the sun (see pages 18–19), the two principal dangers the skin faces are loss of water and loss of sebum.

Loss of water

Despite the skin's natural barriers, water evaporates from it quickly in any atmosphere with low humidity – in hot or cold dry weather, particularly if it is windy, or in a centrally heated room. If this moisture is not replenished the skin feels rough and dry, becomes less supple and has a tendency to crack, which allows bacteria to penetrate so that the skin may become inflamed.

Another rather paradoxical cause of dehydration is immersion in water. This happens because the water within the skin moves through the protective membrane in the epidermis in an attempt to dilute the tap water surrounding the body. The stronger the solution of minerals and salts in the water, the more water the skin loses – so hard water is particularly dehydrating.

The best way to prevent the skin drying out is to use lashings of moisturizer as often as possible, all year round, not only on the face but on any skin that is often exposed. Hands need as much protection as possible since they are sure to suffer both from exposure and from immersion in water (see pages 81–82 for further information on hand care). Remember also that the throat is usually exposed to the elements nearly as often as the face. The legs may also need occasional moisturizing.

A moisturizer cannot put water back into the skin for any length of time as it is virtually impossible for it to penetrate further than the outermost layers of the epidermis. The small quantity of water that does enter the skin is lost very quickly through evaporation. However, a well-designed moisturizer does the much more important job of slowing down the rate of dehydration by acting as a barrier to water loss, in the same way that sebum does. Water is replaced from below eventually, so provided evaporation of moisture diminishes, the skin works towards rehydrating itself; for a further discussion of moisturizers for the face, see pages 21–22.

Loss of sebum

Anything that strips part of the protective film of sebum from the skin's surface allows moisture to escape from the skin more rapidly. Soaps and detergents, which are efficient defatting agents, therefore encourage dehydration. Removing sebum also disturbs the skin's natural acid balance, or pH, rendering it more susceptible to infection. On a scale of 0–14, of which the first half denotes acidity, the second alkalinity, the skin's pH averages about 5. Harsh alkalis tend to neutralize the acid mantle that helps to maintain the skin's defence against bacterial invasion. Many products in everyday use are alkaline, including all detergents, as well as most soaps and many shampoos and bath additives. In general, the more they lather, the more alkaline they are.

It makes sense therefore to use a mild soap for the hands and body and a cosmetic cleanser for the face. This is not because the face is special but because the coating of sebum is particularly important to an area that loses moisture continually through exposure; for further information on cleansers and soap for the face, see pages 20–21. Look among the products that state their pH for one close to or under 5. For the bath, avoid foamy or bubbly additives, since these will almost certainly be alkaline, and use a bath oil instead – while this will do the skin no particular good, it will not harm it either.

What not to worry about

Skin care is the kind of controversial area where myths take root easily. There is no medical evidence that any of the following are bad for the skin: lack of exercise; lack of sleep; smoking; dirt or dust; make-up; coffee; rich food. Alcohol and spicy food do not damage normal skin, but they may affect red or broken veins on the cheeks and round the nose, which can be temporarily accentuated and gradually worsened by anything that causes the capillaries to expand and the skin to flush, including sudden temperature changes.

Bath or shower?

A long soak in the bath can be very pleasant; it relaxes the muscles and has a mildly tranquillizing effect. Immersion in water is less beneficial for the skin, however, than for the inner woman, for a bath can dehydrate the skin, leaving it feeling taut and looking wrinkled, especially in areas where the water is hard. The longer the bath and the hotter its temperature, the greater the dehydration is likely to be. Counter this after coming out of the bath, when the skin is dry and cool, by applying a moisturizer: either use a product marketed for the face or a special body lotion. Warm it first by pouring some out into the palm of your hand.

Showers are held to invigorate rather than calm and can certainly have a stimulating effect. There is no real danger, either, that the skin may become dehydrated, since it is not permitted to soak in the water. In all other respects, the choice of bath or shower is a matter of personal preference.

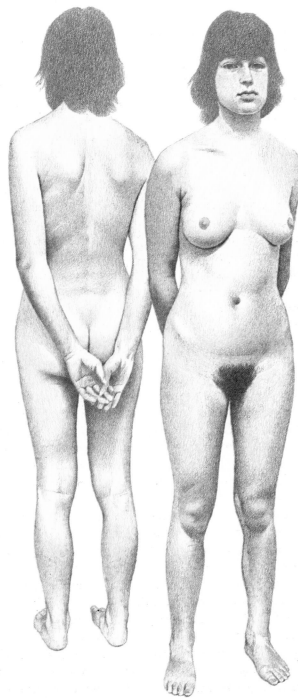

Upper back
Counteract oily tendency by regular washing; a loofah may help you to reach more easily, but do not scrub too hard as this will overstimulate the sebaceous glands.

Elbows
Areas of callus, the skin's protection against friction. Moisturizing makes the skin feel smoother, but cannot diminish the callus.

Hands
Regular moisturizing is important. Keep nails clean with a nailbrush and manicure regularly.

Upper thighs
A pad of fat is a female characteristic and does not differ from fat elsewhere. Massage cannot affect this: the only cure is diet and exercise or cosmetic surgery.

Backs of knees
Surface veins tend to show if standing for long periods is a habit; wear support hose to help circulation.

Heels
Areas of callus are common. Use a pumice to remove this hard, dead skin.

Throat
Moisturize regularly as the skin is often exposed. Keeping body weight stable helps prevent a sagging double chin.

Underarms
Wash regularly; an anti-perspirant-deodorant helps prevent sweating and odour.

Bust
A sensitive area, which needs the protection of a bra during vigorous exercise, in pregnancy or if the breasts are large.

Abdomen
This is the thinnest skin so stretch marks are likely if there are sudden weight changes.

Vaginal area
Apocrine sweat glands function from puberty onwards, so good hygiene is important to prevent odour.

Knees
Like elbows, these often develop calluses.

Feet
A regular pedicure keeps the feet looking good. Comfortable shoes minimize friction and the development of hard skin and corns (calluses).

Sun and the Skin

Although the source of some of our vitamin D depends on the skin being exposed to daylight, I am strongly opposed to baring the skin to the sun. Where sun-worshipping is the issue, the price of a beautiful tan is too high.

The dangers

Ultra-violet rays are harmful to the skin – some more harmful than others (the most harmful wavelengths are 290 to 320 mµ). Only people with very dark or black skins can produce enough melanin to screen off these harmful rays totally.

The damage sunlight can inflict depends directly on the length of exposure to it. In small doses (ten minutes or less) sun simply irritates the skin, making it hot and slightly red. Higher doses lead to inflammation and to swelling. Even greater exposure results in burning, with all its classic symptoms of blistering and peeling. Excessive exposure to sunlight damages the skin to such an extent that it can no longer perform its normal functions – if the damage is severe enough to prevent temperature control, it can lead to sunstroke. This is extremely serious, as the temperature may rise so high that normal body metabolism is impaired. People have been known to die as a result.

A more long-term danger of sunbathing is that it makes the collagen bundles in the dermis disintegrate and finally split. The skin loses its suppleness and firmness and begins to wrinkle – just as it does in ageing. Nothing can be done to slow down, cure or prevent this sequence of events, unfortunately, once exposure to the sun has caused them.

A beautiful experiment by Professor of Dermatology Sam Shuster showed beyond doubt the ageing effect of sunlight. Four small specimens of skin were taken: one from the bottom and one from the forearm of an octogenarian, and one from the same sites in a teenager. Taking into account the normal effects of the ageing process, the collagen in the skin from the old man's bottom matched that in the skin from the teenager's forearm and bottom; but in the sample from the old man's forearm the collagen had disintegrated far more. The only explanation for this difference was that the skin on the forearm had been exposed to 80 years of daylight, whereas that on the bottom had been covered by clothing. This experiment is worth remembering before you strip off on the beach for a spell of sun-worshipping.

By far the most powerful reason for restraint in sunbathing, however, is that exposure to the sun stimulates the skin to undergo malignant change and hence encourages skin cancer. It takes many hours of exposure to the sun to trigger off this change – and white-skinned people living in countries such as Australia, where the number of sunlight hours a year is high, reach the danger level much more quickly and are more likely to get skin cancer than people in countries such as the United Kingdom, where sunshine is a comparative rarity. Black skins produce melanin so efficiently that black-skinned races do not run the same risk of contracting skin cancer, no matter how much they are exposed to the sun.

Skin conditions

People with vitiligo (patches of skin with no pigmentation) or chloasma (patches of skin with over-pigmentation) should avoid the sun. The former burn easily and the latter darken and become more obvious. Dermatitis is another reason to take care: the affected skin is already dry and sunshine, by drying it out further, makes the condition worse.

Acne sufferers, by contrast, can benefit from exposure to the sun. One way of unblocking the outlet of the sebaceous gland is to make the skin peel slightly. This is the basis of ultra-violet radiation therapy for acne and exposure to natural sunlight achieves just the same end. As the dead layer of skin peels from the surface, it takes with it the cells blocking the outlet of the sebaceous gland, allowing the gland to become normal.

Psoriasis is the other skin complaint that may be helped by sunbathing. The cause of this condition is overproduction of new cells in the basal layer; once these large numbers of cells reach the outer horny layer of skin, they pile up into scales. If the affected skin is given a dose of natural or artificial ultra-violet radiation just sufficient to make the skin peel, the scales peel off.

Protection from the sun

Many products on sale today simulate our own natural sunscreen, melanin, if applied to the skin.

These substances can protect the skin from the harmful effects of ultra-violet radiation in two ways: by scattering all light rays that hit the skin (a sun-shade) or by selectively absorbing light of harmful wavelengths (a sun-screen). Zinc oxide, titanium dioxide or calamine lotion applied in a thick layer act as an efficient sunshade, but most people find these unacceptable for cosmetic reasons and sunshades have generally been abandoned nowadays in favour of sunscreens.

The first generation of sunscreens contained such chemicals as para-aminobenzoic acid, tannic acid and phenylsalicylate in a cream base. More recently substances called benzophenones have proved to be effective. It is a basic principle in medicine to use only one drug at a time and not to mix drugs with similar actions, so start with either a para-aminobenzoic acid or a benzophenone and stick with the product unless it proves unsatisfactory.

The degree to which a sunscreen protects the skin is roughly indicated by its 'sunscreen index' or protection factor, on the accompanying instructions. A protection factor of two means that a person using the product should be able to sunbathe for about twice as long before burning as without it; a protection factor of six lets you sunbathe for about six times as long. Protection factors generally lie between two and nine, but some go even higher. (Obviously, the higher the protection factor, the more efficient the sunscreen.)

Apart from the ingredients of the sunscreen used, the extent to which these products can protect skin depends on:
• the intensity of the light.
• your personal sunburn threshold.
• the frequency with which the product is applied.
Whatever product is used, it should be applied liberally to all exposed parts before going into the sun and every two to three hours during sunbathing.

Guide for sunbathers

The fact that sun harms the skin will not deter some people from pursuing a suntan. Here are some guidelines for those who still believe that brown is beautiful.

• Know your own skin. Each person has an individual limit so far as suntan goes. Attempting to overstep this limit is pointless and harmful. People with fair skin will burn after only a brief spell in the sun; they will never go a deep brown colour no matter how cautiously or zealously they set about sunbathing. Even with dark skins there comes a point at which further exposure to intense sun will burn the skin. If you know from bitter experience that you blister and peel after only a short while in the sun, be especially careful to protect yourself with a high protection factor sunscreen.
• Start slowly. Initially even those with fairly dark skin should begin by sunbathing only for half an hour at a time, while fair people should limit themselves to ten minutes in the sun. Work up to longer periods by stretching the sessions by ten or fifteen minutes each day.
• Avoid the midday sun: ultra-violet radiation is at its most intense around noon and the sun's rays have less distance to travel before hitting the skin when the sun is directly overhead.
• Always use a sunscreen. Apply it often, to all exposed parts of the body, and remember to re-apply it after swimming. Use more when on the beach or skiing: sand, water and snow all reflect ultra-violet light on to the skin and make it more liable to burn.

Fake tans

It is possible to look bronzed and healthy without also running the risk of burning, wrinkling and rendering the skin more susceptible to cancer. The simple solution is a fake tan.

Most artificial tans contain dihydroxyacetone, a chemical that attaches itself to the keratin cells on the surface of the skin and gradually turns a browny-orange. The colour may take several hours to develop, which makes it difficult to apply the tan evenly, and it fades gradually over a few days as the skin sheds its dead cells.

Avoid suntan cosmetics that contain an artificial tanning agent plus a sunscreen. A sunscreen has to be applied liberally if it is to protect the skin, while a liberally applied fake tan can look unnaturally dark. For this reason it is much better to use two separate products rather than try to combine them.

Facial Skin Care

Far more attention is lavished on facial skin than on any other part of the body – with good reason. Not only is a clear, healthy complexion essential for an attractive face, but the skin needs particular care as it is constantly exposed to the assaults of sun, wind and central heating, all of which can dry it out (see pages 16–17). So it is important to compensate for dehydration by regular moisturizing and to follow suitable cleansing and toning routines for your skin type, which will not dry the skin more than necessary.

Facts and fictions

Unfortunately, the subject of facial skin care is beset with misunderstandings and misconceptions. There is no evidence that creams containing hormones, vitamins or collagen are of special benefit to the skin, nor that moisturizing ingredients such as mink or turtle oil are more beneficial than the cheaper oils used in standard moisturizers. Nor are there medical grounds for preferring products prepared solely from 'natural' or 'organic' ingredients such as fruits or herbs: synthetic ingredients cleanse efficiently and preservatives reduce spoilage of the product.

The sweat glands open on to the skin's surface and these are what many people mean by the term 'pores'. The sebaceous glands (see pages 12, 14), which open on to the hair follicle rather than the skin, may also be referred to as pores. The common belief that it is somehow medically undesirable to cover these openings for long periods with make-up is quite unfounded, as is the belief that skin can be harmed by dirt on its surface. The covering would have to be as impermeable as paint for it to stop the sweat glands from functioning and the outlet of the sebaceous gland can be blocked only from inside, so neither blackheads nor acne can be exacerbated by make-up or dirt (see page 26). The skin does need to maintain equilibrium with the oxygen in the air, but neither make-up nor dirt will discourage it from doing so; assiduous cleansing is therefore not essential in maintaining the health of the skin. Nor can the pores be 'refined' or 'closed' as no product applied to the skin's surface can affect its structure.

Nothing that is applied to the skin can prevent or banish wrinkles (see page 13). Innate dryness of the skin cannot affect their formation, nor can heat, although sunshine does cause wrinkling and ageing. Anti-wrinkle creams can tighten up the skin for a few hours but they dehydrate it, too, and can have only a very transient effect. Broken veins, a hereditary trait, cannot be caused by scrubbing, or washing with very hot or cold water, although these may worsen them or hasten their appearance in someone predisposed to them. Nor can they be prevented from developing by assiduous moisturizing or by avoiding soap and water, although this will help to keep the overlying skin in good condition. Electrolysis treatment designed to coagulate the capillaries is a possible option for anyone seriously worried by red veins, but should be carried out only by a dermatologist or cosmetic surgeon (see page 215). However, it is simpler and safer to use a densely covering foundation (see pages 206–207).

Soap versus cleansers

Cleanliness may not be a biological necessity, but it is certainly a social virtue – and an elementary beauty aid too, for there is nothing to be gained by hiding an attractive skin under grime and leftover make-up. Even after one day, a skin that has not had make-up on it will be dirty, for the dust and grime in the atmosphere cling to the grease on the skin – as cleansing with lotion and cotton wool will show. Skin that has had make-up applied should also be carefully cleansed, for although cosmetics do not harm or stain the skin, stale make-up looks and feels unattractive.

For cosmetic and aesthetic reasons it is a good idea to cleanse at least once a day, though cleansing more than two or three times a day may irritate the skin. Always cleanse before applying cosmetics in the morning or renewing them for the evening, as make-up is most successfully applied to a freshly cleansed and moisturized surface. Many women also feel more comfortable and attractive if they remove cosmetics at night. As explained on page 15, the best times of day to cleanse are first thing in the morning and early afternoon. Few have the opportunity to cleanse thoroughly in the middle of the day but if foundation is not worn, a toner applied with cotton wool can create an instant feeling of freshness. If time allows, moisturizing dry skin, or

INNATE :- inborn , COAGULATE :- to change from fluid to solid state curdle, clot, set .

assiduous - constant, careful attention, assiduity
∨ persevering & diligent

the dry areas of a combination skin, in the middle of the day helps to keep it smooth and soft.

For the reasons given on page 16, washing with water and soap defats and dries the skin. It is therefore a good idea to use a lotion or cream for cleansing, whether or not make-up is worn. The only exception to this rule is in cases of acne or very oily skin, when it is desirable to strip away some of the excess sebum gently. Furthermore, ordinary soap is not designed to dislodge cosmetics – a further cleanse with lotion and cotton wool would show a surprising amount of make-up still on the skin. Cleansing lotions and creams on the other hand are formulated to dissolve the oils, pigments and waxes in cosmetics and are wiped off with cotton wool or tissues; they are available in a wide range of textures and forms. Choose a non-perfumed, allergy-tested one if your skin is at all sensitive.

For those who prefer to wash their face despite the dangers of dehydration, there are cream-on, wash-off cleansers, which are worked into a lather and then washed off. Non-fragrant cleansing bars, which look like soap but contain none of the harsh ingredients found in most soaps, can also be used. They do not normally form a lather but are gently worked over the skin with water and rinsed off.

Use the same methods for cleansing and moisturizing the eye area as for the rest of the face unless removing waterproof cosmetics. Special cleansing creams, oils or oil-impregnated pads are also available – an oil-based cleanser is essential for waterproof mascara (see page 199).

Toners

Any lingering traces of cleanser, stubborn make-up or dirt can be removed with a skin toner after cleansing. Toners also leave the skin feeling cool and refreshed and are a convenient way of cleansing the face in between fullscale cleansing routines. There are various kinds of toner, the main difference being the amount of alcohol in the liquid solution. Skin tonics and fresheners are the mildest and are usually devoid of, or contain very little, alcohol. These are most suitable for dry and sensitive skin, but can be used on other skin types too. Astringents are stronger preparations and may contain ingredients such as methol and camphor; they are particularly useful for oily skin

as they help to remove excess oil. Do not, however, use anything too astringent as this will make the skin sting and dry it out.

Moisturizers

These are available in a range of forms and textures – watery solutions, emulsions, creams and oily solutions. Watery solutions have a rapid but short-lived moisturizing effect, as the water added to the skin cannot be held there and so evaporates quickly; thus the kinds of moisturizer that sink most easily into the skin give only very temporary benefit. Emulsions are mixtures of water and oil: some products are made as water-in-oil emulsions, some as oil-in-water ones. The latter contain a smaller proportion of oil and so are absorbed into the skin more easily and can be applied under make-up. However, the purpose of the oil is to hold the water in the skin and so emulsions with a higher percentage of oil are effective for a longer time. Nevertheless, the thickest, oiliest emulsions are unpleasant to use and, as they do not easily sink into the skin, tend to rub off on to clothing or pillowcases.

Only the thicker creams and lotions stand much chance of slowing down water loss. The ideal moisturizer is therefore the thickest that can be absorbed by the skin and yet does not leave it feeling dehydrated after a few hours. The most efficient are the creams constituted of fatty acids and alcohols to imitate so far as possible the water-conserving properties of sebum. They are not as sticky as oily emulsions. While it may be necessary to wear a light moisturizer beneath make-up, try to use a heavier creamy type whenever possible – at night, for example, or when make-up is not being worn.

Oily solutions that do not contain water cannot moisturize the skin and, although many moisturizers try to make a selling point of the oils they contain, it is quite safe to ignore such claims when deciding which brand to buy. Although the oils in the moisturizing emulsions help to hold water in the skin, oil in itself cannot keep the skin soft and flexible without the aid of water. For it is water, not oil, that gives skin its suppleness and smoothness, as the following experiment demonstrates. Two pieces of dead skin were taken and allowed to dry out completely. One was immersed in water, the other in oil, and the condition of both pieces was checked a short while later. The skin taken from water was so pliable that it would bend under a 10 g ($\frac{3}{8}$ oz) weight, while the piece that had been in oil was so rigid that even a 100 g (4 oz) weight was not sufficient to bend it. Oil supplied to the skin's surface does not function as an effective shield in the way that the natural oil, or sebum, produced from within does, so it is hard to see how moisturizers, soaps or creams could be worth buying purely for their oil content.

Skin Types

Most of us think we know our facial skin type, but it is easy to be mistaken when constantly treating it with cleansers, toners, moisturizers and make-up, the effects of which could give a false impression. The basic structure of the skin does not, of course, vary from type to type, but only the extent to which the sebaceous glands are stimulated to produce sebum and the areas of the face in which they are most active; the skin's inherent ability to retain or lose water also varies.

Skin types cannot be altered permanently but they can be kept temporarily in check with a suitable skin care routine. To discover your type, first cleanse your face thoroughly, removing all traces of make-up, but do not tone or moisturize. Leave the skin to settle for a few hours without cosmetics. Examine it carefully in natural daylight, using a good mirror or a magnifying one.

Oily skin

The main hallmark of an oily skin is an overall shine: the skin is often sallow and its texture may be coarse – that is, the openings of the sebaceous glands, or pores, may be particularly noticeable. The shiny look is caused by overproduction of sebum (see page 14). While it is often besieged with spots and blackheads at puberty, oily skin can be a blessing as the excess sebum helps to prevent the skin from drying out.

Oily skin tends to attract dirt and dust more readily than dry skin. It benefits from water, so washing with a soapless cleansing bar or a wash-off cleanser is the ideal cleansing method, although some people with very oily skin may be able to use ordinary soap satisfactorily. Light, non-greasy, liquid cleansers may also be used.

Although oily skin benefits from the defatting action of soap and water or cleanser, over-harsh treatment of the skin strips it of too much oil and stimulates the sebaceous glands to produce yet more sebum, creating a vicious circle. A two-minute gentle massage morning and night with the fingertips, using soap or cleanser and water, is the most the skin should be subjected to. After cleansing, remove excess oil with an astringent. Very oily skins need no extra moisturizer but a skin that is only slightly oily may benefit from occasional moisturizing, especially in dry climates. There may also be drier areas, such as the lips, throat and outer parts of the cheeks and forehead, which do need regular moisturizing.

Combination skin

The most common skin type is a combination skin with an oily central panel or T-zone embracing the forehead, nose and chin, and areas of dryness on the cheeks, round the eyes and on the throat. Black skins tend to have greater extremes of dryness and oiliness.

Ideally, two skin care routines should be followed, with two sets of products, as oily skin benefits from washing whereas dry skin does not. However, unless the contrast between the dry and oily areas is very marked, it is simpler to use a milky cleanser over the whole face. The tonic used for the central oily panel should be diluted for the dry areas. Moisturize these areas often.

Dry skin

The skin literally looks dry and sometimes flaky and often feels taut. Because of the lack of protective sebum, it reacts to extreme weather conditions. The skin overlying broken veins is often dry as the capillaries lie near the surface, encouraging more rapid moisture loss. It is less likely to develop pimples than oily skin but tends to become readily chapped or roughened in dry atmospheres.

All products should be mild and toners should be alcohol-free; a rich, creamy cleanser should be used. It is essential to moisturize the face, throat and skin around the eyes regularly and lavishly. If you wear make-up, use moisturized foundations over a moisture base, which is applied after, and is heavier than, ordinary moisturizer.

Cleansing

Cleansing the face regularly leaves the skin looking and feeling its best. Greasy skin, in particular, benefits from gentle, regular cleansing and toning. Types and textures of cleansers vary greatly (see page 21); instructions are given here for a cream that is wiped off. Always use light, gentle movements when cleansing, toning or moisturizing. You will need: hair tied back; cleanser; tissues or cotton wool (cotton balls).

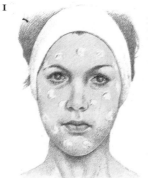

1 Pour a little cleanser into the palm of one hand and dot it generously all over the face with the other hand. Gently work it in with the fingertips, taking particular care round the eye area. Cover the entire face, right up to the hairline.

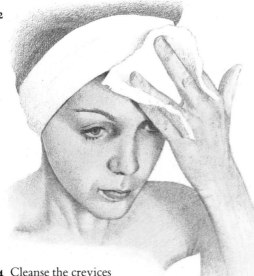

2 Make a square pad from cotton wool or a tissue and wrap it across the underside of the third and fourth fingers. Starting at the forehead and working down each side of the face, remove the cleanser with light, upward strokes.

3 Wrap a fresh tissue or pad of cotton wool round the index finger and cleanse the area round the eyes, with light and gentle strokes.

4 Cleanse the crevices round the nostrils with a fresh tissue or cotton wool pad wrapped round the index finger.

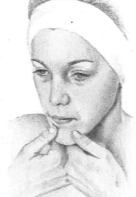

5 To cleanse the dips and curves of the chin, clench the fists, rest both index fingers under the chin and place the thumbs on each side of it. Work in a little extra cleanser with circular movements of the thumbs. Remove with cotton wool or a tissue.

Toning

This second step in the routine is pleasantly refreshing. Toner may leave the skin tingling but it should not be so harsh that it stings – if necessary, dilute it with water. For the choice of toner for your skin type see pages 21–22.

Apply toner immediately after cleansing, on a pad of slightly damp cotton wool. Smooth it over the chin, cheeks, nose and forehead, using fresh cotton wool as necessary. Do not apply it to the lips or eye area as it could irritate the skin and dry it out too much.

Eye creams

The skin around the eyes has very little fat and supporting tissue to keep it supple and plump and so needs gentle handling and lavish and frequent moisturizing. There is no benefit in using special creams as the structure of the skin is the same as elsewhere. Avoid creams containing lanolin (wool fat) as this can make the skin puffy and swollen. Crow's-feet form because of constant wrinkling of the skin when we smile or laugh, but unfortunately no anti-wrinkle cream can cure them or prevent them from forming.

Moisturizing

This third step in the skin care routine is essential to keep the skin from drying out. Moisturize whenever your skin feels in need of it, but at least once a day if your skin is dry; oily skins naturally need less help to seal in the internal moisture. It is particularly important to moisturize in a dry climate or when living in centrally heated rooms. Moisturizing can be combined with facial massage (see pages 176–177). For the choice of moisturizer see pages 21–22.

1 Tip some moisturizer into the palm of one hand and dip the fingers of the other hand into the lotion for a few moments to warm it so that it spreads easily over the skin. Dot the lotion all over the face.

2 Slowly and lightly smooth the moisturizer all over. Return to the centre of the forehead and, pointing the fingers towards each other, press gently. The fingers' warmth helps the skin to absorb the lotion and the pressure is most relaxing. Move the fingers slightly apart and repeat; work towards the hairline.

3 Apply a little moisturizer to the eye area, dotting it on with the little finger, which fits most easily into the crevices and hollows. Try not to pull or stretch the skin or smudge the cream or lotion into the eye itself. Repeat at the end of the routine.

4 With one hand on each cheek, work the moisturizer into the skin, stroking upwards with the three middle fingers from the jawline out to the ears.

5 Work the lotion into the skin at the jawline, chin and around the mouth, using the three middle fingers as in **4**. If necessary, blot any excess lotion from the face with a tissue. To prevent the lips becoming dry and chapped, apply a lip salve.

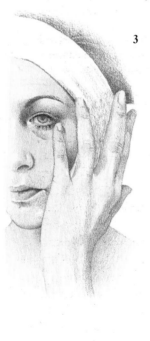

Facial Treatments

Applying a face mask
The mask can be applied to both face and throat. You will need: hair tied or pinned back; a large complexion brush (optional); an eye mask or cotton wool pad cut into the shape of one, soaked in rosewater or skin tonic; a mask.

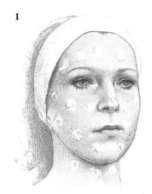

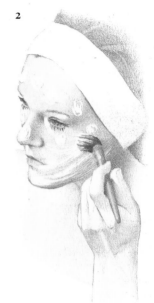

1 Using the fingertips, cover the face and throat with dots of the mask mixture; work up to the hairline but leave blank an area of about 2.5 cm (1 in) around each eye and do not cover the ears or lips.

2 Spread the mask evenly on the throat and face with the complexion brush, working upwards and outwards.

3 Fingertips may also be used to spread the mask. They are especially effective over the bridge of the nose and around the chin and nostrils.

4 Place the soaked eye mask or cotton wool over the eyes and relax for 10 to 15 minutes. Remove mask according to the manufacturer's instructions.

A myriad of special treatments are available that promise to improve on routine cleansing, toning and moisturizing; but many are of doubtful benefit. Medicated products containing anti-bacterial agents should be avoided under normal circumstances as they are unnecessary and may cause allergic reactions. Cleansing grains and facial scrubs are advocated for oily skin. But if used regularly these stimulate the sebaceous glands into producing more excess sebum and may even spread infection where there are spots or acne. Facial saunas leave the skin feeling soft and revitalized, but the excessive sweating dries it out and so they are inadvisable for dry or combination skins. There is also a wide range of electrical aids for facial beauty treatments – vibro-massagers, moisturizing massagers, battery-powered cleansers and the like – which can be regarded as gimmicks or luxuries.

Face masks or packs cleanse the skin and increase the blood flow to it, leaving it feeling fresh and smooth; but despite the exotic ingredients that many contain, from avocados to witch hazel, they can do no more (see page 244). Most are formulated to give help to specific skin types. Masks consisting of thick pastes and creams that harden on the skin are usually oil-absorbers: as the mask tightens, the sebum and the dead surface layers of the skin combine with the mask and are rinsed off with it after treatment. Some contain sulphur, which has a direct chemical reaction on keratin, loosening it and facilitating its removal; these should never be used on dry or combination skins. Softer cream masks, containing fatty ingredients such as egg yolk, wheatgerm or vegetable oils, are designed for dry skins. Brush-on, peel-off masks, with rubber, wax or plastic bases, are usually sticky and transparent, and are especially suitable for combination skin. They set to form a kind of skin over the face, which is later peeled off; there is no need to rinse. Avoid using face masks before a big occasion as any irritation of the skin may cause a few spots to appear. If your skin is spotty or has acne, avoid using them altogether as the mask may spread bacteria. They may also irritate skin overlying broken veins.

A–Z of Skin Problems

Abscess (boil, folliculitis)

Definition: Localized inflammation in the skin with collection of pus. An abscess involving a hair follicle is called folliculitis. (See also Stye, page 51.)

Description: Localized swelling, redness and tenderness, ultimately with a core of pus formed at the centre.

Cause: Nearly always invasion by bacteria.

Prevention: Do not squeeze spots; do not pick or scrub skin (scrubbing for longer than 45 seconds releases bacteria from the lower levels of the skin on to the surface instead of cleaning it).

Treatment: 1 Apply hot poultices to bring abscess to a head.
2 Break skin with a sharp sterile instrument and release pus with gentle pressure.
3 Dress with cetrimide antiseptic cream if small; if large, consult a doctor.
4 If recurrent, use a soap containing cetrimide and get instructions from a doctor about using an antiseptic in your bath water – never use it otherwise.

Acne

Definition: Blackheads plus tendency for the skin to be excessively oily and spotty, commonest in puberty.

Description: Blackheads, small pustules and tendency to develop deeper inflamed spots.

Cause: Blockage of the exit from the sebaceous gland, leading to rupture and release of sebum into the deeper layers of the skin, causing inflammation which becomes secondarily infected.

Prevention: Cannot be prevented because due to:
1 High levels of the hormone androgen circulating at puberty and possibly at other times.
2 Overgrowth of the cells at the neck of the sebaceous glands in response to the high levels of androgen.

Treatment: 1 Meticulous cleansing of the skin. Acne is the one condition in which you should use soap brought to a lather and massaged into the skin for two minutes: the aim is to de-fat the skin. Wash at least three times a day with soap and water.
2 Use an anti-bacterial cleanser.
3 Obtain special acne creams from a doctor – do not use proprietary ones.
4 There is no need to cut out particular foods from your diet – they do not have the slightest effect on acne.
5 Wear a thick-textured make-up to cover the spots. It will not make the acne

any worse, and it will improve morale.
6 Consider sun treatment (see pages 18–19).

Allergy

Definition: Production of antibodies to any substance that the body interprets as foreign, leading to an inflammatory reaction in part or all of the body, which may range from mild, e.g. nettlerash, to very serious, e.g. shock.

Description: The commonest and least dangerous allergy is hay fever, with running nose, sore, itchy, runny eyes and sneezing due to contact with grass or flower pollen to which the body has become sensitive. The worst allergic reactions may involve the digestive tract (with diarrhoea and severe abdominal pain), the heart and the kidneys and may threaten life.

Cause: Anyone may become allergic to anything at any time. It is possible to eat eggs for years and become allergic to them at 50. There are recorded cases of allergy to contact with water.

Prevention: Avoid the allergen.

Treatment: 1 Desensitizing injections (ask a doctor).
2 Antihistamines from a doctor.
3 Strong local anti-inflammatory agents such as steroids, on prescription.

Blackheads (commodones)

Definition: Plug of cells at exit from sebaceous gland.

Description: Firm mass of keratin and sebum blocking the hair follicle. (This is black only because keratin turns black on exposure to oxygen and is nothing to do with dirt.)

Cause: Due to overgrowth of the cells of the sebaceous duct in response to male hormones circulating in the blood.

Prevention: Cannot be prevented.

Treatment: 1 Warm and moisturize the skin with warm water, a hot bath or steam.
2 Squeeze the blackhead.
3 Leave entirely alone.
4 Follow preventive measures as treatment for Acne above.

Blisters

Definition: Sharply circumscribed collections of free fluid.

Description: May be on a base of inflamed skin; variable in size ranging from pearly droplets to several centimetres, depending on the cause.

Cause: Small blisters are commonly seen in cold sores, shingles, burns and reactions to drugs. They can be caused by friction.

Prevention: Protect areas where friction is likely, e.g. wear two pairs of socks or use special sponge pads to lessen the likelihood of blisters on feet.

Treatment: 1 Do not burst the blister – it is the body's way of protecting itself.
2 If the blister bursts, keep it clean and dry and cover it with a dry gauze dressing.
3 If the blister goes on to a scab, do not remove the scab; let it fall off.

Broken veins

Definition: Tiny capillary blood vessels near the surface of the skin.

Description: Usually found on the cheeks and the thighs, where capillaries are nearest the skin surface. Appear 'broken' because with ageing the blood circulates through these capillaries very slowly and tends to stagnate; may be of a bluish tinge.

Cause: An inherited trait.

Prevention: Cannot be prevented.

Treatment: Electrodesiccation by an expert may work (see page 215). No other treatment does any good. To avoid making veins more prominent, take the following precautions:
1 Skin overlying small broken veins is thin and tends to be delicate – moisturize it regularly.
2 Avoid highly spiced food, e.g. curry.
3 Do not face direct heat.
4 Try to avoid marked temperature changes.

Chapping

Definition: Small cracks in the skin, sometimes painful.

Description: Commonest in the skin of exposed parts such as hands, fingers and lips.

Cause: Usually preceded by drying out, scaling and roughening of the skin plus undernourishment such as occurs when extremities are cold in the winter.

Prevention: Keep exposed skin warm and well moisturized.

Treatment: 1 Keep the hands out of water.
2 Wear gloves outside.
3 Use lashings of moisturizing creams and lotions.
4 Wear lip salve at all times.
5 Use hand cream every half hour or so.

Chilblains

Definition: Painful, itchy spots, usually on the backs of the legs, ankles, hands and feet, that occur in winter.

Description: Reddish, purplish lumps that are painful when exposed to the cold and exquisitely itchy when the skin becomes warm.

Cause: Hypersensitivity to the cold, making the blood vessels contract down, causing soreness, and then dilate up again, causing itchiness when warmed.

Prevention: Keep the susceptible parts covered and warm in cold weather.

Treatment: Wear warm clothing and boots. Try thermal insoles inside footwear. Sometimes creams containing nicotinic acid can help through their rubefacient powers.

Chloasma — white skin.

Definition: Brown patches in the skin, frequently on the face and the neck.

Description: Coin shaped patches of pigmentation, often appearing in pregnancy or in women taking the Pill.

Cause: Thought to be a reaction to the sex hormones oestrogen and progesterone (or progestogen in women on the Pill).

Prevention: None; the tendency is inherited.

Treatment: 1 Nearly always goes away of its own accord in 9 to 12 months.
2 Avoid direct sunlight: when exposed to the sun, the patches turn darker.
3 Wear shady hats.
4 Use sunscreen creams.

Crow's-feet See Wrinkles.

Dandruff See page 33.

Eczema (dermatitis)

Definition: Dry, red, scaly patches in the skin, which may weep when acutely inflamed.

Description: Can start in infancy, sometimes accompanied by asthma. The predisposition may remain for life, although many cases of infantile eczema are better by the age of seven. In adults, usually coin shaped red patches of dry skin, which wax and wane according to the general state of health and emotional strain. May go into acute phases, with weeping and blistering, or may be a one-off acute attack with severe inflammation, blistering, scaling and scabbing.

Cause: Predisposition to develop eczema is inherited; can be triggered off by decline in general health or emotional strain. One-off acute attack may accompany a sore throat or may be due to contact with an allergic substance, e.g. hair dye.

Prevention: None.

Treatment: 1 Mainstay of treatment consists of creams and tablets prescribed by a doctor.
2 When the condition is bad, avoid all contact with water or soap.
3 Use emollient creams often.
4 Try to avoid stress, strain, overwork, anxiety.
5 Make sure you get a good night's sleep.

Freckles

Definition: Small collection of melanocytes (cells that produce melanin, the pigment in the skin).
Description: Small brown flecks, usually in those parts exposed to sunlight, e.g. the bridge of the nose and cheeks. Will fade over time.
Cause: Melanocytes' response to exposure to sunlight, i.e. tanning effect in tiny patches of skin.
Prevention: Try a sunscreen if freckles bother you.
Treatment: Never interfere, only camouflage.

Impetigo

Definition: Infection of the skin with streptococcus.
Description: Bright yellow scabs, usually around the mouth and face.
Cause: Streptococcus, which lives on all skins but in children may cause an infection when the integrity of the skin is lost. Highly contagious in school children.
Prevention: Good standard of hygiene and immediate treatment when a case is detected.
Treatment: 1 Meticulous hygiene. Separate soap, flannels (wash cloths) and face towel.
2 Specific treatment from a doctor.

Itching

Definition: Delicious irritation in the skin.
Description: Pricking sensation that demands scratching.
Cause: Inflammation (e.g. dermatitis), infection (e.g. lice), nervous tension, worry, chronic scratching (e.g. the itch/scratch/itch cycle).
Prevention: Prevent the underlying condition. Never continue to scratch the skin no matter how it itches.
Treatment: 1 Cooling lotions such as calamine.
2 Creams containing tar, a potent anti-itch application, from a doctor.
3 Antihistamines.
4 If it prevents sleep, possibly sleeping pills (if your doctor thinks it appropriate).
5 Potent skin creams from a doctor for treatment of the underlying condition.

Milia See Whiteheads.

Moles

Definition: Large collections of melanocytes in the skin.
Description: Flat or raised brown patches, possibly containing hairs.
Cause: During development of the skin, melanocytes collect together in small patches.
Prevention: None.
Treatment: 1 Never interfere.
2 If mole gets larger, itchy, inflamed, swollen, visit a doctor immediately.
3 Removal by cosmetic surgery (see Excision page 215).

Nits

Definition: Infection of the head with head lice or the pubic region with pubic lice.
Description: The affected part becomes very itchy.
Cause: The head louse and the pubic louse are specific to human beings and infection is by contact. The adult lice lay eggs at the root of the hair, to which they are cemented and therefore difficult to remove. This distinguishes them from dandruff.
Prevention: Treat all discovered cases promptly and treat all contacts at the same time.
Treatment: 1 Treat with one of the anti-louse preparations available on the market.
2 After treatment, remove the dead eggs from the hair with a fine tooth comb.
3 Repeat seven days later if itching has not subsided.
4 Treat all members of the family.

Ringworm

Definition: Fungal infection of the skin or scalp.
Description: Round, reddish, scaly patches, which are irritating; if in the scalp, they may cause baldness.
Cause: A fungus contracted from animals (e.g. cows, mice, cats) or other human beings.
Prevention: Treat all contacts of discovered cases promptly.
Treatment: Obtain specific treatment from a doctor promptly – do not treat yourself.

Scabies

Definition: Infection with the mite acarus.
Description: Very itchy rash, nearly always on the hands and fingers. May affect the elbows, ankles, feet and toes.
Cause: A mite, acarus. Very infectious, contracted by contact.
Prevention: Treat contacts of all discovered cases promptly.

Treatment: 1 Obtain specific treatment from a doctor and use it over the whole body.
2 Make sure everyone in the family and every contact is treated simultaneously.

Spots

Definition: Inflammation of skin.
Description: Red pimples or spots, very often on the face and shoulders.
Cause: May be part of acne (see page 26). Appear in many women during the week before menstruation due to high progesterone levels: very common in adolescence when hormone levels are swinging about erratically. Not caused by rich diet.
Prevention: None if the cause is hormonal or if the tendency to develop spots is inherited.
Treatment: 1 Unless a blackhead or pus is present, never squeeze. (Squeezing only pushes the bacteria further into the skin and spreads them out so that the spot becomes bigger, harder and lumpier.)
2 Allow pus to develop: when it does, gently expel it.
3 Do not use proprietary antiseptic creams; the skin heals itself just as quickly.
4 Cover up an unsightly spot with heavy tinted make-up – it does no harm and may make you feel better.

Stretch marks See pages 77–78.

Vitiligo — dark skin

Definition: Absence of pigmentation of the skin, usually in patches.
Description: White patches.
Cause: Congenital absence of melanocytes in those patches of skin affected.
Prevention: None.
Treatment: 1 Protect skin from sunlight, by wearing shady hats and sunscreens. Patches of vitiligo are very sensitive to sunlight and burn easily.
2 Camouflage with make-up.
3 If severe, consult a dermatologist.

Warts

Definition: Virus infection of the skin.
Description: Well circumscribed rough lumps, varying in size from pinpoint to 2.25 cm (1 in) in diameter or possibly more. Very often affects the fingers and hands, soles of the feet (verrucae), very troublesome if around the genital and anal area.
Cause: A very infectious virus about which not much is known. Some people seem to be immune; those who have a tendency to

catch it very often have sweaty skin.
Prevention: Cannot be prevented.
Treatment: 1 Do not try patent wart cures.
2 Go to a doctor for specific treatment.
3 Wait two years for your body to build up antibodies that will kill the virus.

Whiteheads (milia)

Definition: Small white spots.
Description: Tiny rounded and raised spots usually over the bridge of the nose, the upper cheeks and under the eyes.
Cause: Cysts in sebaceous or sweat glands, where sebum secretion is low. The gland does not burst as in acne, but the sebum becomes thick, hard and white.
Prevention: Cannot be prevented.
Treatment: 1 With a sterile needle prick the skin over the whitehead and very gently squeeze out. Cleanse skin with cetrimide antiseptic cream.
2 If not troublesome, leave alone.

Whitlow

Definition: Infection of the nail fold.
Description: Swelling, pain and redness around cuticle and nail margin.
Cause: Entry of bacteria into the skin around the nail due to trauma (continual picking of the nail, sogginess of the skin due to constant immersion in water, or bad hygiene).
Prevention: Do not allow any of the above to happen.
Treatment: 1 If minor, is self-curing (but painful).
2 If pain is severe, do not interfere but seek help from a doctor: the whitlow may need to be opened under local anaesthetic.

Wrinkles

Definition: Thinning and folding of the skin, most commonly on the face.
Description: The appearance of lines, bags, folds and loose skin, very often around the eyes (crow's-feet) and mouth (laughter lines).
Cause: Disintegration of collagen with age or through chronic exposure to sunlight.
Prevention: The tendency to develop wrinkles or conversely to have a young-looking skin is inherited. There is nothing that can be applied to the skin or taken by mouth to prevent wrinkles.
Treatment: 1 Avoid anti-wrinkle creams that tighten the skin: they dry the skin out and the tightening lasts only a few hours.
2 Cosmetic surgery (see pages 222–223) or, for fine lines round mouth, dermabrasion (see pages 214–215).

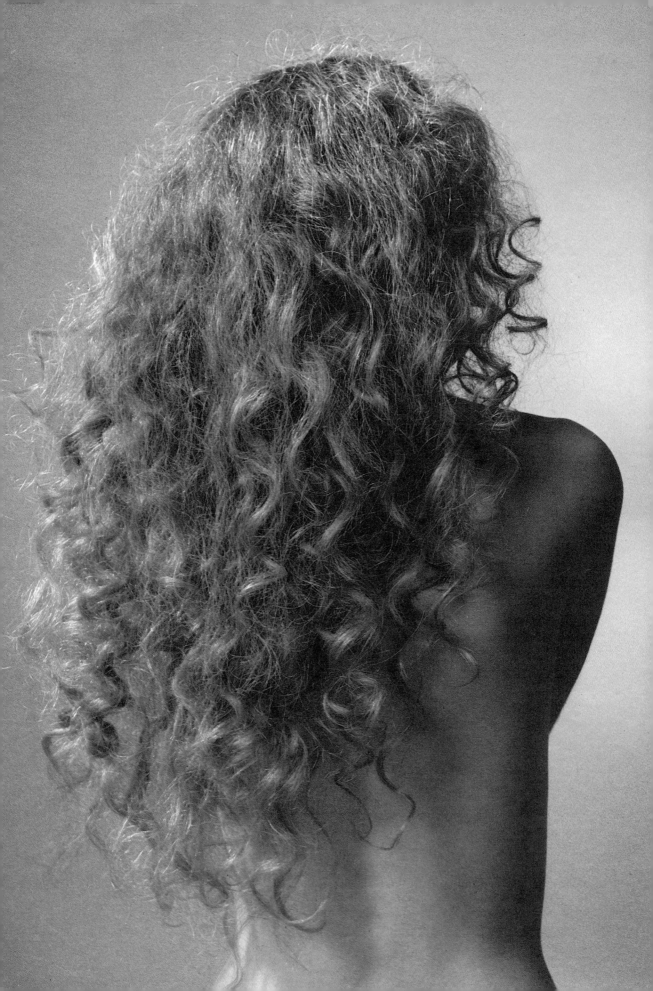

Hair

The hair root is the fastest-growing organ in the body: hair on the scalp, for example, grows at an average rate of 0.4 mm a day (roughly $\frac{1}{2}$ inch a month). Hair cells are formed in the matrix of the hair root, which is situated in the deepest part of the hair follicle. Hair grows as a result of a continuous process whereby new cells are formed, mature and finally die, moving upwards as they do so. The hair shaft – the only bit of hair that is visible – is composed of keratin, shares the skin's slight acidity and is entirely dead. In this and many other respects it much resembles the nail, another horny appendage of the skin (see page 82).

The rate at which the hair cells in the matrix reproduce is greater than that of any other tissue in the body, with the possible exception of the bone marrow. Such a highly active tissue is understandably liable to react to illness or stress: if these are severe enough to interfere with the rate of cell division within the matrix, the result may be an immediate slowing-down of hair growth.

There are four different types of hair: scalp hair, discussed here in detail; eyebrow and eyelash hair, whose function is mainly protective; underarm and pubic hair, which clearly marks out and embellishes the genital organs; and fine, short body hair, whose main function is insulation.

How hair grows

Hair does not grow at a constant rate. In the first place, its growth is seasonal – it grows faster in summer than in winter. Second, hair does not grow indefinitely. The growth phase for each individual hair varies from person to person. It generally lasts for between two and six years – but it may go on for much longer, as the fact that some people have hair long enough to sit on indicates. When the growth phase ends, the hair follicle enters the resting phase of its cycle, which lasts for a few months only. The old hair, known as a club hair, stops getting longer and simply remains in the follicle until a new hair forms underneath and pushes it out. We lose club hairs all the time without noticing it – in the region of 20 to 100 each day. Fortunately the growth/resting cycles are not synchronized in adjacent follicles.

Hair growth is under hormonal control. The male hormone testosterone governs the development of hair that appears after puberty, including beard and body hair and hair in the armpits. This applies to both men and women, although in women the female hormone, oestrogen, generally prevents hair growing on the chin and encourages it to grow on the head. Occasionally, women may develop signs of male-patterned baldness at the menopause when oestrogen levels drop; treatment with oestrogens has been successful in restoring hair growth.

What hair looks like

Hair colouring is produced by a row of melanocytes located at the tip of the hair follicle. The melanin they produce is deposited in the horny cells as they move upwards from the root and the hair colour depends on how much melanin is formed while the hair cells are growing. As a person gets older, the melanocytes become less active – hence the appearance of grey or white hairs. These are just as healthy as hair that still has the tint of youth.

Natural hair colour and all the other characteristics of hair growth, such as curliness, oiliness and thickness, are hereditary. In Caucasian races, the genes for dark hair and wavy or curly hair generally dominate those for blonde or straight hair. This means that someone who inherits a gene for dark hair and one for curly hair will end up with dark curly hair even if she also inherits genes for blonde straight hair. The rules that govern inherited traits are exceedingly complex, however, and dominant genes vary from race to race. In some African races, for example, spiral hair, which forms coils of progressively smaller diameter, tends to dominate straight hair, but helical hair, which has coils of constant diameter, is also frequently found.

It is possible to change the appearance of your hair by using an artificial colourant or a perm (see pages 44–46). With a colourant, a chemical film is applied to the hair shaft. The depth to which the dye penetrates into the hair shaft determines how long the artificial colour lasts. Some colourants shampoo out within weeks; others change hair colour permanently, until the hair is cut off. A perm operates by breaking the chemical bonds that hold the keratin scales of the hair shaft together and then rehardening them in a different

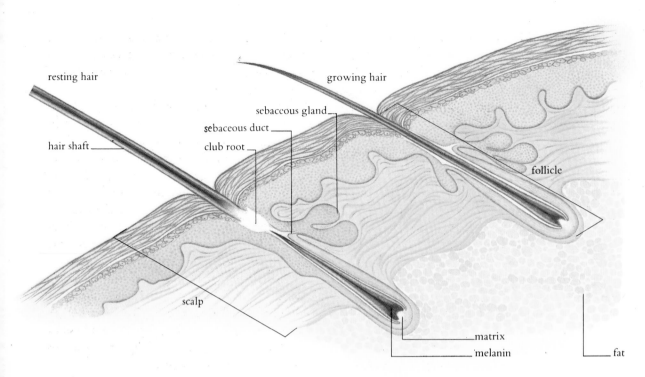

resting hair

growing hair

sebaccous gland

sebaceous duct

hair shaft

club root

follicle

hair shaft

scalp

matrix

melanin

fat

form. Traditionally, perms and chemical hair dyes always consisted of strong alkalis and as such they offered a massive insult to the hair's natural acidity. More recent formulations include buffering agents that are claimed to protect the natural acidity of the hair and are low in ammonia. This may limit to some extent the harm these preparations may inflict on the hair, but they are still best used with caution. Inexpert use of either can temporarily damage the hair, making it go dull, frizzy or even break off close to the scalp. So either go to a well qualified professional hairdresser for these treatments or follow the manufacturer's instructions scrupulously at home.

An additional reason for caution in using hair dyes is that laboratory tests on animals have revealed that there is a possible link between certain chemicals many dyes contain and cancer. In the United States the Food and Drugs Administration has ruled that dyes containing one particular derivative of coal tar, 4-MMPD, must carry a warning to this effect. In these circumstances it may make sense, if you use these dyes at all, to do so only for streaking the hair (see page 45), so that the chemicals do not touch the skin and hence are not absorbed into the body. A vegetable dye such as henna is probably safer to use, and kinder to the hair, than a chemical colourant.

Disturbance of hair growth

All the hair follicles a person will ever have are present at birth. Follicles that die are not replaced and never again produce a hair. It follows that any condition that destroys large numbers of the follicles makes the hair permanently thin. This is what happens in male baldness and in certain rare scarring diseases of the scalp. Proprietary hair restorers will do nothing whatsoever to help these conditions: nothing can make a dead hair follicle produce new roots.

Illness, prolonged drug therapy or emotional stress can also affect hair growth and quality, so that patches of thinning hair appear; however, this condition – called alopecia – is usually only temporary for quite often the result is simply to shorten the hair's life cycle so that it enters its resting phase prematurely. Rather than cause hair loss, illness may make the hairs thinner in diameter, more liable to split and so less shiny.

If a serious illness sends the majority of hairs into a simultaneous resting phase, their loss will show up as thinning of the hair or even as bald patches; but within a matter of months, the new hairs should grow through. Pregnancy, a very dramatic event physiologically, can have this effect too: it is quite common for a new mother to experience some degree of post-partum hair loss, a worrying phenomenon. When the hair regrows (and this may take up to two years), it may have different characteristics from before – it may grow wavy or straight, for example, instead of curly. This is simply a reflection of the immense impact that pregnancy and child-bearing have upon a womans' body. There is, unfortunately, no specific treatment for this condition, but it is advisable to treat the hair and scalp as gently as possible during the period of regrowth.

Hair conditioning

It is extremely difficult to bring about a lasting change in the condition of anything dead. So the results of most attempts to condition the hair shaft – a completely dead, inert structure – are superficial and transient. It is worth bearing in mind that, given its average growth rate, hair that is more than 30 cm (12 in) long has been dead for around three years.

It is possible, however, to make the hair look better. On healthy hair, the scales of keratin lie smoothly one on top of the other, so that they overlap. With neglect or mistreatment, the scales become curled at the edges, distorted or even disconnected. Hair in good condition has scales rather like the tightly overlapping feathers on a bird's wing, while hair in bad condition has scales like a bird's wing when the feathers are ruffled. A conditioner can smooth the scales and so improve the hair's appearance (see page 38).

Nevertheless, to improve the physical condition of the hair in any sense that goes beyond the merely cosmetic, it would be necessary to affect the hair-forming organ itself, which lies well beneath the surface of the scalp, at the time the hair was actually growing. Because the hair mirrors the general state of body health so faithfully, the best hair conditioner of all is to get and stay healthy.

The scalp

The outer layer of the skin on the scalp, like that of all skin, is composed of dead keratin cells and is slightly acid. If it is irritated in any way – by vigorous shampooing or the application of strong alkalis, for example – it responds by increasing production of keratin. Because of the hair these dead cells are not so easily shed as they are from the rest of the body. Someone who has dandruff, a condition in which the keratin cells build up until they show as tiny whitish flakes, does not have a disease: the condition is simply a variation of normal skin growth.

It follows from this that dandruff should be treated extremely gently: too vigorous, frequent shampooing may exacerbate it. Anti-dandruff shampoos containing selenium should be regarded with particular caution. Applied more frequently than once every two weeks, selenium may act as an irritant to the scalp and make the dandruff worse. It may even exacerbate seborrhoeic dermatitis, in which the scalp weeps and the scales become crusted and yellow. Dermatological clinics often have to treat cases of seborrhoeic dermatitis entirely caused by over-zealous use of anti-dandruff shampoos. To improve the condition of the scalp, it may simply be necessary to cut back on the use of anti-dandruff shampoos and to treat the scalp more gently.

A final point: dandruff is not infectious and so it is quite unnecessary to use a medicated shampoo (that is, one that contains antiseptic).

What to look for in a shampoo

Because the scalp needs to be treated gently, it makes sense to use as mild a shampoo as possible. In this respect it is impossible to beat a baby shampoo. If this does not suit you, look among the makes that state their pH (a measure of acidity/alkalinity) and choose one that is around pH 5. This will be very close to the normal acidity of the scalp.

I can think of no good reason for using a medicated shampoo. An antiseptic is called for only if an infection is present and anyone with a scalp infection is in need of a doctor, not of a medicated shampoo.

Hirsutism

Excess hair (known as hirsutism) arises from a combination of two factors: overproduction of the male hormone testosterone and oversensitivity of the hair follicle to testosterone. The result can be anything from a few hairs around the nipple to a distressing amount of facial hair. There is no simple do-it-yourself treatment to remedy this condition permanently. For ways to cope with both excess facial and body hair, turn to pages 46–47.

Equipment and Accessories

Equipment for grooming hair can be divided into two groups: the items used for everyday brushing and combing and those needed for setting and drying wet hair. The choice of equipment depends on the hairstyle – modern, well-cut styles need a minimum of attention apart from drying and brushing, whereas more complicated styles, particularly for longer hair, need a carefully executed setting pattern, or 'pli', and close attention paid to the way they are brushed out.

Many people think that prolonged, arm-aching brushing sessions with sharp-pointed bristle brushes are essential to maintain sheen. In practice, such brushing may do more to damage hair than to improve its condition and with greasy hair, it will spread the excess sebum, or oil, along the shaft faster. Nor will vigorous brushing help dry hair, as this is caused by lack of moisture rather than of oil. Test brushes or combs against the palm of the hand before purchasing – the tips should be smooth, rounded and fairly long, so there is no danger of splitting hairs or scratching the scalp.

Choice of equipment is particularly important when dealing with hair that is wet, as its water-absorbing property lessens its ability to stretch; if it is treated roughly or harshly, it may break or split. Always use a comb or a rubber-cushioned brush with wide-spaced, smooth plastic bristles rather than a harsher natural bristle brush. A wide range of heated appliances is available for helping to dry hair after shampooing and for 'locking in' curls or waves. These aids include styler-dryers with various attachments to create different effects, heated rollers for use on dried hair and various types of hot combs, brushes and tongs. Equipment such as this, which requires heat to be concentrated on one spot, tends to dehydrate the hair, so it is inadvisable to use it regularly; however, some heated rollers and tongs are equipped with special water-misting or conditioning devices to overcome this problem.

All items that are in use on the hair and scalp should be kept meticulously clean – they should be washed every time the hair is shampooed and the same shampoo can be used for cleaning them. To clean a brush, remove all the hairs and dirt with a comb or the tail of a comb and then apply soap or shampoo; both combs and brushes can be cleaned with a nailbrush.

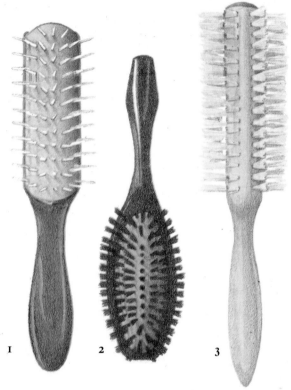

1   2   3

Brushes

Rubber-cushioned brush (1) with well-spaced, smooth, plastic bristles. Ideal for most hair textures, suitable for wet hair, simple to clean; comes in various sizes. Bristle or bristle-mix brush (2) achieves a closer-textured result for shorter, wavy or curly hair; may be used to style damp hair.
Round bristle styling brush (3) used on damp hair to form curls or to straighten the hair when blow drying.

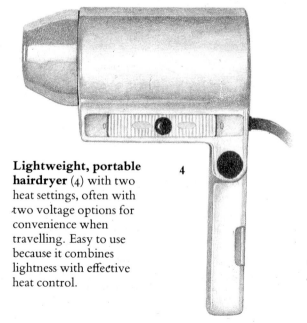

Lightweight, portable hairdryer (4) with two heat settings, often with two voltage options for convenience when travelling. Easy to use because it combines lightness with effective heat control.

4

Combs

Styling comb (5) with teeth spaced closely together at one end, wider apart at the other. Daily grooming aid for fine or straight hair.
Tail comb (6) with metal tail for sectioning off the hair when putting in rollers or blow drying.
Long-toothed comb (7) for very thick, curly hair. Used to give volume and bounce by lifting hair rather than smoothing.

Rollers

Soft sponge roller (8), available in different sizes, for a loosely curled effect. Comfortable to wear and so ideal for overnight sets.
Plastic mesh roller (9) with wired frame and inner, removable brush to grip the hair. Available in many different sizes, this is used by professionals for all kinds of sets, as it holds the hair in place most efficiently.

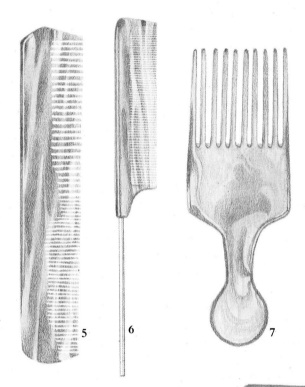

5 6 7

Hair pins

Straight hair pins (10) for anchoring rollers. The pin is pushed into the roller at a 45° angle to rest along the contour of the scalp.
Metal clips (11) for making single, round pincurls. The hair is wound into shape and the clip placed diagonally across the curl.
Plastic-tipped grips (12) or fine hair pins (13) can be used to make pincurls or to anchor twists, rolls and chignons. Available in different shades to match hair colours.

Heated styling wand

(14) for making curls and waves on dry hair. The strands to be curled are held in place under the central clip and are wound round the wand. Also used to straighten frizzy hair or kinks.

Heated styling brush

(15) for use on dry hair to add bounce, volume and lift to any hairstyle and to help straighten frizzy hair.

Heated rollers

(16) give a quick, all-over set to dry hair which, although not as long-lasting as a wet set, can achieve good results. Some have conditioning features.

14

15

16

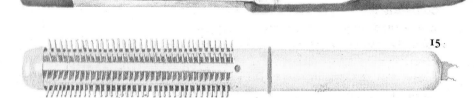

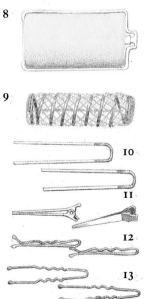

8

9

10

11

12

13

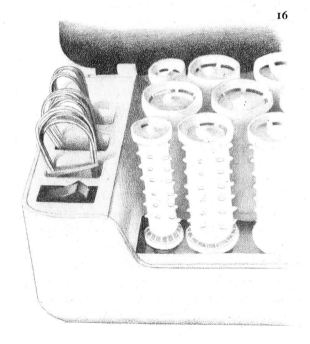

The Cut and the Style

When choosing a new hairstyle, many women select a picture from a magazine and show it to their hairdresser. There are obvious limitations that are often overlooked – for example, straight, fine hair cannot easily be coaxed into a halo of thick curls, even with the aid of a perm; and hair that is naturally springy and curly will never adapt to a sleek, straight bob. A good stylist always spends some time with a new client before her hair is shampooed, not only to discuss the effect that she wants to achieve, but to study the way her hair grows, its length, texture and weight. He should take time to explain to her exactly what can – and cannot – be achieved with her particular head of hair, but at the same time should be able to adapt his techniques to fulfil her hopes as far as possible. It is important that the chosen style suits not only the client's hair but her lifestyle, and that its upkeep does not require the expenditure of more time and money than she can afford.

Look for a stylist who is sympathetic and skilled; personal recommendation or a prior visit to a salon are good bets. Skills in hairdressing vary widely and unfortunately a high price does not guarantee good results, nor is there any foolproof way of predicting whether a stylist's personal tastes will coincide with the client's. A good salon should have a specially trained receptionist who is able to discuss all aspects of the work done there, who can be extremely helpful about price scales and who can arrange free 'consultation' appointments with a stylist when necessary. It is important to have the best possible cut, for hair, unlike a mistaken fashion purchase, has to be worn every day.

Cutting techniques

Hair may be either 'club' cut or 'graduated'. In a club cut all the hair is cut to approximately the same length; in practice, underneath or top hair may be cut slightly shorter, according to the type of style required. In a graduated cut, the hair is cut in layers so that the length graduates from shorter to longer from top to bottom. This effect may sometimes be achieved by using a razor instead of scissors, according to the preference of the cutter. Graduated cuts achieve a lighter, curlier effect than club cuts. Both techniques may be used on one head of hair; but the important part of the stylist's skill is integrating a head of hair so that

each section helps form part of an entity. For instance, hair may need to be cut slightly longer on one side of the head if it has a tendency to curl in the opposite direction to the one that is wanted.

Whatever method is used, the hair is always cut wet and may be re-cut when it is dry. The only exception to this rule is very thick or curly hair, which the stylist may want to do a preliminary rough cut on when dry to see how it behaves. Ideally, a haircut should make the shape of the final style obvious even when the hair is roughly dried and shaken into place.

A cut is at its best for approximately six weeks only, for, as the hair grows, the style becomes out of balance. However, it is always inadvisable to attempt to cut your own hair, or even to trim a fringe, or bangs, as this may ruin the overall shape and effect of the cut.

Choosing a style

Hairstyles change so rapidly that they are often considered as a fashion accessory rather than as a perfect frame for any individual face or face shape. There are one or two considerations, however, that should be borne in mind when choosing the shape or length of a new hairstyle. Round or plump faces tend to look better with a style that is cut no shorter than jawbone length. Square faces need a shape that softens the jawline, either with the hair brushed away from the face or with softness in the form of curls at chin level. Generally, a very short cut will suit only the most perfect bone structure and so the shape of the ears, neck and head must be considered carefully and great care must be taken to compensate for any features that are less than perfect. Very short hair can be more difficult to manage than a longer, softer style as the effect can be flat and dull if the texture is fine; it also requires more frequent visits to a salon. Very long, loose hair, on the other hand, usually suits only the young. As a woman matures, the ageing process begins to show on the face as a series of downward planes. Downward movement in the hair exaggerates this, so styles should be softer and fuller as a woman grows older. Very straight hair is also unflattering to an older face, unless swept up into an elegant chignon or French pleat, which can look most effective (see pages 42–43 for instructions).

Shampooing

Ensuring that hair is clean and shiny is the most important step in hair care. Choose a shampoo from a reputable manufacturer to suit your hair type (see page 38). The active cleansing ingredients vary considerably in quality. A shampoo should cleanse thoroughly without irritating or de-moisturizing the scalp – this is more important than the acid/alkali balance (for an alternative view on the choice of shampoo, see page 33). It should not be necessary to use much shampoo to get good results, nor should shampooing leave the hair 'squeaky clean', as this indicates that too much oil and moisture have been removed. Such additives as herbs and fruit or protein do not affect the hair's condition.

Really greasy hair may be washed once a day but it is inadvisable to shampoo more than once or twice a week if your hair is dry, as over-washing can rob the hair of moisture. Dry shampoos, made of a grease-absorbing fine powder, help to make hair look fresher when there is no time to wash it.

You will need: a brush or comb with widely spaced teeth, a spray attachment, mixer tap or shower, and shampoo.

1 Brush or comb hair thoroughly to loosen dirt and dead skin cells from the scalp. Wet the hair with the spray, so the underneath layers are saturated with water as well as the top ones.

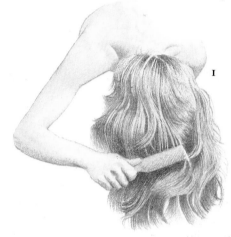

2 Pour a small amount, roughly a teaspoon, of shampoo into the palm of the hand.

3 Massage the shampoo gently into the roots with the fingertips, covering the whole of the scalp.

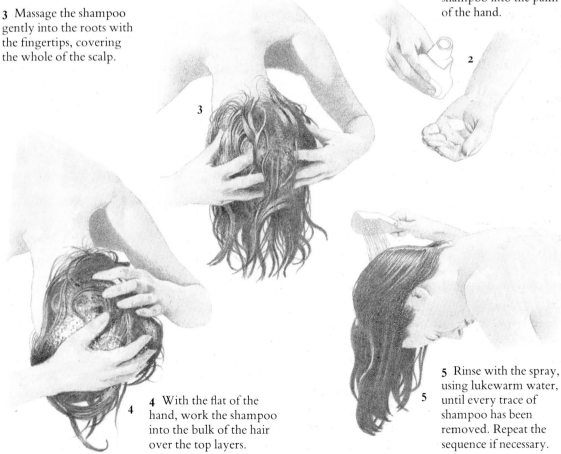

4 With the flat of the hand, work the shampoo into the bulk of the hair over the top layers.

5 Rinse with the spray, using lukewarm water, until every trace of shampoo has been removed. Repeat the sequence if necessary.

37

Conditioning

As tap water is mildly alkaline, hair that is dried straightaway after shampooing may become charged with static electricity, making it flyaway and difficult to manage. Our grandmothers resolved this by adding vinegar or lemon juice to the final rinsing water to neutralize the alkalinity. A modern-day equivalent is to use a cream rinse or conditioner after every shampoo; in addition to stabilizing the pH value of the hair, these include light-reflective ingredients, which coat the length of each hair to increase shine and gloss, as well as adding bulk. A cream rinse or conditioner also helps to smooth down the outer layer, or cuticle, of the hair. This swells and flaps open when any alkaline substance, such as hard water, shampoo, dye or a perming solution, touches it. By making it smooth again, a conditioner helps to make each hair more light-reflective and prevents penetration of anything harmful to the inner core. The cuticle also helps 'seal' each hair to guard against water evaporation, the major cause of dryness. It is damage to this water-preserving cuticle layer rather than to the inner structure of the hair that is the main danger when chemical treatments, such as perms or permanent colourants, are used.

Range of products

Conditioners and cream rinses come in differing strengths and range from wash-off varieties to 'hair packs' designed to work with heat to penetrate and soften damaged hair. As the instructions for such products vary considerably between one manufacturer and another, it is always advisable to study them closely for time and method of treatment before using any new product. A conditioner is usually composed of various emulsions of oils or waxes that are not water-soluble, so a fine coating is left on the hair when the conditioner is rinsed off. Recent developments have included 'oil free' conditioners, which can be used on greasy hair without risk of aggravating the build-up of oil.

However, any shine-restoring product has only a temporary effect in maintaining condition, since the hair is dead when it leaves the scalp and cannot be mended or renovated. Such products cannot cure split ends, which are quite natural; the only remedy is to have them cut off. But a conditioner or a cream rinse, chosen according to the hair's type, texture and condition, is an important adjunct to a good programme of care and should not be skimped or ignored.

Common hair conditions

- Combination hair

Hair that is oily at the scalp and dry and brittle at the ends may be caused by over-zealous washing with the wrong shampoo when the natural state of the hair tends towards greasiness. Using a milder shampoo – one based on high quality wash-active ingredients, which clean gently without demoisturizing the scalp – and conditioning the ends counteracts the dryness.

- Dry hair

A mild shampoo should be used, followed by a conditioner formulated for dry hair. Hair should be trimmed regularly to eliminate split ends, which may travel up the length of the shaft, giving a roughened, brittle appearance. The condition of the scalp and the condition of the hair can be quite different: the scalp can be oily, while the hair is dry because over-washing has removed the moisture from it. Hot oil treatments may be helpful where dry hair is accompanied by a dry scalp: the oil temporarily seals the surface of the skin and hair, so that no moisture can escape, allowing time for the natural moisture to restore itself. Warmed olive oil should be massaged into hair and scalp, which should then be covered with a towel for an hour; remove oil by first applying neat shampoo, then gradually adding water.

- Fine hair

It is particularly important to use a conditioner regularly on this type of hair to counteract the static, which makes it flyaway and difficult to control; a conditioning rinse helps to add bulk.

- Greasy hair

This condition is caused by an over-abundance of sebum from the sebaceous glands, which lie next to the hair follicle (see pages 12, 14). The sebum is spread along the shaft by the matting of the hairs and friction of one against the other. There is no way of suppressing the over-activity of the sebaceous glands so the hair needs to be washed more regularly than normal since its greasy state attracts dirt more quickly. Dry shampoos are particularly useful and effective for greasy hair.

Blow Drying

Used correctly, a hand-held dryer and a styling brush can create a wide variety of bouncy looks and can even help straighten hair that is too frizzy or curly. It is important to keep the stream of air moving rapidly over each section and to keep the dryer at least 15 cm (6 in) away from the hair, to avoid dehydration. Use this method if your cut determines the shape of the style you want; but if the hair has been permed to give additional curl or volume, allow it to dry naturally or give it a roller set. Other methods of drying, mostly used in salons, include infra-red lamps to give a naturally dried look in half the time and hooded dryers, which dry a roller set evenly. Hair with a natural curl can be left to dry in its own time.

You will need: a tail comb, metal clips, a round styling brush to curl hair up or under or simply to give lift and bounce to an uncurled style, and a hand-held blow dryer. After shampooing and conditioning, wrap the hair in a towel for ten minutes. Gently comb or brush it to straighten out any tangles.

1 Rough hair all over until it is only slightly damp.

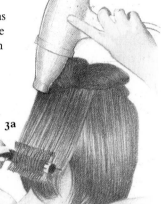

2 Using the tail of the comb, divide the top layers of hair into sections: one or two at each side and one at the back. Twist each bunch and clip it up on the top of the head.

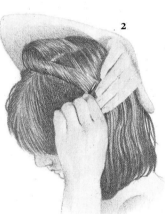

3 Dry the underneath sections of first the back (a), then the sides (b): stretch the hair slightly as you brush, following the strokes of the brush with the dryer. Brush from underneath to curl the hair in, from above for flicked-up curls.

4 Unpin the top section at the back and gradually blend the two layers as you dry. The more you lift the hair away from the head, the more bounce the finished style will have.

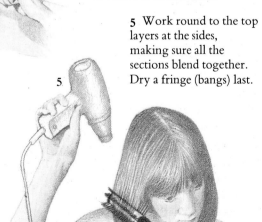

5 Work round to the top layers at the sides, making sure all the sections blend together. Dry a fringe (bangs) last.

..., rollers give ... they are essential ... een permed. Hair ... l more tightly and ... rs than hair that is ... Quite small sections of ha... ... (2 in) across, should be used on e... ... ke sure you have enough rollers before yo... ...etting. If too much hair is bunched on to an individual roller, the finished effect will be uneven.

There is a wide variety of setting patterns, but generally, crown, back and side hair is rolled downwards. However, the direction in which the hair is rolled is not as important as the way in which the curl is brushed out. For example, hair that has been rolled under can be brushed out in the opposite direction to create a flicking-up effect. Unless the setting pattern states otherwise, start putting in rollers at the top, then work round the lower sections from one side to the other.

A triangular hairnet helps keep rollers in place while the hair is being dried, either naturally or with a hairdryer. Make sure that the hair is completely dry before removing the rollers – try unwinding a test curl from the back of the head, where the hair grows at its thickest, and feel for dampness before unwinding the rest of the curls. If they are unwound too soon, the final result will be frizzy and hard to manage.

After removing all the rollers and clips, brush through firmly to smooth out any curl lines. Then brush lightly into shape, forming curls and waves with the tail of a comb. A hair spray will keep this kind of style in place and help to protect it in a damp atmosphere; remember that the spray should be held at least 15 cm (6 in) from the head.

Setting a pincurl
Suitable for short strands at the hairline. Wind the strands from tip to root, like a snail, and secure them flat against the head with a metal clip placed diagonally across the curl. Do not bunch too much hair into one curl and try not to twist the strand as you curl it. A whole head can be set in small curls, but this takes some time.

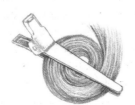

How to put in rollers
You will need: rollers, straight-sided roller pins and a tail comb. Dry hair with a towel until just slightly damp. A setting lotion helps hold the set and protects the hair from a damp atmosphere when it is dry. Modern setting lotions are easily washed out and do not build up a coat that attracts dirt.

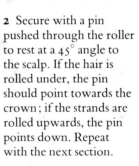

1

2 Secure with a pin pushed through the roller to rest at a 45° angle to the scalp. If the hair is rolled under, the pin should point towards the crown; if the strands are rolled upwards, the pin points down. Repeat with the next section.

1 Using the tail of the comb, divide off a triangular section of hair with the apex furthest from the crown. Comb the section carefully, holding it at 90° to the head and making sure the ends are as even as possible. Place the ends against the roller and wind the strands firmly and evenly down to the scalp. Do not pull or wind too tightly, as this can weaken the roots, causing temporary hair loss if repeated often.

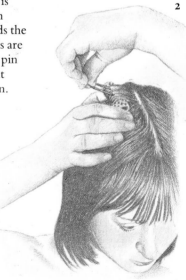

2

Setting with rollers

A wide variety of effects can be achieved according to the number and size of rollers used and the direction in which they are wound.

For body and bounce

Use medium-sized rollers. Working upwards from the neckline, roll the hair at the sides and back downwards, dividing the sides into two sections. Roll the central section of the fringe (bangs) forwards.

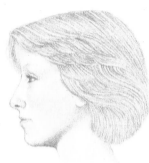

  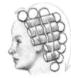

For a fuller wavy set

Wind the two sections at the nape of the neck downwards on to narrow rollers. For the middle layers, use a row of narrow rollers placed vertically rather than horizontally along the scalp to give more bounce; roll the hair towards the face. With the top layers make a side parting and roll the hair down on larger rollers.

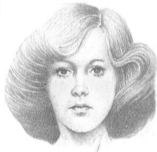 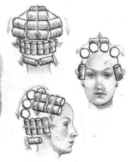

Using a heated styling brush

For use on dry hair only. Curl a few strands of hair on to the brush, lifting from the roots for a fresher, fuller look at the same time as creating loose curls. Hold momentarily while the wave develops, carefully unwind the section and start on the next.

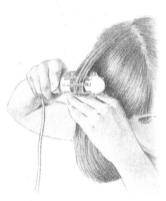

Setting with heated rollers

These are always used on dry hair. Although the rollers are electrically heated and thermostatically controlled to maintain a certain temperature, over-use may contribute to hair damage and dryness, so they should be regarded as an occasional, emergency aid. Some models have conditioning mist features, which help to prevent dehydration.

When the rollers are hot, the hair is wound on to them in the same way as with wet hair and ordinary rollers; but because the rollers are made of solid plastic, which cannot be pierced with a standard pin, special wide pins that encircle the rollers are used to hold them in place. Some sets come in full head packs of 20 or more, others have fewer rollers. When using only a few, begin with the underlying layers of hair, removing each roller as it cools, re-heating it and starting again on a top section.

Damage may be caused to the hair by the sharp spikes on some rollers; hairdressers often file these down and cover the roller with a layer of foam. Care should always be taken, too, when using heated rollers near the hairline – a piece of cotton wool placed between roller and skin prevents any danger of burning.

Setting with styling tongs and brushes

Styling tongs and brushes are used on dry hair and work in the same way as heated rollers, but treat only one area at a time. They are ideal for curling small sections such as flicked-back sides or fringes (bangs). Although their effect is not as long-lasting as an ordinary roller set, or a well-executed blow-dry set, they are quick and convenient to use. A styling brush is particularly effective for giving body and bounce to limp hair. The brush can be held horizontally or vertically and the hair wound under or outwards depending on how the curl is intended to fall.

As they do not heat up to a very high temperature, they are unlikely to damage the hair unless used daily; but always proceed with caution when using heated appliances and remember to use conditioners after every shampoo. Some setting lotions now incorporate a heat-protection shield and are well worth using if heated appliances are needed for your style.

Classic Styles

Classic hairstyles
Before following the directions for any of these styles, set your hair with conventional or heated rollers to give bounce and movement to the whole head, rolling hair downwards on to large rollers. A three-way dressing table mirror will give an accurate view of the back and sides of the styles.

2 Still twisting the hair, coil it down in a circle around the covered band; secure with pins, holding up the loose ends.

Woven chignon
1 Carefully brush or comb hair back to the nape of the neck, ensuring that it lies smoothly, and secure it in a ponytail with a covered elastic band. Divide the ponytail into three even sections and lift the lefthand one towards the left ear. Pin across the section just above the covered band so that most of it is still hanging free.

Simple chignon
1 Brush or comb all the hair up on to the crown and, without pulling too tightly so the strands lie evenly, secure into a ponytail with a covered elastic band. Using both hands, gently twist the ponytail.

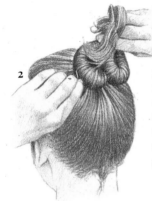

3 If your hair is long, form a second smaller coil above the first. Tuck the loose ends into the centre of the coil and pin carefully so none of the grips show.

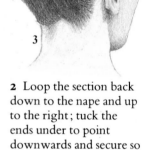

2 Loop the section back down to the nape and up to the right; tuck the ends under to point downwards and secure so that the pins are covered.

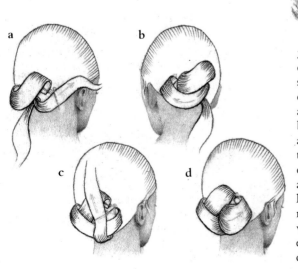

3 Divide the remainder of the ponytail into two sections. Following the directions shown by the arrows, pin the righthand bunch up to the right (a) and then loop it over to the left (b). Lift the central bunch straight up and pin it under the first loop (c) and take it to the right (d), to create a woven effect. Tuck in the ends, pinning them down if necessary.

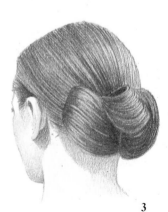

French pleat

This can be positioned on either side or the back of the crown.

1 For a pleat on the right side, bring the hair from the left over the top of the head to the right, brushing or combing it so it lies smoothly. Pin in place with a line of grips running from front to back; leave the ends hanging loose.

2 Brush or comb the back section up to the same position.

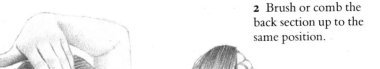

3 Pin in place, so the grips are parallel with those in **1**, and leave the ends loose.

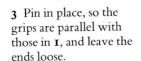

4 Lift up the hair on the righthand side and all the loose ends. Grasping them all together, twist them slightly and comb or brush through.

5 Roll the hair down on to the crown over the pins, tucking all the ends under. Secure just under the top edge with a line of pins so that the hair forms a smooth roll on the righthand side of the head.

6 The final effect is elegant and understated, with the hair swept up in smooth sections to form simple lines.

Perming and Colouring

A permanent wave can add lift, curls, waves and volume to hair that is naturally fine, limp or lank, creating a style that would be difficult to maintain with rollers or any of the other setting aids available. Judicious use of hair colour can enliven the dullest, drabbest natural shade. But both these processes, with the exception of the temporary water-colour rinses, involve a long-term change in appearance and it is worth looking closely into what they entail, how they affect the hair and what they can – and cannot – do.

Perming

As explained on pages 31–32, the initial step is to break down the chemical bonds between the keratin scales of the hair shaft and this is done by applying a permanent waving solution. The hair is thus left in a soft, almost plastic state and is re-formed by winding round curlers or rollers. A neutralizer is then applied to counteract the chemical process, so that the links between the keratin molecules mould themselves into the new shape and stay curled permanently. Although the effect gradually wears off as the hair grows and becomes heavier, a perm usually holds its shape until the hair is cut off.

Hair should always be trimmed before a permanent wave treatment and some hairdressers like to cut it again afterwards to give a more natural, soft effect. Using a perm on hair that is already broken or damaged, either by rough handling or by the use of other chemical agents such as bleaches or dyes, may cause it all to break off close to the scalp. A perm should never be used on a scalp that is known to be sensitive to strong ingredients or that is in any way sore, scratched or infected. Perms can greatly improve greasy hair because, as well as adding more volume, they also lift the hair slightly away from the scalp and so help to prevent the sebum travelling up the shaft so quickly. It is important to obtain professional advice if your hair is in poor condition. In any case, a test strand should always be treated in advance and a patch test done for allergy.

Home perming technology has advanced to the stage that the new ammonia-free perms are as good as any that are used at the hairdresser's and they are, of course, far less expensive. However, the professional is paid for skill, judgement and training in applying the solution, neutralizing it correctly and winding just the right number of rollers of the right diameter in the right directions. It can be tricky putting in the rollers at exactly the correct angle, particularly at the back of the head, so ask a friend to help with a home perm if possible. It is essential to stick rigidly to the manufacturer's instructions, since research chemists experiment, test and improve products such as these continually and instructions may vary from one batch to the next of even a familiar home perming product. After-perm treatment should consist of using gentle shampoos and plenty of conditioners to counteract any adverse effects on the keratin layer. Approach colouring or re-perming with great caution.

A perm can also be used in reverse to straighten naturally frizzy or curly hair, but again caution should be observed. African hair, for example, is already quite weak and lacking in elasticity. Wrongly applied, a straightening treatment can cause extensive breakage, as the stresses imposed on unwinding the links of the hair chemically are far greater than those caused by winding it into a curl. Home straightening is not recommended.

Permanent tints

These are the only colourants that can radically change the hair's natural shade, as they penetrate the core of each hair, removing the pigment and replacing it with a new shade. They require the addition of a liquid or powder oxidant, such as sodium perborate, to develop the colour, and so all permanent tints require pre-mixing of two solutions or a solution and a powder. Ammonia is often included in the dye to assist this process of oxidation. The action of the ammonia on the hair causes the scales of the cuticle to open, facilitating the entry of the dye into the core; the action of the ammonia on the oxidant also causes more rapid liberation of oxygen and therefore quicker activation of colour development. These dyes can be shampooed in; or they can be applied with a brush or swab to dry hair divided off into sections.

The result of a permanent tint is indeed permanent until the hair is cut off; new growth has to be retouched accurately without any of the new colourant overlapping on to the previously treated hair. It is therefore important to select the right colour. Many people use these tints for covering up grey hair, which they do very effectively. However, as the hair loses pigment and becomes grey, the skin also becomes paler, so restoring the hair to an approximation of its original colour may look too severe.

Despite the suspicion that the coal tar derivative commonly used in these dyes may have carcinogenic properties (see page 32), there has as yet been no firm scientific evidence that they cause cancer in human beings, and many people would be loth to abandon them without very hard evidence of this link. The same derivative may also cause allergic reactions, so always perform a patch test on the inside of the elbow or behind the ear before applying a whole-head tint, allowing five full days for a reaction to show; this is also a wise precaution before using other types of dye. A strand test can also be helpful in indicating what to expect from the finished result.

Semi-permanent colourants

The dyes used in most semi-permanent colourants penetrate and adhere to the outer layer, the cuticle, but they differ from permanent colourants in that there is no chemical bonding between the colour and the hair, so the colour gradually washes out after two to eight weeks. It is not possible to alter the colour of the hair radically with these products and they are not always successful in covering grey hair. They work best when they enhance or lift the natural colour – reddish tones on brown hair, blue tones on black hair, golden tones on fair hair.

They usually incorporate a conditioning agent so that the hair looks shinier and healthier. They are applied like a shampoo, with the lather left on the hair for a stated length of time, then rinsed off. Because the colour gradually washes out there is no need to retouch. They can be used safely after perming or bleaching, although a strand test might be advisable beforehand, as the porosity of the hair after chemical treatment affects the amount of colour it takes up.

Temporary tints

These are often called rinses because they are usually put on the hair after shampooing. A light film of colour coats the outside of the hair cuticle and is removed by the next shampoo. These dyes are often made from food colourants or vegetable extracts and are used for slight alterations in colour – toning down blonde hair that looks brassy, highlighting red tones in a permanent tint, freshening up hair that has been permed. A disadvantage ·is that, being water-soluble, the colours are rain-soluble too and may also rub off on to sheets, clothes and collars. But as they are the safest, most predictable form of colouring, they are ideal for anyone who wishes to experiment.

Bleaching and lightening

Anything that lightens the colour of the hair by even one shade is a bleach; these products range from mild brighteners, which simply lighten the hair a little, to strong bleaches, which can turn brunettes into blondes. Bleaches work in much the same way as permanent tints but, instead of deepening the shade, they strip a little or a lot of the hair's own colour, depending on the strength of the product used. The effects are permanent until the hair grows out. Whereas mild bleaches, usually in cream or shampoo form, are safe and easy to use on fair hair that has dulled, the stronger types are more tricky to use safely and any complete colour change using bleaches should be left to a professional. Radical colour changes usually involve two stages, as bleached hair may need a toner to soften any brassy or reddish effects.

Streaking and highlighting

One of the most effective ways of making the hair look fairer, without the root-retouching problems of a whole-head bleach, is to add streaks or highlights to the hair (highlighting is also known as frosting) or to add colour just to the tips. There are two methods for tipping and highlighting – home kits are available. In the first, the strands of hair to be dyed are pulled through a perforated plastic cap with a crochet hook, leaving the rest of the hair and scalp protected. In the second, sections of hair are dyed in strips of aluminium foil, which takes a little longer and is more effective for tips; this method is also used for streaking. Apart from bleaches, any colour lighter than the natural hair colour may· be used to highlight; some colourists use a combination of highlights for a beautifully natural, dappled look.

Henna

A vegetable-compound hair colourant that adds glorious rich red tones to dark or brown hair, henna also conditions the hair, giving it an extra lustre. Black henna is obtainable for very dark hair. The effects of henna resemble a permanent tint – the colour fades with time, but does not wash off with repeated shampoos. Some hairdressers are wary about perming hennaed hair, as the reactions are unpredictable. Always buy henna from a reputable source.

Wigs and hairpieces

If you want to change the appearance of your hair temporarily without perming or colouring, then a wig or a hairpiece can create the illusion of an instant change of length, texture or colour. Do not expect to fool anyone though – fashion wigs and pieces are essentially fun. Modern wigs are made entirely of acrylic fibres, which give a good approximation of the appearance and texture of real hair but which are inexpensive and can be cleaned easily by washing. They may have inbuilt curl, they can be cut to any length that is desired and they usually have stretchy lightweight net bases so that the wig fits all head shapes easily and is comfortable to wear. Long pieces or plaits can be pinned on to short hair and then wound into, say, a chignon or a ponytail for a different hairstyle; but this will look effective only if the join between the hairpiece and the natural hair is concealed by the style. Again, these pieces are made from acrylic fibres and come in such a wide variety of shades that it is easy to find one to match every shade of natural hair colour. Wigs can also be a valuable aid for anyone who, for example, is considering having a perm and wants to know how her hair would look – trying on a range of curly styles can give a preview of the effect.

For people who, through illness or accident, have little or no hair of their own, wigs or hairpieces may be recommended as prosthetic devices. Great care is then taken to match up the 'false' hair with the patient's own. The wig or piece is made of real hair rather than acrylic and is carefully fitted, as comfort is the prime consideration. The disadvantage is that real hair must be cleaned rather than washed and needs colouring regularly to preserve the original tint.

Body Hair

Hair grows all over the surface of the body, with the exception of the palms of the hands and the soles of the feet. This soft downy hair, which is called vellus hair, is never a problem in youth. But with age, the vellus hairs may become coarser and darker – a problem that is particularly apparent on the upper lip and chin of some women after the menopause. It is thought that the male hormones produced by or ingested into the body have a cumulative effect and, as oestrogen supplies diminish, hair growth becomes heavier. Excess hair problems in younger people may be associated with an endocrine disorder.

Many women like to remove the hair covering their legs and armpits for cosmetic reasons. It may be argued that removing underarm hair is also conducive to good hygiene as the hairs act as a trap for sweat; however, regular washing should cope with this problem.

While there are several methods of temporary hair removal, electrolysis, which destroys the root by chemical reaction, or short-wave diathermy, which destroys it with heat, are the only means of removing hair permanently. Each method bears examination as there are arguments for and against each and some methods are much better suited for some parts of the body than others. It is generally unwise to use deodorants or antiperspirants on underarms for 24 hours after depilation, as they may irritate the skin.

Shaving, plucking and cutting

These are the most widely used methods of temporary hair removal. The disadvantage of plucking is that it may distort the hair root; nor is it suitable for a large area. Shaving and cutting chop the hairs at the surface of the skin, leaving a blunt edge, which quickly feels scratchy and prickly, and so they are not methods recommended for the face for purely aesthetic reasons. There is, however, no truth in the notion that shaving makes the hair grow back thicker or faster but to keep the skin smooth, it is generally necessary to shave at least once or twice a week. Provided the razor is sharp and carefully handled and the skin is well wetted and primed with soap, this method gives quick, smooth results for the minimum of expenditure and is particularly suitable for underarms and legs. Electric razors also give good results and have the advantage that they can be used outside the bathroom with a minimum of preparation; special models designed to deal with female body hair are also available. Lightweight disposable razors are easy to wield round tricky areas such as the ankle bone or the front of the shin where the skin is thin. After using a razor, apply a body lotion or cream.

Depilatory creams, lotions and aerosols

The chemicals in these products dissolve excess hair, giving much smoother and longer-lasting results than shaving or cutting. However, some people may be allergic to one or other of the ingredients, so it is worth doing a patch test when using a depilatory for the first time. Most products are stringently tested and are safe for the face provided the skin is not unusually sensitive. Depilatories are smoothed on to the skin, left for a stated amount of time and then the hairs are rinsed off with the cream. It is important always to follow the manufacturer's instructions on the length of time that the cream or lotion is left on the skin in order to avoid irritation.

Waxing

A thin film of heated wax is applied, allowed to cool slightly and then ripped off in strips, taking the hairs with it by tearing them out from the root. The advantages of this method of hair removal are that large areas can be treated in one session, that it leaves very soft, smooth skin and that the hair takes longer to grow back than with other methods and is fine-ended as it grows through. It does not, however, discourage regrowth. Hair has to grow to a certain length before it is suitable for waxing, which may not be aesthetically acceptable to some people, and the treatment may occasionally give rise to ingrowing hairs, which need attention before they can be waxed again. The main disadvantage is that unless the wax is applied skilfully and heated to exactly the right temperature, the process can be very painful. Trained personnel in salons will wax legs, underarms, lips, chin or 'bikini' hair; but home waxing kits are also available. There are also methods involving cooled wax or re-usable wax strips, which are applied to the skin cold.

Permanent hair removal

The only methods that remove hair permanently are short-wave diathermy and electrolysis, both of which destroy the hair root and surrounding cells so that no hair can grow at the particular site again. Short-wave diathermy destroys the root by means of heat; electrolysis destroys it with a chemical reaction produced by a galvanic current. Fine hairs may require only one treatment; coarser hairs may need several but will grow progressively finer after each treatment until they disappear altogether. Both these methods use extremely fine needles introduced into each hair follicle – a process that requires specialized training since the operator needs a highly developed sense of touch and considerable skill in order to judge the requirements of each follicle. It is therefore important that permanent hair removal by diathermy or electrolysis should be carried out by a trained operator in a reputable salon or clinic. Kits for use at home are available but should be avoided. Because only a few hairs can be treated in any one session, these methods are chiefly reserved for removing facial hair, where very good results can be obtained. The treatment can be painful and is fairly expensive, especially as several visits are necessary even for a relatively small patch of hair; it may make the skin temporarily red and sore, but many clients find it the best solution for facial hair.

Abrasion

Pumice stones, emery mitts and other roughening agents can be used to rub off unwanted hair, but this method is not popular, largely because there is the danger of over-abrading the skin and making it tender and sore. It is most suited to the legs, providing the hair is rubbed off fairly gently. Regrowth occurs at approximately the same rate as for shaving and cutting.

Bleaching

This method is most effective for a light growth of dark hair and can be used on the face or the body. A cream or liquid bleach is applied to the skin and rinsed off after a stated time. The bleach may weaken the hair and encourage it to break off, but unfortunately it may also irritate the skin, so always do a patch test first.

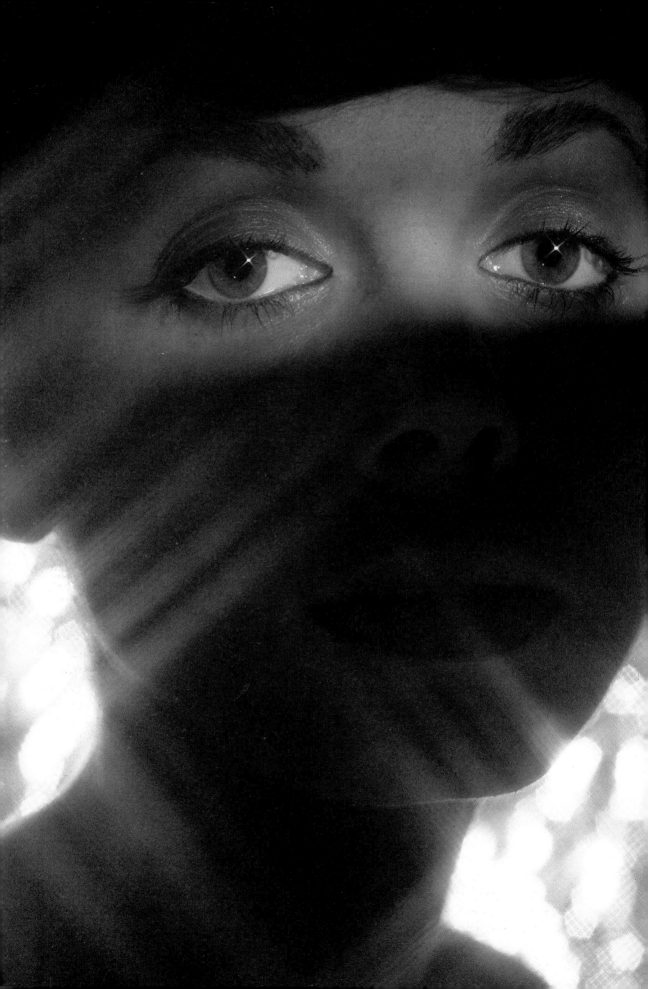

Eyes

Two completely spherical organs, the eyes lie within the orbits – protective bony hollows in the skull – and are further cushioned from injury by being embedded in fat. The eyelids and eyelashes provide additional protection and lessen the likelihood of foreign bodies entering the eye.

The eyeball is filled with a jelly-like substance called humour. It has a tough, opaque outer coat (the sclera), which becomes transparent at the front, where it is known as the cornea. The inner coat of the eyelids (the conjunctiva) is reflected over the front of the cornea. It too is transparent and so allows light rays to enter the eye through the pupil, a central gap in the iris.

The iris contains muscle fibres arranged in a circular and radiating pattern. When the circular fibres contract, the pupil gets smaller, and when the radiating fibres contract, the pupil dilates. The iris contains varying amounts of pigment, which give the eyes their colour. Blue eyes have little pigment, brown eyes much more. Eye colour is inherited: each parent passes on one gene relating to it to their child. Because the gene for blue eyes is recessive, anyone who inherits genes for both blue and brown eyes will have brown eyes, not blue. Eye colour varies with race, brown eyes being more common among dark-skinned races.

Just behind the pupil is the lens, the size of which is controlled by the ciliary muscles. The job of the lens is to bend the rays of light entering the eye so that the image of the object seen is focused on the back of the eye (the retina). The lens is long and thin when focusing on distant objects, thick and fat, as a result of the contraction of the ciliary muscles, for looking at objects close to. As we grow older, the eyeball tends to change shape and the ciliary muscles can no longer work as quickly and efficiently as in youth. As a result, the image of the object being looked at does not always fall on the retina and it may therefore appear blurred. This is why even those who have good eyesight in youth may need to wear spectacles by their late forties or early fifties.

The retina is the light-sensitive part of the eye and it is made up almost entirely of nervous tissue. Some of the nerve cells are responsible for detailed vision and colour perception, while others are more sensitive to movement. The latter enable us to some extent to see in the dark.

In the outer corner of the upper eyelid are the tear, or lacrimal, glands. They open into the eye through ducts running along the edge of the upper eyelid. The tears they secrete keep the eyelid lubricated and are swept regularly over the eyeball by the eyelid's blinking action. Blinking also causes tears to be sucked into the inner corner of the eye, from where they drain away into the lacrimal sac and from there into a channel that leads to the nose – this explains why weeping tends to make the nose run. Tears constantly bathe the eye therefore, which helps to keep it clean and to wash away anything harmful. As well as salt, tears contain lysozyme, which is one of nature's most powerful anti-bacterial substances and helps to keep the eye free from infection.

Each eye has three pairs of muscles, which can move it up and down and right and left. Normal binocular vision is a consequence of having all these pairs of muscles perfectly synchronized and balanced in each eye. When one muscle in one eye is stronger than the opposing muscle in the other eye, the result is a squint.

Sun and the eyes

Some years ago many people believed that it was unwise to wear sunglasses because a degree of exposure to the sun was deemed necessary to strengthen the eyes, whereas wearing sunglasses was thought to weaken them. This is a myth. Recent research, indeed, suggests that chronic exposure to sunlight may promote the development of cataracts in the lens. In view of this, it makes good sense to wear sunglasses in strong sunshine. Tinted prescription lenses are worth while for those who would otherwise have to use ordinary spectacles for work in bright sunlight. If ordinary daylight makes you squint, photosensitive lenses (the kind that darken and lighten according to the strength of the light) are worth considering.

One of the reasons why bright sunlight can be uncomfortable is because of the way light hits the retina from all directions simultaneously, thus creating a glare. This glare is reduced if the rays of light are polarized (bent before entering the eye), so that they reach the retina from one direction only. Glass that polarizes light is often used in spectacles and car windscreens for this reason.

Eye Care

'Tired eyes'

It is a myth that reading too much or reading in poor light can strain the eyes. The eyes are made to see and sight does not strain them. Even when we are doing close work, we tend automatically to rest our eyes by glancing up every now and then, and this allows the ciliary muscles, which control the shape of the lens, to relax. Special eye exercise routines are therefore quite unnecessary. (If, however, you would like to try out some exercises for the eyes, turn to pages 146 and 177.) It is possible for the eyes to become sore and dry after close work as a consequence of our forgetting to blink often enough. In this instance the remedy is simply to blink a few times: this sluices the eyeball out with tears and cures the dryness.

'Palming' – the practice of cupping the hands over the eyes to rest them – will do no harm, but shutting the eyes for a few seconds every now and then is just as effective a method of refreshing and relieving them.

No eye lotions or eye drops come anywhere near tears for bathing the eyes. So the best way to bathe them is simply to have a good cry. The second best way is to dissolve a teaspoonful of salt in a glass of water and, with (clean) fingers or a dropper, put two or three drops into each eye. This can be repeated four hours later if need be. Do this only if the soreness has been caused by some foreign body in the eye. If the eye is sore for no obvious reason and is red and bloodshot, consult a doctor straight away. The cause may be an infection, which needs antibiotics. As a general rule, do not put anything into the eyes for longer than a few days without consulting a doctor. Any condition that persists may prove serious unless the proper treatment is given promptly.

Despite the fact that tears are good for the eyes, a long bout of crying may make the tear glands overwork and leave the eyes feeling sore and swollen. Cold water compresses on the eyelids should help to relieve the discomfort. I have found no evidence that lotions containing vegetable extracts (such as cucumber) are any more efficacious than plain water. It does no harm, incidentally, to rub the eyes, provided that there is no foreign body in either of them and that rubbing them does not cause any pain.

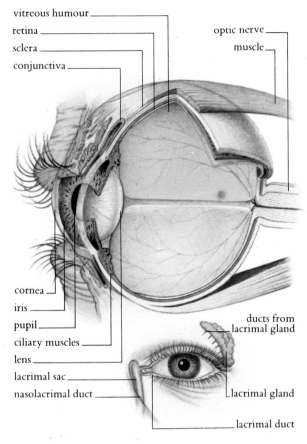

vitreous humour
retina
sclera
conjunctiva
optic nerve
muscle
cornea
iris
pupil
ciliary muscles
lens
lacrimal sac
nasolacrimal duct
ducts from lacrimal gland
lacrimal gland
lacrimal duct

Skin care for the area around the eyes

Treat the skin around the eyes gently, for although its structure does not differ from the skin on the rest of the face, it has very little subcutaneous fat and muscle. As it also covers a hollow in the skull bones, it has little support and therefore tends to stretch and wrinkle all too easily (see pages 23–24 for skin routines for this area). Ordinary moisturizer is just as good as special eye cream, no matter what exotic and expensive ingredients the latter may lay claim to. Avoid any eye cream that contains lanolin (wool fat): this can make the skin puffy and swollen.

The dark rings that some people get under their eyes are caused by extra skin pigmentation. This is accentuated by the fact that the skin in this area lies over a hollow in the bone and hence tends to be in the shadow. Several sleepless nights will make the circles look darker still because the muscles in the face will be relaxed as a result of fatigue, so having the unfortunate effect of making the hollows under the eyes appear deeper and more pronounced than usual.

Spectacles

Fashion has long since overtaken function where spectacles are concerned, but ideally they should have the following features:

• a good, balanced shape – not too high above the eyebrow or too much of the frame below the eye and not much wider than the face.

• fairly light in weight. Heavy spectacles can make the ears and nose sore and may even stretch the skin on the nose so that it wrinkles.

• a good fit – the arm of the spectacles should be expertly fitted so that it grips the ear gently and stops the spectacles sliding down.

Contact lenses

There is an increasing vogue for contact lenses nowadays. Two types are available: hard and soft. The comfort and length of time for which the lenses can be worn depends on how much oxygen they allow to reach the conjunctivae – when too little gets through, the eyes become sore and the lenses have to be removed. Some modern hard lenses allow enough oxygen through to make them comfortable to wear for up to a day (they must be removed at night, however). Some soft lenses also have to come out at night; others (extended wear lenses) can be left in for several months without discomfort, but should be removed and cleaned at least once a week.

Where expense and durability of the lenses are crucial considerations, the hard type have advantages, but soft lenses are generally more comfortable to wear, at least initially. A slight tint on the lenses makes them easier to keep track of and can change eye colour too.

Common eye complaints

• Blepharitis

This is a form of seborrhoeic dermatitis that inflames the hair follicle of the eyelashes and makes the eyes look red-rimmed. It is usually part of dermatitis of the scalp, ears and other greasy areas (it is not related *per se* to dandruff). Do not try to treat blepharitis with proprietary creams – consult a doctor.

• Bloodshot eyes

The bloodshot look is caused by dilatation of the capillaries in the conjunctivae. The eyes may be sticky too and the eyelids crusted with 'sleep' upon waking. The cause is often an infection (invariably so if the eyes are also sticky), but some people have bloodshot eyes for no apparent reason. In the older age group, another possible cause is glaucoma, an increase in pressure within the eyeball. Whatever the cause do not use eye drops. Consult a doctor or – if the eyes are not painful or sticky – ignore.

• Conjunctivitis

When the conjunctivae are inflamed, the eyes feel sore, prickly and itchy and look red and weepy. The cause may be an infection, a foreign body or glaucoma (rise in pressure within the eyeball). Do not try to treat with proprietary preparations – consult a doctor. As a temporary remedy, bathe the eyes with a solution of one teaspoon of salt dissolved in a glass of water (use an eyebath).

• Foreign body in the eye

Because the eyes are so well supplied with nerve endings, even a speck of dust under the eyelid can feel like a boulder. Try the method shown below to remove the intruder. If that fails, go straight to the nearest hospital casualty department, or emergency room, for expert attention.

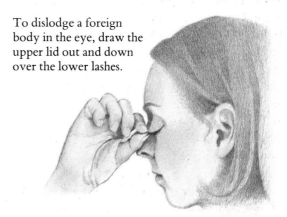

To dislodge a foreign body in the eye, draw the upper lid out and down over the lower lashes.

• Stye

This is a form of folliculitis centred on an eyelash. A red spot appears at the base of the eyelash and a pustule may eventually form there. If the eyelash can be removed, the pus will drain away. Styes are caused by bacterial infection and may arise as a result of blepharitis or seborrhoeic dermatitis. Treatment is to remove the eyelash if possible and let the pus drain away naturally. Consult your doctor for specific treatment – do not use proprietary eye ointments, which may contain mercury, or eye drops.

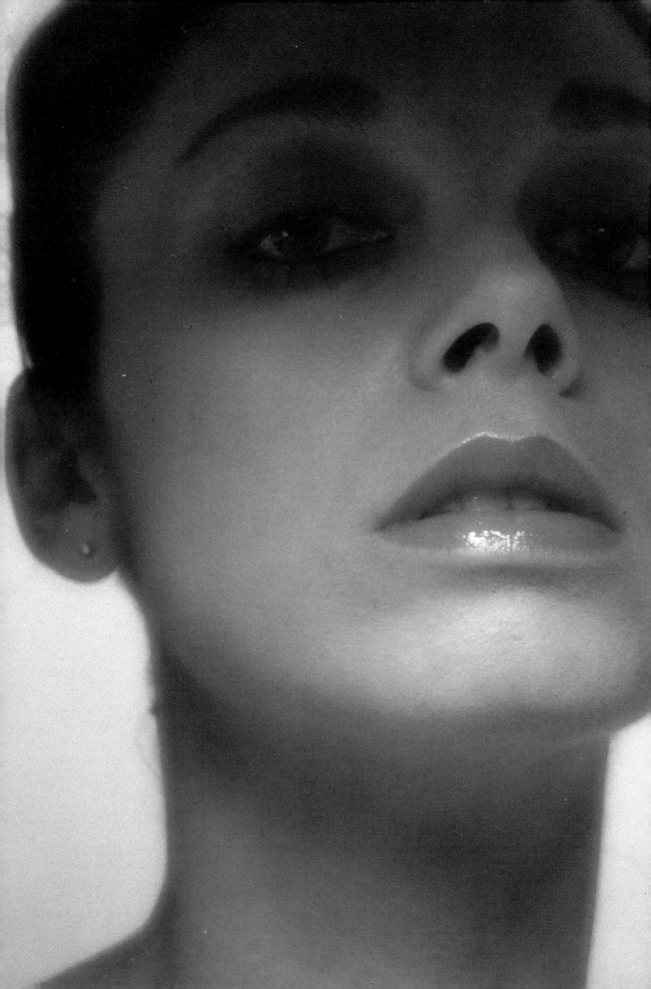

Ears, Nose and Mouth

The ear has three parts: the inner ear, the organ of balance, buried deep within the skull; the middle ear, associated with hearing; and the external ear, including everything from the ear drum, or tympanic membrane, outwards.

The external ear

The outer part of the ear consists of the pinna, which funnels sound waves towards the ear drum, and the external auditory canal, which runs towards the ear drum. The skin lining the external auditory canal is rich in hair and grease glands, both of which help to protect the ear drum from injury or infection. The hair does this by preventing small, light foreign bodies finding their way through the canal to the ear drum, and the normal activity of the grease glands coats the walls of the canal with thick, reddish-brown wax. This wax has strong anti-bacterial properties and is part of the canal's self-cleansing mechanism. If the inside of the ear is irritated (by some foreign body, for example), the glands respond by producing an extra quantity of wax. Exactly the same process is set off if the wax is removed.

It follows that it can do only harm to try to clean out the inside of the ear with cotton wool buds or to scratch out the wax with hair pins or even a judiciously used finger nail. The presence of wax in the canal is normal and beneficial to the ear. If so much wax should be produced that hearing becomes impaired, get a doctor to syringe it away rather than make any attempt to clear the blockage yourself.

The middle ear

The real organ of hearing, the middle ear, is encased within the bones of the skull. It is filled with air and connects with the throat via the Eustachian tube, which keeps the air pressure within the middle ear the same as that in the atmosphere. When there is a sudden change in altitude, and therefore a change in atmospheric pressure, as happens at take-off in an aeroplane, the equilibration of atmospheric pressure with that in the middle ear through the Eustachian tube is not immediate and the ears 'pop'. Swallowing hard or sucking a boiled sweet or candy are two generally effective ways of relieving this unpleasant sensation.

Sound waves travel down the external auditory canal to the ear drum, which begins to vibrate. This in turn causes three tiny bony ossicles within the middle ear to vibrate, passing sound waves on to the nerve endings in the hearing apparatus, the cochlea. From here they are passed on as electrical impulses to the brain.

The ears, nose and throat are anatomically one interconnecting system. One consequence is that a nasal infection such as the common cold can develop into sinusitis and a sore throat can easily become an infection of the middle ear, producing earache, particularly in children.

The inner ear

Within the inner ear is a system of semi-circular canals arranged at right angles to one another around a central sac. The canals are filled with fluid, which flows if the position of the head is altered. Messages are transmitted to the brain about the direction of the flow, enabling it to interpret body movement in any plane.

Ear piercing

This is very unlikely to damage the ear or to cause any infection provided that it is done by a competent person and the holes are properly cared for afterwards. First, keep the newly pierced skin meticulously clean: wash it at least once a day (preferably more often) with soap and water and follow this up by dabbing the skin on both sides of the ear with surgical spirit. Second, keep the tiny holes free from scabs by rotating the sleepers in the ear frequently – at least twice a day, but every half hour if you can remember.

To keep newly pierced ears open, wear earrings two or three times a week for the first year.

Common ear complaints

- Deafness

Two entirely different mechanisms may be the cause of deafness. The first is stiffening of the bony ossicles within the middle ear so that they can no longer transmit sound waves to the cochlea properly. This condition can be alleviated by a hearing aid, which amplifies sounds. The second cause of deafness is deterioration of the nerve endings in the cochlea. This is not amenable to any kind of hearing aid.

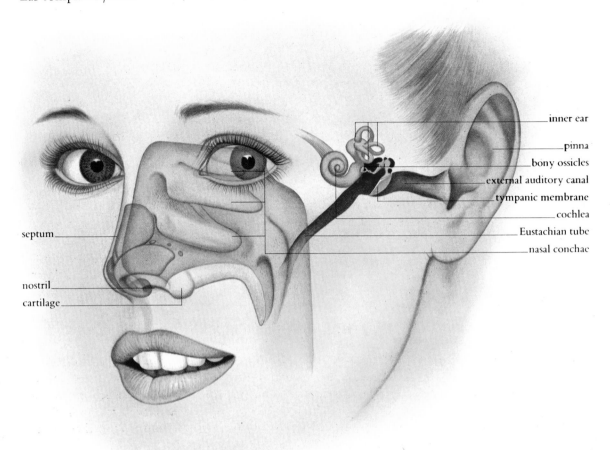

septum

nostril

cartilage

inner ear

pinna

bony ossicles

external auditory canal

tympanic membrane

cochlea

Eustachian tube

nasal conchae

Sometimes slight deafness may be caused by a build-up of wax blocking the external auditory canal. Do not try to remove the wax yourself – you may damage the canal. See a doctor for treatment.

• Dizziness (vertigo)

This is very often due to some abnormal cause working on the inner ear. Violent movements from side to side or backwards and forwards can produce it – hence seasickness is a common cause. In this case the dizziness arises from the brain's attempts to reconcile conflicting messages about body position: those that reach it almost instantly from the eyes and those that travel much more slowly from the inner ear. Other possible causes are getting up suddenly from a hot bath or from a sitting or lying position – here the dizzy feeling is due to a temporary shortage of blood to the brain. For recurrent dizzy spells, it is advisable to consult a doctor.

• Earache

The commonest cause of earache is inflammation in the middle ear. If the Eustachian tube becomes blocked, a rise in pressure in the middle ear follows. This is very painful because the middle ear is rigidly contained within the bones of the skull. High temperature, nausea or vomiting and headache are commonly associated with this un-pleasant condition.

For treatment, consult a doctor without delay. Sometimes a recurring earache is not due to disease of the ear at all but to bad teeth. This type of chronic infection should show up on a dental X-ray.

• Ringing in the ears (tinnitus)

Occasional ringing in the ears is nothing to worry about but persistent tinnitus (generally accom-panied by dizziness and loss of balance) can be part of an inner ear complaint known as Ménière's syndrome. It rarely starts before middle age and can be treated with diuretics (drugs that eliminate water from the body). Always consult a doctor about persistent ringing in the ears.

• Sticking-out ears

A woman can generally disguise her ears by adapting her hairstyle. If the ears are a real source of misery, it may be worth having them pinned back. This type of cosmetic surgery is known as otoplasty. It is relatively inexpensive and is generally highly successful (see page 224).

Nose

The visible part of the nose is formed from the nasal bones and cartilage, divided by the septum. Nothing short of cosmetic surgery can alter its appearance. It is lined with skin in which there are numerous hairs that help to prevent foreign bodies from entering the nose. Just inside the nostrils is a highly sensitive area of skin containing many tiny capillaries (blood vessels). If injured, this area may bleed quite profusely. In some people the overlying skin is extremely thin, producing a tendency to suffer from nosebleeds (see below).

The nasal cavity is a cave-like opening behind the nostrils and its surface area is augmented by three folds called the conchae. The large surface area helps the nose carry out one of its crucial functions, that of warming and moistening the air before it enters the bronchial tubes and lungs. In the highest part of the nasal cavity are the nerve endings of the sense of smell.

The skull bones surrounding the nasal cavity have hollows known as the nasal sinuses. In health, these hollows perform very useful functions in that they help to make the skull bones of the face light in weight and also act as resonance boxes, giving a pleasant quality to the voice. During a cold the mucous membrane lining the sinuses may become infected, giving rise to a painful condition known as sinusitis (see below).

For comfort, the lining of the nose and air passages should be kept moist. The surfaces are lubricated by mucus produced from glands within the skin and this helps to moisturize the air that is breathed in. Drying out of the lining for any length of time causes an itchy, prickly sensation inside the nose. Even fierce central heating is not on its own sufficient to damage the lining if the air is humidified, but a transpolar flight, where air is constantly filtered and recirculated, can make the inside of the nose feel sore. If this is very uncomfortable, it may help to smear Vaseline inside the nose in order to stop it drying out.

The nose is an extremity and in cold weather lack of a good blood supply may make it go red or blue. Rubbing or pinching it may improve things temporarily but disguise with tinted make-up is the only real solution.

Common nose complaints

● Common cold

The common cold is a virus infection. The symptoms can be treated but not the cold itself. A proprietary medicine available over the counter will work as well as anything a doctor can prescribe. If you have a high temperature stay inside (not necessarily in bed) and drink plenty of fluids. Two soluble aspirin every four hours can do wonders for a headache or sore throat. If the cold develops into bronchitis or severe sinusitis (see below) or if there is an underlying condition, such as heart or chest disease, which would be made worse by a cold, consult a doctor.

● Hay fever

See Allergy, page 26.

● Loss of the sense of smell

This rare condition can occur as a result of injury or chronic infection in the nose. Since the sense of smell is responsible for about 80 per cent of the sense of taste, this means missing out on many of the subtle flavours in food. Sadly, there is no treatment.

● Nosebleeds

Some people have a patch of skin just inside the nostrils on the inner side where the tiny capillaries are very near the surface and therefore vulnerable. If this area is injured, the nose bleeds. The tendency for this to happen is exacerbated by picking at the skin just inside the nostril, so avoid doing this.

During a nosebleed keep the head forwards so that the blood is not swallowed (it can irritate the stomach and cause vomiting). Apply pressure on either side of the nostrils with thumb and forefinger until the bleeding stops. If the nosebleeds are frequent and embarrassing, the doctor may recommend cauterizing the area – a treatment that is normally effective.

● Sinusitis

As a result of a cold, the membranes lining the sinus cavities may become inflamed and start to secrete mucus. If infected, this produces a yellow nasal discharge and a nasty pain, due to a rise in pressure within the sinus cavities. Treatment is difficult (because the sinuses are fairly inaccessible) and also quite lengthy (maybe six weeks on antibiotics). If this remedy fails, a sinus washout may be tried.

Mouth

A multi-purpose organ of extraordinary interest, the mouth is bounded at the front by the lips, which are highly specialized and extremely sensitive as a result of their rich nerve supply. They are important sexually, because they redden to give a signal to the opposite sex during sexual arousal, and important for survival because we feed through them. The walls of the mouth cavity are formed by the muscles in the cheeks, the roof is formed from the hard and soft palates and the tongue fills the floor.

The most interesting parts of the mouth medically – the teeth and gums – are of great importance from the beauty standpoint also: we show them off to some extent each time we smile or speak.

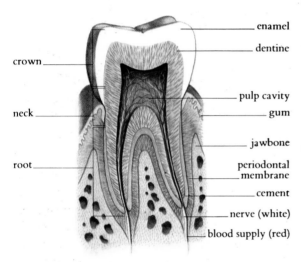

Teeth

A tooth has two outer layers. The outermost one is composed of a hard, insensitive substance called enamel. It may be naturally white in colour or naturally yellowish – if the latter, then no amount of frequent or careful brushing will make the teeth white. Beneath the enamel lies the tooth's second coat, a much softer substance called dentine. If the enamel wears away to expose this layer, toothache begins. Inside the tooth is a pulp cavity containing blood vessels and nerves, reaching right up into the roots. The roots themselves are embedded in the jawbone in a thin, hard covering of cement. They have a narrow channel at their base (the apical foramen), through which the blood and nerve supply can reach the

pulp cavity. The periodontal membrane, which lies between the cement and the jawbone, has a separate nerve supply from that of the pulp cavity; hence a totally dead tooth may still hurt.

We all have two sets of teeth over a lifetime. The primary teeth come first, erupting through the gums in the first and second years of life. They are being formed in the baby's jawbone well before birth (see page 230 for what a mother can do to help her child develop strong, attractive teeth). These primary teeth are gradually replaced by permanent ones, which arrive in the period between the ages of five or six and 25. There are 20 primary teeth and up to 32 permanent teeth, but some people never get their wisdom teeth, the last four molars.

The gums

For healthy teeth, it is essential to have healthy gums. In developed countries many more teeth are lost through gum disease than through tooth decay. The process begins with some injury to the gum margin – probably caused by the build-up of plaque (see Looking after the teeth and gums, below). The gum margin loosens and pockets form in which bacteria multiply. Infection follows, making the gum margin soft and spongy. The tooth is no longer firmly seated and becomes loose. Finally the gum margin recedes still further and the tooth, which may be perfectly healthy, becomes so loose that it has to be removed.

Looking after the teeth and gums

The great enemy of healthy teeth and gums is plaque, a film that forms upon the teeth and that is made up of bacteria and soft material formed from saliva and bacteria. The worst offenders are sweet, starchy foods, drinks sweetened with sugar and sweet snacks between meals. The plaque starts off as a soft, sticky substance but it gradually becomes rock hard due to the deposition of calcium. It forms a nutritious medium for bacteria, which damage the enamel, so encouraging decay. Plaque also irritates and erodes the gum margin.

The first step towards keeping teeth healthy is therefore to discourage plaque. Cutting down on sweet foods and drinks helps. The more of these there are in the diet, the more important it is to brush the teeth thoroughly and frequently –

Brushing your teeth
1 From the gum margin, brush downwards with a flick of the wrist for the top teeth, upwards for the lower, cleaning the front of every tooth.

2 Clean the inner sides of the teeth, again brushing the top teeth downwards and the bottom teeth upwards, with the same flicking motion of the wrist as in **1**.

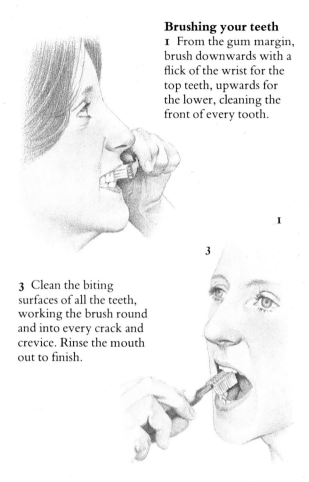

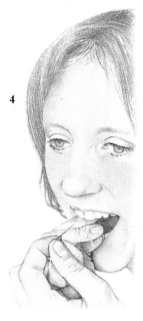

3 Clean the biting surfaces of all the teeth, working the brush round and into every crack and crevice. Rinse the mouth out to finish.

4 Use dental floss to keep the gaps between the teeth free of plaque. Wind a good length of floss round the middle finger of each hand and guide it gently with the index finger and thumb down the edge of the tooth from the gum and then up again. Do not saw to and fro – this may harm the gum.

preferably every time you eat one of the offending foods, but certainly each morning and evening. Toothpaste is not necessary – it just makes brushing more pleasant. Dental floss, used as shown above, can help to get rid of stubborn food particles between teeth and thus also discourage plaque formation. To see how much plaque collects on the teeth between brushings, try using a disclosing tablet once in a while before your tooth-cleaning routine (follow the manufacturer's directions for use). The plaque shows up as a bright red or green colour. It is usually quite a shock to see the extent of it. Check again after brushing the teeth to see if all the stains have been banished.

It is important to use a technique that suits you when brushing your teeth (see **1** above). Note that vigorous seesawing movements backwards and forwards or from side to side should be avoided: they can damage the gums. A short scrubbing technique, however, is efficient.

Take care when buying a toothbrush. Nylon is preferable to bristle as bristle splits and loses its shape quickly. Choose a brush with a small head, which is easy to manoeuvre round the teeth, and one with a straight rather than a serrated edge so that it is less likely to scratch the gums. Above all, the toothbrush should be soft: a hard, spiky one is likely to irritate the gums. Change toothbrushes every month or so: after around 60 brushings any toothbrush will show signs of wear and become less efficient.

Regular dental check-ups are the second important step in any programme for healthy teeth and gums. Two checks a year should be enough for most adults, three a year for a child. During pregnancy, try to visit a dentist at least twice. This is not because the baby may take calcium from the mother's teeth if her diet does not supply enough – this is a myth (unlike the theory that calcium from the mother's bones may be depleted). The gums tend to suffer during pregnancy, however, and may become soft and swollen. An extra dental check-up is a good idea for that reason.

Fluoride

The use of toothpaste containing fluoride has been shown to reduce tooth decay among children by increasing the resistance of the teeth to cariogenic foods such as chocolates and candies. A few tests have shown that similar toothpastes cut down tooth decay among adults, who tend to eat fewer sweet foods and have fewer sweet drinks. It has been proved that traces of fluoride in the diet make the teeth resist decay and it is possible to have fluoride painted directly on to the teeth.

There is no objective evidence linking fluoride with the development of cancer.

Mouth hygiene

As long as you are eating and drinking regularly, brush your teeth frequently and do not dry your mouth out by breathing through it for any length of time, there is no need to take any other measures to ensure mouth hygiene. In normal circumstances, mouth washes are not necessary – use one only if the doctor recommends it. Gargling may help the spread of bacteria and can do more harm than good.

Smoking can cause bad breath. The most efficient remedy – apart from giving up smoking – is to camouflage the smell with mints or cachous (see also Common mouth problems, below). Discolouration of the teeth due to smoking can be remedied by a visit to the dentist for descaling; brushing by itself will not remove the yellowish scale once it has built up over a few months.

The tongue

A muscular organ, the tongue is attached at its base to the lower jaw. Much of it is covered by a membrane, which owes its velvety appearance to tiny projections (papillae) all over its surface.

The tongue helps when food is being masticated, makes swallowing efficient and facilitates clear speech. Its principal function, however, is to convey tastes – it is almost entirely covered with taste buds. The four basic tastes – sweet, sour, salt and bitter – are detected by different areas of the tongue. Sweet tastes are identified with the tongue tip, sour tastes with the edges, bitter tastes at the back and salty tastes at the tip and edges. Flavours – variations on these basic themes – are appreciated mainly through the nose. With the nostril pinched it is impossible to tell grated apple, for example, from grated onion.

The tongue is not a particularly good indicator of the body's health. A doctor often asks a patient to stick her tongue out simply because this makes it possible to look at the back of the throat. At the same time the doctor can see whether or not the tongue or gums look pale, denoting anaemia.

A brown, furry-looking tongue is not a sinister phenomenon: the 'fur' is made up of cells that have collected on the tongue's surface quite naturally. Their presence simply indicates that no food or drink has been taken in the past few hours (salivation, eating and drinking normally carry the cells away). A long spell of breathing through the mouth dries the skin of the tongue out, which is why the tongue may feel furred on awakening when a heavy cold has made it difficult to breathe normally through the nose.

Common mouth problems

● Abscess (tooth)

The root of a molar, which may lie 2.25 cm (1 in) beneath the jawbone, can be infected if chronic tooth decay penetrates the living pulp at the centre of the tooth. The infection travels along the hollow root to its tip, where it is halted by the bone. The condition is acutely painful because the collecting pus cannot expand into the rigid bone. Instead it normally spreads under the gum, giving rise to a tender, soft swelling.

Treatment is in two stages. First, the pus is released, either by puncturing the gum or by opening up the tooth. Second, the root is treated and then the tooth filled. Despite the agony, never have the tooth removed. With modern dentistry a completely dead tooth can serve well for 30 years.

● Bad breath (halitosis)

The usual causes of bad breath are: not eating or drinking, bad teeth, infected gums, mouth ulcers, smoking and alcohol. However, some people suffer from halitosis for no traceable cause. It may indicate a stomach complaint – but this may be simply because when the stomach is upset, the appetite for food or drink tends to wane.

If bad breath is traceable to some specific cause, the treatment is to eliminate the cause. If not, the only solution is to disguise it with mints, cachous or chlorophyll sticks or tablets.

• Bleeding gums

Gums will bleed easily (during tooth-cleaning routines, for example) if they are inflamed or swollen. The commonest cause is plaque. Treatment is to keep the plaque at bay (see Looking after the teeth and gums, pages 56–57). For recurrent bleeding, see Gingivitis, below.

• Chapped lips

Lips generally become chapped only when the weather is cold (hampering the blood supply to the skin of the lips) and the lips are allowed to dry out. The best form of treatment is lip salve: it forms an insulating layer, which stops the lips from getting too cold, and it also helps prevent moisture loss. Ordinary lipstick is almost as good.

• Cold sores

Caused by a virus related to chicken pox, cold sores occur on the lips (or the genitals) and can be transmitted by kissing. The virus lies dormant in the skin until a rise in skin temperature – caused perhaps by ovulation, a fever or sitting in the sun – awakens it. The typical itchy spot progresses to a blister and then a scab. People who develop them in strong sunlight should smear sunscreen cream on their lips before going out.

Idoxuridine cream (available from a doctor) may help if applied before the spot actually appears. Once the spot has formed, it takes ten days to clear no matter how it is treated. Some authorities recommend surgical spirit to dry the scab; others suggest Vaseline to keep the skin soft and supple. Neither remedy makes much difference, so use whichever makes you more comfortable. Never use spirit of camphor: this damages the cells in the skin.

• Gingivitis (inflamed gums)

A descriptive term for sore, red, swollen, inflamed gums, gingivitis is nearly always caused by an infection. The condition needs specific treatment from a dentist or doctor – do not try to treat it with a proprietary medicine.

If the condition becomes chronic it is very difficult to eradicate and may go on to pyorrhoea, which puts the teeth in jeopardy. The treatment consists of antibiotics in severe cases; gingivectomy (cutting away the inflamed margin); the use of dental floss or dental sticks to harden the gum margin; careful and regular tooth brushing (see page 57).

• Mouth ulcers

An aphthous mouth ulcer, commonly linked with psychological stress, starts as a sore patch on the inside of the mouth, enlarges to form a painful yellow crater and then slowly heals. The whole process takes ten to 14 days and no proprietary medicine will speed things up. An injury caused by a jagged tooth, or some other sharp object, can also produce an ulcer if it becomes infected (and it generally does, since the mouth is such a bacteriologically dirty place). If you get crops of ulcers, consult a doctor – and avoid acid foods until the mouth has healed.

The chin

One of the areas of the body where sebum secretion in the skin is high, the chin is part of the central greasy panel of the face. For this reason it is prone to blackheads and spots, particularly in adolescence and the week before menstruation. Guidance on how to deal with these skin complaints is on pages 26–29. Never scrub hard at oily skin – doing so only makes the area oilier, as the sebaceous glands are stimulated to produce extra sebum.

Many people are troubled by sagging fat beneath the chin. This double chin is nearly always part of generalized overweight. It is not a necessary part of ageing, nor is it caused by sleeping on too bulky a pillow – thin people can grow older and sleep on piles of pillows if they wish without getting a double chin. So the easiest way to avoid this problem is to stay as close as possible to an ideal weight. Someone who already has a double chin will have to shed at least 9.5 kg (20 lb) before the fat on the neck can be affected. Skin that sags badly round the jawline can be treated by cosmetic surgery (see pages 222–224).

Special care when applying cosmetics to the face and chin can help prevent a sagging jawline. Always put cosmetics on and take them off with upward movements. For further advice on care of the neck see page 61.

The following isometric exercise may help to keep the muscles in this area in trim. Tense the muscles of the face, neck and chin as if trying to push forwards hard against an obstacle. Do this ten to 12 times in succession several times a day (in private as it distorts the face).

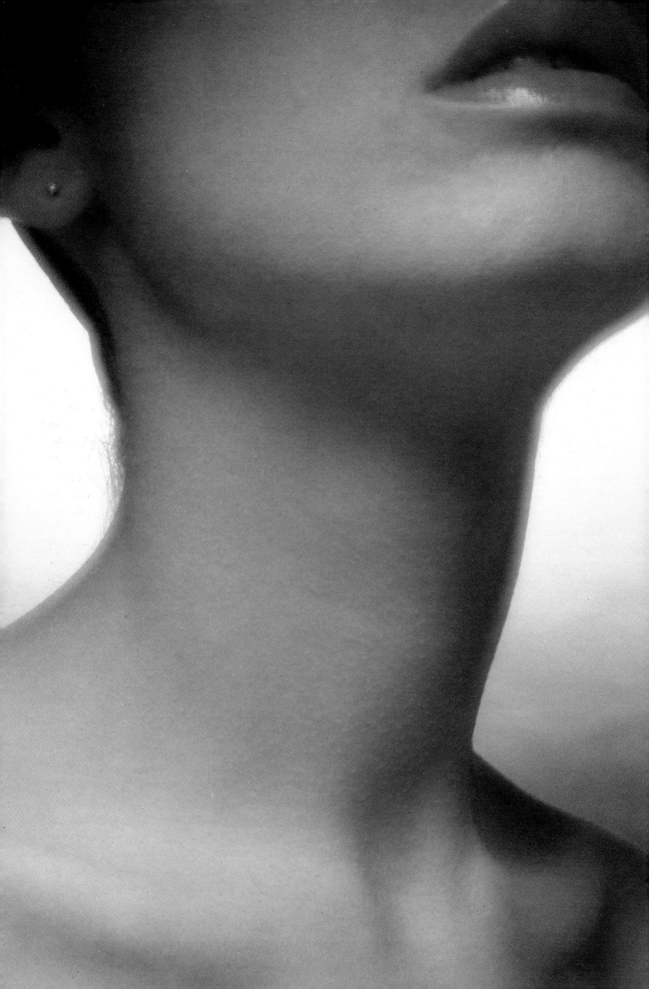

Neck and Throat

Many women spend time and money on face and hair treatments, but neglect their necks and throats, taking their youthfulness for granted. However, a woman's age can be divulged by the condition of her throat long before the years reveal themselves on her face. For, as the throat is often exposed to the weather and is usually washed with soap and water, it tends to become dry. Ideally, it should be included in facial cleansing and toning routines; moisturizer is especially important for a soft, attractive skin. Ordinary face moisturizers are effective; the slightly richer type (sometimes called night creams) are better still for dry skin. There is no advantage in using a special 'throat cream' as the skin on the throat is not intrinsically different from the skin elsewhere; nor can creams prevent or cure wrinkles (see page 13).

Good posture is the answer for many neck and throat problems (see pages 130–133). Bad posture throws the body out of alignment and puts extra strain on the spine; this in turn puts the neck at an awkward angle so that the muscles become stiff and tense. The nerve junctions and muscles in the back of the neck can be manipulated or massaged to bring relief from headaches and body tension and the throat can be massaged while moisturizing (see page 177).

When dieting, it is important to watch the state of the neck. In particular, older people who lose a lot of weight tend to lose it quickly from the neck, leaving it looking wrinkled and scraggy. If there are signs of this happening, soft pedal the diet a little and try to lose weight gradually over a longer period. Practised daily, neck exercises (see page 146) help to keep the neck supple. When turning to look sideways, it should be necessary to turn the head only and not the whole body.

Although the length of the neck cannot be altered, its appearance can be improved by careful choice of hairstyle and clothing. A short neck can be made to appear longer with a short hairstyle or mid-length hair swept back off the face, as long hair swamps a short neck. Fringes (or bangs) also tend to minimize face and neck area. High collars and roll-neck sweaters do not camouflage a short neck, but in fact work the opposite way. A classic, open-shirt collar and a V-neckline make the neck look longer and more graceful.

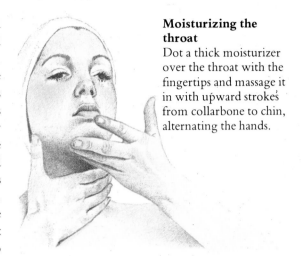

Moisturizing the throat
Dot a thick moisturizer over the throat with the fingertips and massage it in with upward strokes from collarbone to chin, alternating the hands.

Perfume

The back and sides of the neck and the throat are the traditional places to apply perfume. This is because they are the more accessible of the main pulse points, or points where the pulse of a blood vessel can be felt – the others are the temples, the fronts of the wrists, the crooks of the elbows, the cleavage, the front of the groin, the backs of the knees, the inner sides and tops of the ankles. At these points, the warmth of the skin allows the fragrance to blossom on the skin.

Fragrances are based on complex blends of concentrates, which can be natural or synthetic. A selection of these essences is blended to form the high and middle 'notes'; the low or lasting notes are formed by fixatives. The fragrance retains its individual character whether sold as perfume, the true essence of the fragrance, or as the weaker and shorter-lasting eau de toilette and cologne. However, a fragrance may smell different on different skins, according to the variations of the chemistry of the oils and acids that we have on our skin, which are under hormonal control. For this reason, the varying hormone levels in the skin during the menstrual cycle change the smell of the scent; they also affect the sense of smell, so that the perception of scents varies according to the cycle. An oily skin changes the character of a scent more than a dry one, but retains it for longer. As the reaction between skin and perfume is so important, always apply perfume directly to the skin. If, however, this provokes allergic reactions, it should be sprayed on to clothing, under hems or inside necklines as it may stain fabric.

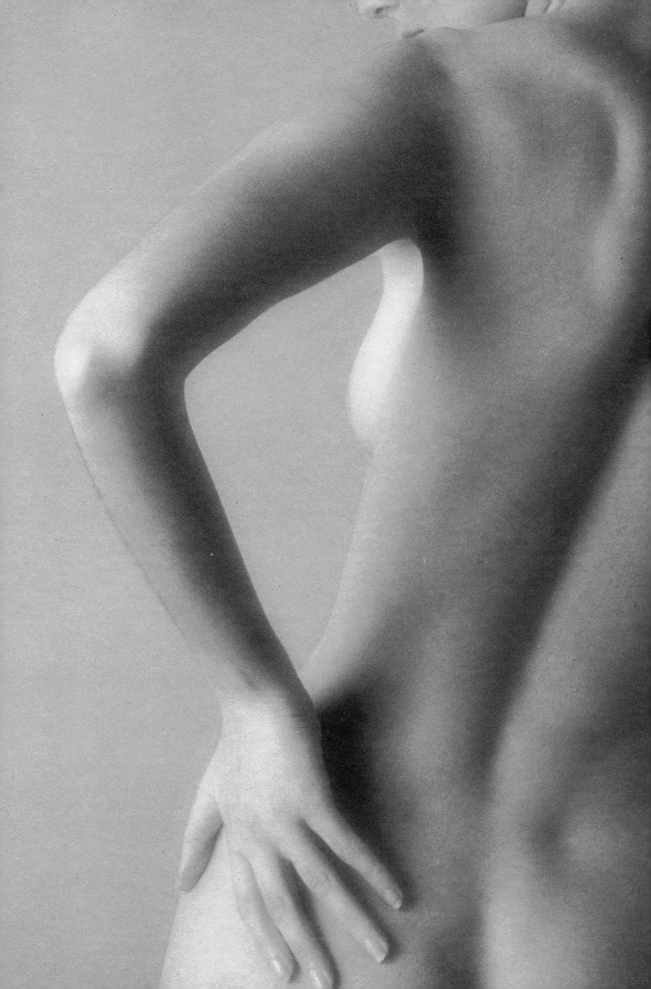

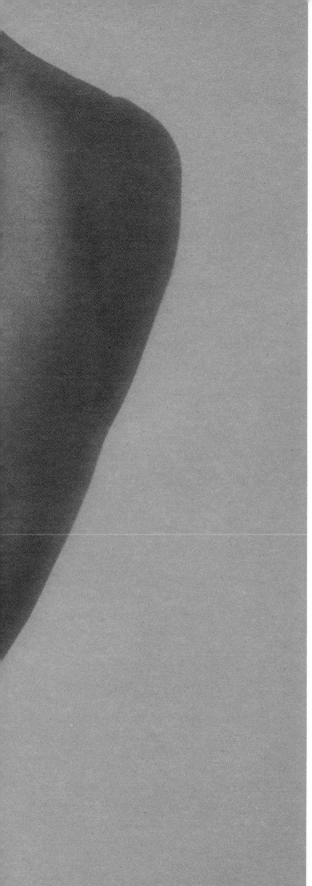

Shoulders and Back

The shoulders and the back are two areas that repay with interest the attention we give them. The pay-off comes in terms of health as well as appearance. Correct carriage of the shoulders is essential for good posture, while a strong, supple back can make an immense difference to the way we walk, look and feel.

Shoulders

These are formed by a freely moving ball-and-socket joint. The ball is the bone of the upper arm (humerus), and the shoulder blade (scapula) and collarbone (clavicle) make up the socket. The shoulders themselves are the outer corners of the shoulder girdle, formed at the front by the two collarbones, at the back by the two shoulder blades.

Good carriage of the shoulders is a very simple way to improve the appearance of the whole body dramatically. For good posture the shoulders should be held back and down in a relaxed fashion, with the head erect. As well as improving the appearance, this posture helps keep the spine in a good position and thereby minimizes strain (see also pages 130–131).

The skin covering the shoulders is one of the oily areas of the body and blackheads and acne pimples are often found there. Treat these complaints as indicated on page 26. Mild doses of exposure to sunlight can help acne sufferers, but if you try this be particularly careful not to overdo things: the skin on the shoulders seems particularly liable to burn and should normally be protected by a sunscreen if exposed.

Two possible shoulder complaints are recurrent dislocation and 'frozen' shoulder. The former, a fairly infrequent but extremely painful condition, generally arises as a result of injury to the shoulder and can be satisfactorily treated only by surgery. The latter, due to a strain of a tendon running over the shoulder, renders the shoulder immobile, often occurs for no apparent reason, is also very painful and may take several weeks to clear up. Hydrocortisone injections around the tendon may be used to treat this condition.

Back: Spinal column

The spine is a very unstable structure, consisting as it does of 24 small circular vertebrae piled on top of one another, with discs of cartilage (which act

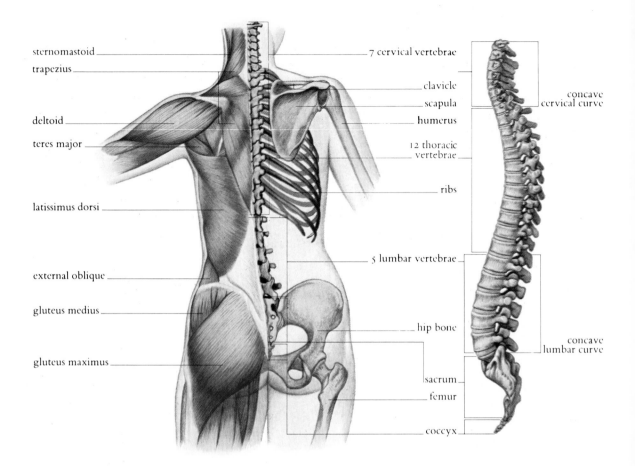

sternomastoid

trapezius

deltoid

teres major

latissimus dorsi

external oblique

gluteus medius

gluteus maximus

7 cervical vertebrae

clavicle

scapula

humerus

12 thoracic vertebrae

ribs

5 lumbar vertebrae

hip bone

sacrum

femur

coccyx

concave cervical curve

concave lumbar curve

as shock absorbers) in between. Through holes in the middle of the vertebrae, just behind the discs, runs the spinal cord, a column of nerves connecting the brain and the lower part of the body. The spine's essential design is more suited to a quadruped than to an upright creature. Considering that the spine was tilted through an angle of 90 degrees when man first began to walk upright, it is something of an engineering miracle that it functions as well as it does.

The spine is held rigidly in position by numerous bands of tough muscle and ligament. Imagine trying to balance 24 small bricks on top of each other without toppling the pile over and you will have a good idea of why these supporting bands are necessary. Awkward posture when performing demanding physical activities, such as lifting heavy objects, overstrains the spine's muscular supports and invites back trouble.

Good posture involves holding the body erect so that the concave curvatures of the vertebrae at the neck and the bottom of the back are not lost. The primary aim when sitting, walking, driving, standing and even sleeping should be to maintain

these natural curves in the back. If the curves are allowed to become convex (as in some of the examples of bad posture opposite) the muscles are put under strain and the spine is weakened. The result is an increased likelihood of a prolapsed intervertebral disc, commonly known as a slipped disc, with severe backache and possibly sciatica (pain felt down the back of the legs) as well.

Once the back has been weakened it rarely has the chance to recover: it would take something like eight weeks lying flat out on boards to recuperate fully from back strain. Since few of us can afford to spend this length of time immobile, it is simple common sense to look after our backs. Following the guidelines opposite on how to perform everyday tasks and actions is a good start – for exercises that will help to strengthen the back and make it more supple see pages 140–141.

Backache

There are many possible causes of backache. Here are the most common.

1　Muscular strain – usually brought on by some unusual activity such as digging the garden.

This cause can be avoided by keeping the muscles toned up with regular exercise.

2 Previous back injury (e.g. bruising) resulting in a permanent weakness. This can give rise to backache after lengthy sitting or standing (especially if posture is bad).

3 A slipped disc – the dramatic outcome of years of chronic weakening of the back (a normal disc does not slip). Maintaining good posture helps prevent this.

Tension and anxiety do not in themselves cause backache, but they can make it feel worse.

Treatment for backache includes rest, massage, heat treatment, painkillers and having a board under the mattress to support the spine during sleep (just as effective as an orthopaedic mattress). A spinal corset, worn for a few hours each day, may also help by resting the muscles in the back – check with a doctor whether this is appropriate in your case. If the treatment is not doing much good, try asking the doctor whether physiotherapy or an orthopaedic specialist might be able to help, or consider going to an osteopath or chiropractor (see pages 237 and 233).

How to use your back
To lift a large or heavy object, bend down from the knees, not from the waist.

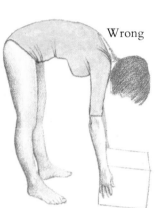

Wrong

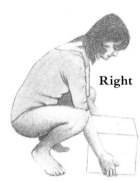

Right

Carry a heavy package close to the body, not out in front of it. Bend at the knees when putting the package down.

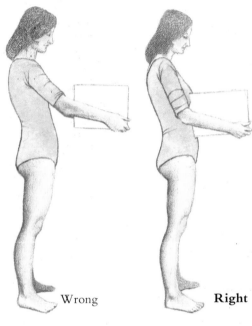

Wrong   **Right**

Kneel right down to do a job at floor level such as cutting out or weeding. Stooping is tiring as well as a strain on the back.

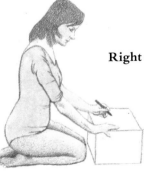

Right

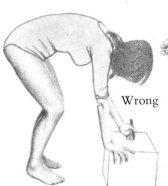

Wrong

To shift a heavy weight such as a big wardrobe, push with the back rather than with the hands. Do not try to move too heavy a weight unaided.

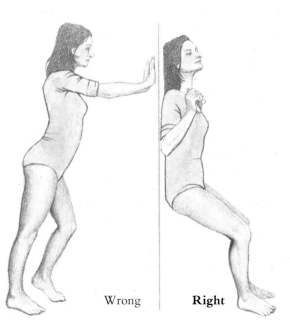

Wrong | **Right**

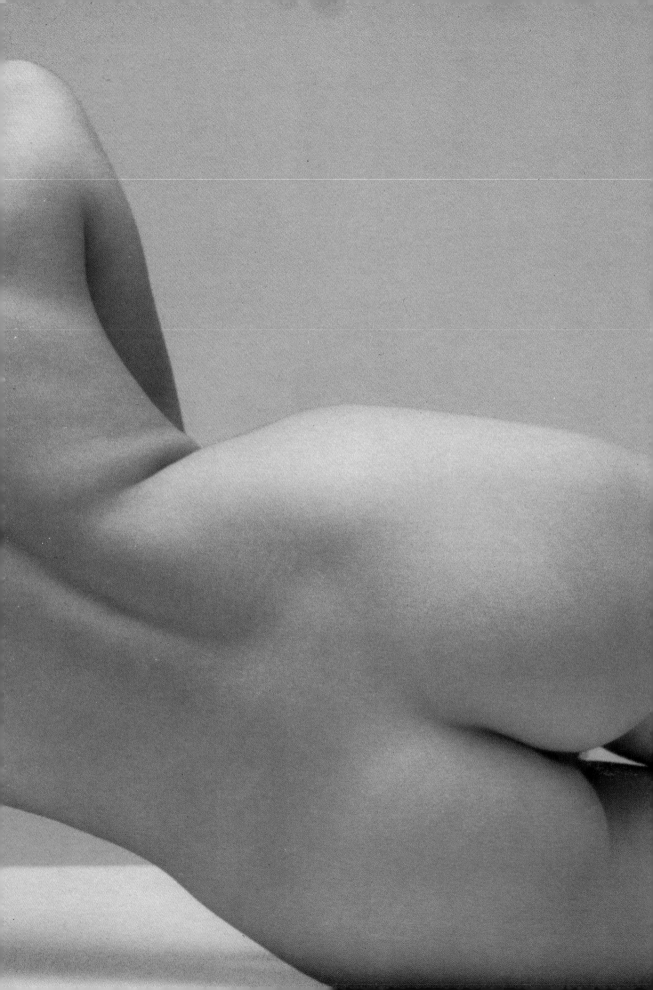

Hips and Bottom

The hip is a highly mobile ball-and-socket joint constructed from the head of the femur (the ball) and the ilium, a bone in the pelvis (the socket). Because of its position and the strenuous job it has to do, plus the fact that it is a weight-bearing joint, it is subject to a great deal of wear and tear. All joints tend to show the effects of age sooner or later: their surfaces grow rough, they become stiff and painful to move (a condition known medically as osteoarthritis). The hip is more likely to get osteoarthritis sooner than other, less well-used, joints and more likely to be a serious inconvenience when it does so (because of the need for it to bear the body's weight with every step). The nerve that supplies the hip joint also supplies the knee, so pain in the knee may be one symptom of damage to the hip. For persistent pain in hip or knee, consult a doctor. In chronic arthritis damage to the hip may be so severe that your doctor may recommend a hip replacement operation; in most cases this operation restores full mobility.

It is not really possible to consider the hips without also considering the pelvis, the shape of which plays an important part in determining hip measurement. Women have wider pelvises than men so that they can accommodate a growing baby inside the womb. Fifty years ago, when it was still quite common for children to suffer from rickets (the result of a diet deficient in vitamin D), some women had pelvises so narrow that childbearing was particularly hazardous for both mother and baby – the pelvic bones had failed to develop properly as a result of rickets. It is rare today for a woman to have a pelvis insufficient to permit childbirth, at least in developed countries where malnutrition is no problem.

The width of a woman's pelvis means that the angle of the thigh bone between the hip and the knee is smaller than it is for a man. This sexual difference shows up in the way we sway our hips when we move and it also accounts for women's tendency to have knock knees.

Both hip and pelvic joints change during pregnancy. To make room for the growing baby and to facilitate delivery through the birth canal, all the ligaments and joint capsules slacken as the pregnancy progresses (this applies particularly to the joint at the front of the pelvis, the symphysis

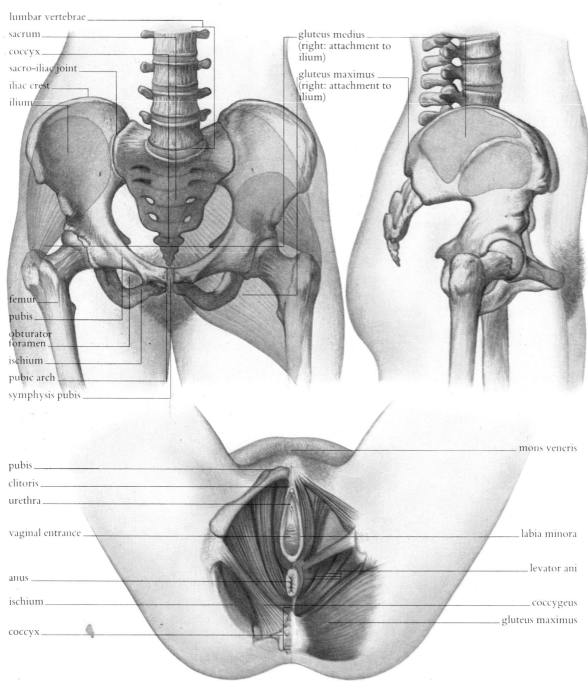

lumbar vertebrae

sacrum

coccyx

sacro-iliac joint

iliac crest

ilium

gluteus medius
(right: attachment to
ilium)

gluteus maximus
(right: attachment to
ilium)

femur

pubis

obturator
foramen

ischium

pubic arch

symphysis pubis

pubis

clitoris

urethra

vaginal entrance

anus

ischium

coccyx

mons veneris

labia minora

levator ani

coccygeus

gluteus maximus

pubis). The joints are less stable and less well supported than usual as a result and the muscles have to work overtime. This is why backache is so widespread among pregnant women.

The pelvic floor

The bottom of the pelvis is closed in by a group of muscles that form the pelvic floor. They support the pelvic organs – the bladder, the bowel and the uterus. If you imagine looking up at the muscles of the pelvic floor from underneath, they would resemble the spread pages of an open book, sloping downwards and inwards from back to front and from the sides to the centre. The three important organs that penetrate the pelvic floor in mid-line are, looking from front to back, the urethra (the opening of the tube from the bladder), the vagina and the anus.

The muscle that is responsible for keeping the vagina supple is the main muscle of the pelvic floor (the levator ani). It can be toned up by doing the following exercise several times a day (more often during pregnancy and immediately after delivery). When passing urine, pull your bottom in tightly to stop the flow. Hold this position while counting to ten and then let the urine flow again. Once you learn the knack, you can practise contracting this muscle at any time.

Bottom

The shape of the bottom is determined by the muscles and fat of which it is made up. The size and shape of the gluteal muscles vary from race to race – in general, negroid women tend to have higher, rounder and sometimes thicker musculature than Caucasian women. Apart from this, the contour of the bottom depends principally on the subcutaneous fat.

It is a female characteristic to have deposits of fat on the bottom (as on the breasts, upper arms and thighs). Curves here are just as much a part of being a woman as broad shoulders and narrow hips are part of being a man. These curves can be attractive, but a bottom that sags with excess fat is another matter – for how to deal with this problem, see below.

Bottoms – like breasts – come in all shapes and sizes and very few conform to the high, rounded shape made so desirable by the media. Some women who are neither fat nor out of condition have wide bottoms simply because nature made them that way (not, incidentally, as a result of too much time spent sitting). Leaving overweight aside, the contour of the bottom is about as amenable to improvement by diet or exercise as the colour of the eyes or hair.

What to do about a sagging bottom

Fat on the bottom responds to the same treatment as fat elsewhere on the body – namely dieting. The treatments advertised by many beauty clinics (electrical therapy, bandaging and so on) will do no good whatsoever. As for massage, the only person who will get any slimmer is the masseuse.

It is possible to uplift fat on the bottom with a firm support such as a pantee girdle, tight jeans or stretch trousers but you should not rely on these to keep your tummy flat as well as your bottom in shape. In general the most hopeful route to a more

attractive bottom is through clever dressing to disguise its shape. Long, loose tops that end below the buttocks are one solution and high-waisted dresses are another. Those with flat bottoms can turn them to good account by wearing clothes that need a slim profile, such as skirts that fit snugly over the hips and then flare out. Capitalizing on your assets is much better sense than making your life miserable in the pursuit of some unattainable ideal.

Cellulite

When a lot of fat is in a position to be pulled downwards by the force of gravity, it may take on a dimpled appearance. When this happens, it is currently fashionable to refer to the fat as cellulite. This type of fat is often seen on the underside of the upper arms, the breasts and the thighs as well as the buttocks. It occurs almost without exception in women and typically afflicts mainly those who are overweight and in their middle years.

The dimpling is a variant of normal fat deposition. It is in no way abnormal and it needs no treatment – indeed it cannot be treated because it cannot be changed unless the underlying fat is lost. This sort of fat is unattractive, is considered ageing and ever since it was called cellulite it has been described in various ways and ascribed to various ingenious causes: abnormal fat, abnormally deposited fat, fat with an abnormally high water content, bad circulation, starchy diet, lack of exercise and even to the overproduction of female hormones.

Claims are made that everything from electrical massage to diuretic therapy will cure cellulite. This is erroneous. The only thing that will almost certainly improve the dimpling is dieting. If the fat is lost, the dimples diminish.

Dieting is rarely mentioned because it calls for more effort than many cellulite sufferers are prepared to make. Cellulite is, in fact, a fake word for a fake condition. The very existence of a multitude of remedies (some of them exceedingly bizarre) proclaims that none works – they were fashioned principally to satisfy the demand from insecure women for a lazy way out, with just enough pseudo-science to convince them it is worth trying. Sadly, the only thing that is real is the pseudo-science.

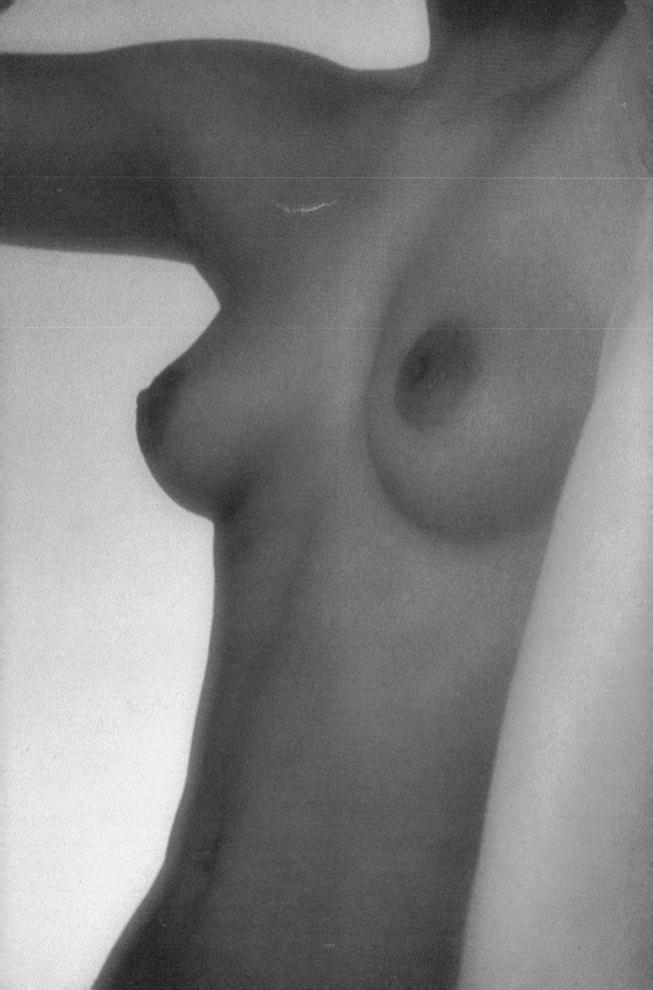

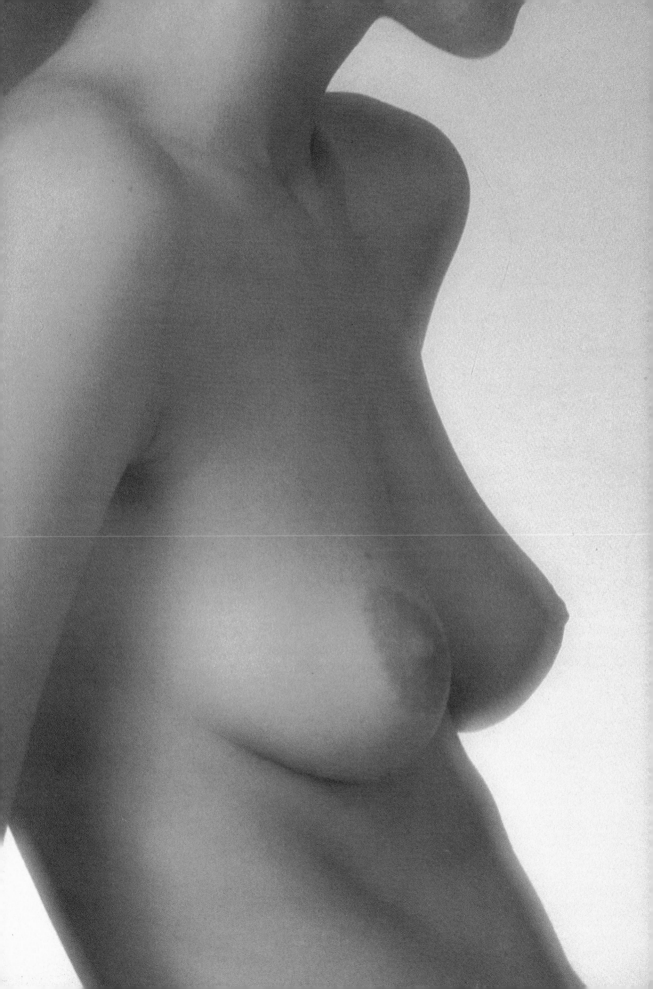

Breasts

There is no such thing as normal-looking breasts: they come in all shapes, sizes and textures. Apart from individual characteristics – even on one woman the right and left breasts may be slightly different – there may be racial differences too. Mary Quant used to have some difficulty exporting her dresses because of national variations in the shape and position of the breasts: apparently oriental breasts point outwards, French bosoms tend to be high and English bosoms rather low-slung. She had to adapt her designs accordingly.

The structure of the breasts

The breasts are almost entirely composed of subcutaneous fat. They contain tens of thousands of tiny modified sebaceous glands, adapted over the millennia to produce milk rather than sebum. Ducts leading from all these milk glands converge into around 20 lobes, each of which has an opening on to the nipple. Surrounding the nipple is a rosy-coloured area called the areola, which becomes red – as the lips do – at times of sexual excitement. There is a rich nerve supply to this area because of its function in breastfeeding babies, and this makes the skin very responsive to touch. It is an erogenous zone not only in women but, rather surprisingly, in men too.

The breasts are supported and attached to the body by suspensory ligaments, strands of fibrous tissue that fade into the pectoral muscles on the chest wall. The breasts themselves contain no muscles – which is why exercises will do nothing to change the size or shape of the breasts, although it is possible to firm the pectoral muscles.

The glandular tissue of the breasts is highly sensitive to female hormones in the bloodstream. As the level of these hormones circulating in the body increases in the years leading up to puberty, the breasts gradually begin to enlarge. When menstruation begins, this enlargement speeds up and is more marked. During pregnancy, hormone levels rise again and the breasts develop further.

Two (genetically determined) factors dictate the size a woman's breasts can attain: the level of hormones in her blood and, even more crucial, the sensitivity of her breasts to those hormones. Breasts that are fairly insensitive to oestrogen will not enlarge no matter how high the level of oestrogen circulating in the blood. This is why some women's breasts get bigger when they take the contraceptive pill while others are unaffected.

It follows from these facts that no exercise routine or course of massage will help to develop a large bust. Hormone creams are no good either, since hormones applied to the skin have no effect upon the internal growth of the breasts. And even if a woman's breasts were small as a result of a hormone deficiency, this would not on its own be a strong enough reason for prescribing hormones to be taken orally. A woman who puts on weight will find that her breasts get fatter just as the rest of her body does; if she slims her breasts will get smaller for the same reason – but no diet will affect the size of the breasts without also affecting fat elsewhere on the body.

The only way to improve the bust naturally is by good posture: simply pulling the shoulders back will make the breasts *look* larger and higher.

Normal changes in the breasts

The breasts react each month to the varying levels of oestrogen and progesterone circulating in the body. As the menstrual cycle progresses and oestrogen is produced, the breast tissue enlarges. Just before menstruation the breasts may feel rather swollen and sore, and the lumpiness apparent at this time is caused by the swollen glands primed to secrete milk. With the onset of menstruation all these changes regress and the breasts return to normal.

If pregnancy occurs, the development of the breasts continues. They enlarge, the glandular tissue becomes more active and the number and size of the veins visible on the breasts increases as the blood supply to the area is augmented. Not merely the nipple but the whole breast may feel sensitive and rather tingly. The build-up of breast tissue by the end of pregnancy may be as much as 0.7 kg ($1\frac{1}{2}$ lb) in weight. A clear liquid known as colostrum is secreted by the breasts in small amounts throughout pregnancy and can be expressed by firm pressure on the areola. When the baby is born a hormone called prolactin is produced, which gives the signal for the breasts to switch to producing true milk in place of colostrum – a change that happens about three days after delivery.

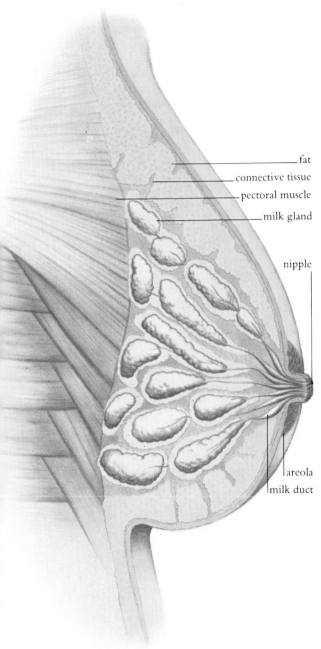

fat
connective tissue
pectoral muscle
milk gland

nipple

areola
milk duct

those that are small and light. If heavy breasts are not supported, the suspensory ligaments stretch. Once this happens, they never return to their original shape and the breasts sag.

A woman with good-sized breasts should help them to retain their youthful shape by wearing a bra of some sort – not necessarily a stiff or heavy one. Some underwired bras that give good support are seamless, filmy and allow the natural contour of the breast to be evident.

Even if you normally like to do without a bra, it is only common sense to wear a firm supporting one when you are pregnant. Go up a size of bra as your breasts enlarge. For breastfeeding there are special nursing bras that open at the front. As long as the ligaments that support the breasts are not overstretched, the breasts should not lose any of their shape or uplift as a result of pregnancy.

Special care for pregnancy and breastfeeding

Apart from making sure the breasts get proper support during pregnancy, it is a good idea to wash them gently with soap and water each day and rub a little moisturizing cream into the nipple area. Inverted nipples – which make breastfeeding difficult – can be corrected by wearing small plastic discs known as breast shells inside the bra in the last two months of pregnancy. Begin by wearing the shells for an hour or two each day and gradually increase the wearing time to a full day; never keep the shells on at night.

Breastfeeding a baby can make your breasts sore from the chomping action of the baby's tongue and gums. An emollient cream or baby lotion rubbed in several times a day should alleviate the soreness and help avert the danger of a cracked nipple. You can help prevent soreness ever developing by making sure the baby leaves the breast gently after feeding. Do this by pressing firmly on his chin – he will automatically open his mouth and your breast can be removed without his tugging at it.

Breastfeeding itself, although it may make the breasts slightly smaller and softer, does not change their shape in any way and should never be blamed if changes do occur. Lack of support for the breasts during pregnancy or afterwards is the cause of loss of shape, not pregnancy or breast-feeding on their own.

Around the time of the menopause, the breasts change again. The level of female hormones in circulation begins to decline and breast tissue along with the tissue of the genital organs starts to thin, sag and become less supple. There is nothing to be done about these changes. Unless they are accompanied by severe menopausal symptoms (see page 78) they are never a sufficient reason for using hormone supplements.

The case for wearing a bra

It became fashionable a few years ago for women to go bra-less. For purely anatomical reasons, this fashion will spoil the shape of all breasts except

Breast Self-examination

Breast cancer is a curable disease if you seek help early enough. To make sure you get help early, do two things.

1 Examine your breasts regularly and frequently – about every two to four weeks. After a bath is a good time to do this.

2 Consult your doctor *immediately* if you find a lump of any kind. Please remember that most lumps are not malignant.

The kind of lump you are feeling for when you examine your breasts should not be confused with the natural lumpiness of most breasts in the week before menstruation. At this time the breasts are enlarged, heavy, possibly sore when squeezed, and feel as if they contain small lumps like orange pips. These are swollen milk glands and they will shrink as soon as menstruation is established. Do not be alarmed if you feel them.

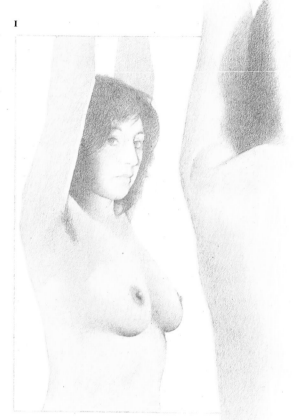

1 Stand or sit naked to the waist in front of a mirror and look at your breasts carefully. Stretch both arms above your head and turn from side to side – this makes the outline of the breasts and any dimpling of the skin over the surface of a lump more obvious. Check the nipples for any change in size, shape, colour or any unusual discharge.

2 Now lie down flat with a folded towel or small cushion under your shoulders. Think of your breast as a circle with four quarters. With your hand held flat and fingers straight, you are going to examine each quarter systematically, working from the outer edge in to the nipple. Use the right hand to examine the left breast, the left hand for the right breast.

3 Stretch the arm you are not using back above your head while you examine the inner quarters of the breast.

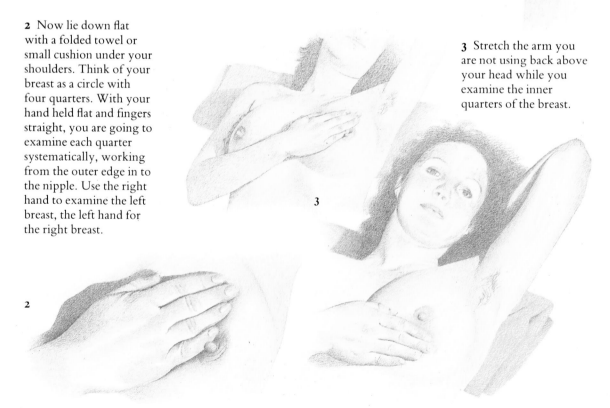

If you find a definite lump – soft or hard, freely mobile or tethered, painful or painless – where there is none in the other breast, do not wait to see if it will disappear. If you find anything at all that worries you, *consult your doctor straight away*. He will examine the lump for himself and if he is suspicious about any of his findings he will send you on to see a consultant – usually within days.

If the consultant is in any way suspicious he will almost certainly suggest removing the lump (a lumpectomy). This kind of operation can normally be arranged speedily so there should be little delay between the visit to the consultant and admission to hospital. While you are still in the operating theatre, the lump is taken to the pathology laboratory where a precise diagnosis of its nature can be made within minutes (a biopsy). Four out of five lumps turn out to be quite harmless.

Even if the lump should be found to be malignant, for early cancer many surgeons do not believe it is necessary to carry out complete removal of the breast (a mastectomy). It is common for one or two of the lymph glands under the arm to be removed for examination to ascertain whether or not the cancer has spread. If it has not, simple removal of the lump and post-operative radiotherapy may be all that is necessary.

By going to the doctor as soon as you find a lump you give yourself the best chance of a full cure and of avoiding an operation that can be psychologically and emotionally extremely hard for a woman to accept.

If your doctor decides that mastectomy is the best treatment for you, be brave and ask for a full discussion about the operation. Surgeons are very sympathetic to your fears and anxieties and will be able to allay many of them. Talking to someone who has had a mastectomy will help to give you confidence before the operation so explore this possibility with your doctor. The prostheses (false breasts) that you can wear after a mastectomy are of a very high quality and are undetectable when you are fully clothed. Some can even be worn to go swimming.

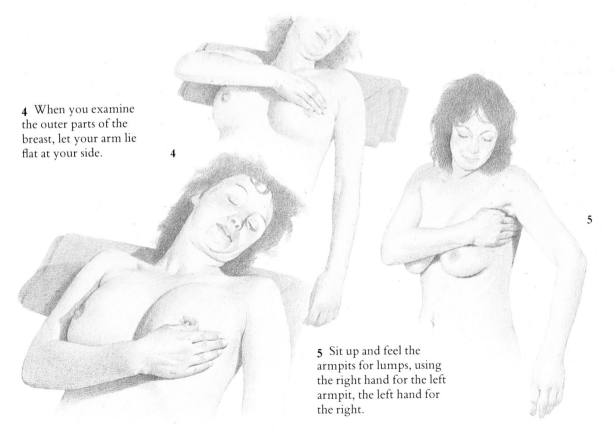

4 When you examine the outer parts of the breast, let your arm lie flat at your side.

4

5

5 Sit up and feel the armpits for lumps, using the right hand for the left armpit, the left hand for the right.

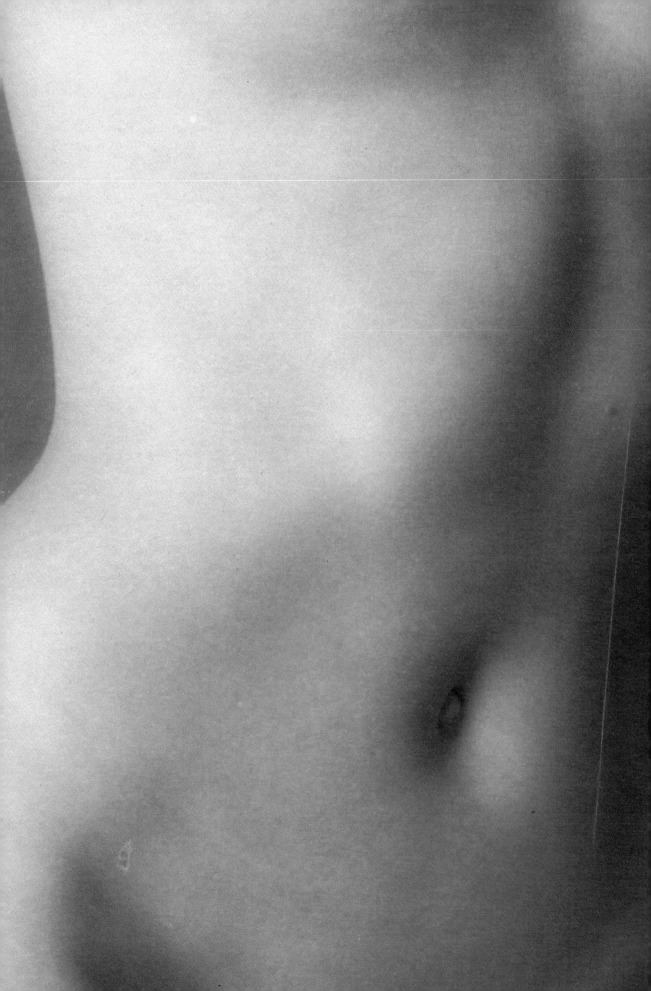

Abdomen and Waist

No woman can do much about the basic figure type she inherits but no one has to have a sagging tummy. If the sag is due to excess fat, no gimmick, such as massage or electric stimulation, will help: the only answer is to diet. If it is caused by flabby muscles, try the exercises on pages 136–137 and try to pull in your tummy several times whenever you remember. Doing this ten times in a row three or four times a day should gradually eliminate the bulge.

The abdominal walls are formed by four fairly thin, sheet-like muscles. The rectus abdominus is the front wall and the external oblique, the internal oblique and the transversus abdominus together form the side walls. The rectus abdominus runs longitudinally like a strap on either side of the navel from the edges of the lowest ribs down to the pubic bone. The internal and external oblique muscles fan out over the rest of the abdomen from the pubis up to the ribs. If these muscles are kept in good condition, the tummy should look trim and flat.

Size of waist is difficult to modify once dieting has done all it can. No exercise can produce a tiny waist unless the figure is naturally petite. Good posture is the only real help: you can cut about 5 cm (2 in) from your waist measurement by straightening the shoulders, holding the head high and lifting the rib cage. This pulls up the skin, fat and abdominal contents and defines the waist more clearly. It also minimizes the midriff bulge from which many of us suffer.

Some people have the impression that fluid retention can cause abdominal distention and weight gain, but in normal circumstances this is not so. However much fluid is taken, the kidneys will be able to eliminate any excess within 12 to 18 hours. It is too much fat rather than too much fluid that makes us overweight.

The exception to this general rule is pre-menstrual fluid retention, which for physiological reasons may lead to a weight gain of up to 6.5 kg (14 lb) that is shed when menstruation begins. Changes in mood at the same time may make a woman irritable, depressed and difficult to get along with, while there may be physical symptoms such as headaches or backache too.

Women who suffer from pre-menstrual fluid retention can help themselves by cutting down their intake of fluids in the week before menstruation. Another good tip is to drink increasingly strong coffee (a diuretic) to eliminate water from the body. Very severe pre-menstrual symptoms may be relieved by injections of progestogen. It is worth consulting a doctor about this if mood swings and depression are making one week out of four a nightmare.

Pregnancy

It is very important to get the abdominal muscles into good shape before pregnancy. The weight of the growing baby inside the uterus puts quite a strain on the muscles as the pregnancy progresses. The better condition you are in beforehand, the better the tummy will look when it is over – and the easier it should be to carry the baby.

It does no harm at all to do exercises during pregnancy provided they cause no discomfort – indeed, it is beneficial to keep the muscles in good shape for as long as possible. In the last few weeks, however, it is wise to avoid any movement that increases abdominal pressure, such as bending down from the waist, since this may make the waters break prematurely.

The muscles of the abdominal wall cope easily with the expansion of the uterus and should become quite firm again within six weeks of delivery if exercised properly (for both ante- and post-natal exercises see pages 147–149).

During pregnancy, the skin on the tummy may darken slightly as part of a general increase in skin pigmentation and a brown line (the linea nigra) may appear, running from the navel down the middle of the tummy. The depth of colouration depends on skin type – brunettes generally go a darker brown than blondes and some women experience no change in skin colour at all. The colour usually fades after the baby is born, but sometimes a faint shadow remains. Darkening of the areola is usually permanent.

During late pregnancy many women find stretch marks (reddish streaks of thin skin) appear on the abdomen – sometimes literally overnight. (These marks may also appear as a result of rapid weight gain, particularly during puberty.) During pregnancy they are partly the result of the skin being stretched by the increasing size of the abdomen – at full term the waist will measure around 102 cm (40 in). The high level of the pregnancy hormones oestrogen and progesterone circulating in the blood also plays an important role, however. If the skin is very susceptible to the hormones, stretch marks will develop and nothing can be done to prevent them. It does no good whatsoever to rub lotions, oils or creams into the skin, no matter what they contain. Once the baby is born the marks usually fade but if necessary they can be removed by cosmetic surgery when child-bearing is over (see page 228).

If the baby is very large, it is quite normal for the navel to evert (stick out). This needs no treatment – in fact it should never be necessary to take special care of the navel: it is a self-cleansing orifice and looks after itself. If it should become red and itchy, a little cetrimide cream, night and morning, should clear the symptoms within 72 hours. If they persist, see a doctor.

Weight gain in pregnancy

It is natural to want to return to normal shape and size as soon as possible after the baby is born. This is a good deal easier to do if weight gain is limited during pregnancy. Opinions vary, however, on what limit should be set. The most severe line is that weight gain should be kept to 8.2 kg (18 lb) or less (this is what the extra weight of the baby, placenta, uterus and amniotic fluid should roughly amount to). Some authorities tolerate as much as 12.7 kg (28 lb) of total weight gain but anything above this figure is agreed to be very undesirable. The best strategy is probably to aim for a fairly low weight gain, but not to worry about going slightly over your limit, provided you are well and eating sensibly (see pages 96–105).

It is worth mentioning here that weight gain should be concentrated in the last six months of pregnancy – the first three months may even see a weight loss, particularly if there is nausea. Many doctors feel it is important to avoid gaining more than 4.5 kg (10 lb) between the twentieth and thirtieth weeks: high weight gain at this time may predispose a woman to pre-eclampsia, which, if unchecked, may endanger mother and child.

Clothes in pregnancy

For the first half of pregnancy there is no need at all for special maternity clothes. Waist and tummy begin to enlarge visibly from around the thirteenth week (counting from the first day of the last period) but for long afterwards can be disguised by ordinary loose-fitting clothes. Even when these get too tight it is still possible to adapt them – and you may feel happier doing this than splashing out on a maternity outfit far removed from your ordinary style of dress. If it suits you to wear jeans, for example, you can wear them virtually up to delivery by slashing the waistband down to the groin in a couple of places, elasticating the gaps, and hiding the lot under a long, loose smock or tunic. By sticking as close as possible (within reason) to a normal style of dress, you may feel less enormous and more yourself.

High heels are definitely not sensible in the later stages of pregnancy. It is hard to balance in them and because they force the muscles to overwork they can make the legs and back ache.

The menopause

At some point – usually between the ages of 45 and 55 for most women – menstruation gradually comes to a halt. The periods typically become scantier and then less frequent, and finally stop. Irregular bleeding is not a normal part of going through the menopause – if this should happen consult a doctor.

The cause of the menopause is the gradual failure of the ovaries to produce the female hormones oestrogen and progesterone. This change can produce very severe symptoms over weeks or many months, including hot flushes, mood changes, tearfulness, depression, irritability, loss of sex drive and pain in the joints. If any of these symptoms is very troublesome, see a doctor. If he takes the view that nothing can be done to help you, do not let the matter rest there: try a menopause clinic.

Taking oral supplements of oestrogen and progestogen (hormone replacement therapy) can produce a dramatic improvement for some women. However, because hormones are potent drugs they should never be considered for the relief of minor or occasional symptoms, and a woman taking them should be closely monitored by a doctor. They should be seen as a way of tiding a woman over a difficult period in her life, not as a long-term solution.

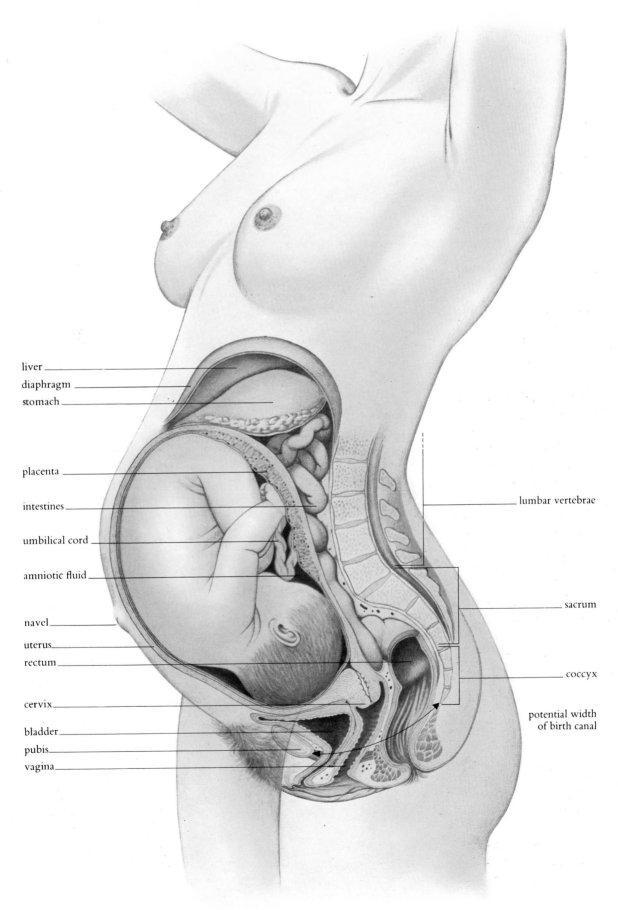

liver

diaphragm

stomach

placenta

intestines

umbilical cord

amniotic fluid

navel

uterus

rectum

cervix

bladder

pubis

vagina

lumbar vertebrae

sacrum

coccyx

potential width
of birth canal

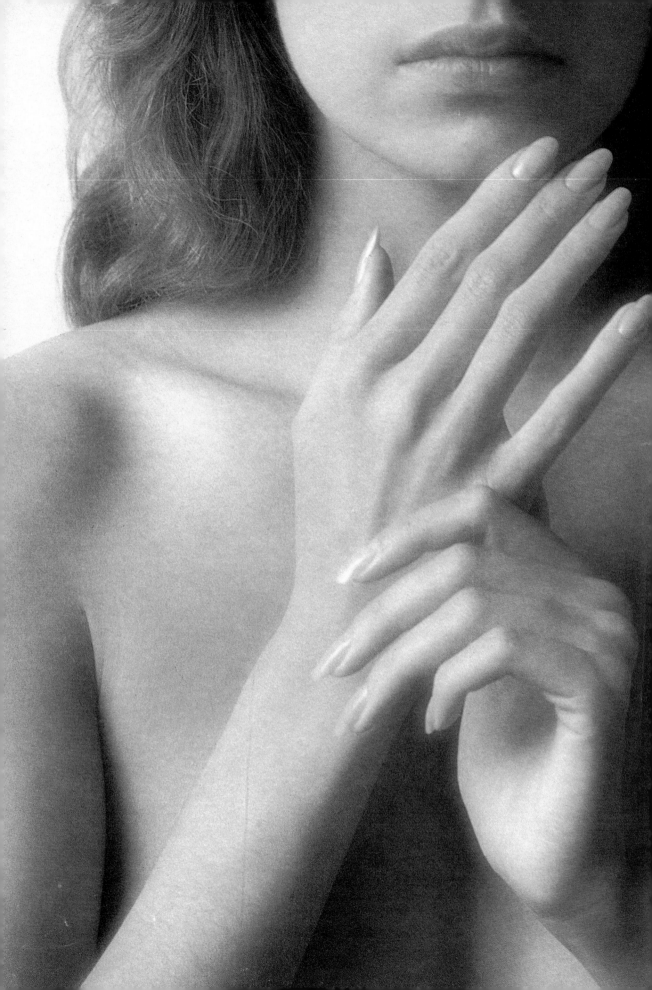

Arms and Hands

The shape and size of the arms and hands are genetically determined. So concentrate on keeping them in good condition, with the skin soft, supple and attractive, and do your best to forget about short forearms and stubby fingers. From the beauty point of view the areas to keep an eye on are the shape of the upper arms, the condition of the hands and the nails.

Arms

When a woman gains weight, one of the first places for fat to be deposited is on her upper arms. This looks ugly and ageing. Worse still, once the fat has been deposited it is very hard to get rid of, even with exercises. Prevention is by far the best cure and that depends on maintaining a slim figure and an ideal weight. It is particularly important to avoid putting on too much weight during pregnancy (see page 78) as excess weight remains after the baby has been delivered, and quite a lot of it will be on the upper arms.

One part of the arm that is fairly easily injured is the elbow. Tennis elbow (so-called because it can arise from repeatedly performing the movement used to produce a backhand drive) can afflict people who have never lifted a tennis racquet in their lives. Many common household tasks, including painting or window cleaning, can give rise to this condition. The symptoms are pain on moving the joint and exquisite tenderness at the point of the elbow. The underlying cause is a strain, tearing or swelling of the muscle or tendons that straighten the elbow. Treatment consists of rest and pain killers. In very severe cases local hydrocortisone injections and ultrasound therapy (see page 241) may be tried.

Hands

More rough treatment is meted out to the hands than to any other part of the body. They are immersed in water, which is itself dehydrating (see page 16), and then defatted by contact with washing-up liquids, detergents and soap powders. Unless measures are taken to counteract this kind of abuse, the hands are bound to suffer.

The first simple rule is to make sure that the hands are properly dried with a towel after every contact with water. The longer the water remains on the skin, the more dehydrating it is. Another

obvious precaution where dirty work is involved is to wear rubber gloves or, for gardening, special gardening gloves. It is important not to keep rubber gloves on for longer than about five minutes, however, as they make the hands sweat profusely. This dries out the skin so that within a few minutes of taking the gloves off, the hands feel hard and dry. If it is really necessary to wear rubber gloves for longer than five minutes, try to wear them over a pair of cheap cotton gloves impregnated with hand cream or lotion. This way the hands are given a beauty treatment every time the rubber gloves go on.

It is worth trying to look after the hands as carefully as the face. Use a mild soap (preferably one that comes close to the skin's normal slight acidity, about 5 on the pH scale). Scrubbing fiercely at dirty areas will make the skin red and sore so try applying a little lemon juice to the stains instead (this should have a lightening effect). When gardening or doing household chores, try applying 'barrier' cream, which is specially formulated to prevent the penetration of dirt, particularly round the nail tips. Most important of all, make sure that the hands are well moisturized. If possible keep a tube of hand cream wherever you work and apply it often.

Hands are in action with hardly a pause all through the day. We depend on them to perform countless tasks, some of them so automatic that they are carried out almost unconsciously. Supple hands are more graceful and expressive than neglected ones, so practise these hand exercises when you can (for others see pages 142–143).

1 Stretch the arms out straight. Rotate the wrists ten times, clockwise, then anti-clockwise.
2 With both hands held palm down, curl the fingers into a loose fist. Slowly turn the palms upwards in a circular movement, while unfolding the fingers. Stretch the fingers out; relax them, then repeat the sequence in reverse.

Some ordinary activities that provide good hand and finger exercise are typing, piano playing and needlework.

The onset of arthritis in the hands may greatly reduce their dexterity and manipulative powers. Provided the condition is not acutely painful, the basic pattern of therapy is a combination of rest and exercise. The exercises, such as those above, are best practised when the hands have been warmed up (by immersing them in warm water, for example) and should always be performed gently – never to the point at which the joints grow stiff or tired. To strengthen the fingers, practise clenching the fists round a cotton reel. At night, it may be easier to rest the hands in a comfortable position in a set of splints. A doctor should be able to advise on how to get splints made up and on where to obtain specially designed gadgets for facilitating everyday tasks.

Nails

The nails and hair have much in common. Both are composed of dead keratin and grow slowly from a living root. Both mirror the body's general health and are often affected by the same diseases.

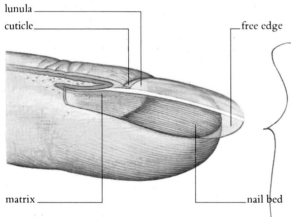

lunula
cuticle
free edge
matrix
nail bed

The nail grows from a nail 'follicle', which runs almost parallel with the skin, just a few millimetres beneath the surface cuticle. The nail rests on a bed of slightly modified skin, to which it is so firmly attached that if the nail is bent back or separated from the finger, the underlying skin comes with it. Part of the root (or matrix) is visible: it lies beneath the half-moon (lunula) at the base of the nail. The matrix is continuous with the cuticle and damage to the cuticle disturbs nail growth. The nervous habit of pushing back the cuticle can be sufficient to produce a ridge in the nail, which shows as it emerges. As well as reflecting this kind of local stress, nails grow at twice their normal rate of 3 cm (1.2 in) a month if persistently bitten.

Anything that has an effect on the body's overall health affects the nails. Emotional stress may show up as thinning, ridging or furrowing. As the nail grows out completely in about $3\frac{1}{2}$ months, a doctor can pinpoint the time of a health crisis quite accurately by examining the nails alone. In a severe illness, profound allergy or long fever, they may be lost altogether.

Contrary to popular belief, vitamin and mineral deficiencies do not cause nails to become brittle or split. These conditions commonly have no traceable cause and do not respond to dietary supplements. So it is no use eating gelatin or cheese, for example, in the hope of improving your nails. Because all the visible nail is dead, it is equally pointless to apply cream to 'nourish' it. The nails' condition can be affected only during their growing stage, which is very short.

Another common nail problem for which there is no treatment is white spots on the nail surface. These may be caused by bangs or knocks to the matrix and they grow out with the nail.

What will improve the nails is proper care and attention. Brittle, chipped and peeling nails look ugly and are unnecessary. Brittleness and peeling are commonly caused by immersing the hands in water and detergents, thereby drying out the nails. Once this has happened, misusing the nails will make them chip at the edges. The remedy is to wear rubber gloves if the hands are to be in water for more than a short while, and to take sensible care not to put the nails under a lot of stress. Colourless nail polish or a liquid nail strengthener, applied to the tip of the nail, provides a protective shield and helps prevent flaking.

Another common problem is discolouration, which can be caused by ill-health, anaemia or smoking, among other things. Pink nail polish can sometimes leave a stain – the yellow dye in the polish leaks out and penetrates the nail plate. To avoid such staining, apply a base coat before putting on polish; the only way to remove existing polish stains is to stop using polish and allow the nails to grow out. Try rubbing lemon juice around the nail tips for other stains.

A regular manicure of the kind shown on pages 84–85 will prevent many unattractive faults developing in the nails. Hangnails, for example – tiny painful tears in the cuticle and surrounding skin – commonly happen only when the cuticles have been neglected, so that as the nail grows, the

Applying false nails

False nails are a useful temporary camouflage for unsightly nails, but they should not be worn daily as they involve total coverage of the nails and adhesive has to be used. They can either be applied singly or as a complete set.

You will need: an emery board, false nails, special adhesive and adhesive remover, both of which come generally with the nails, and a cotton bud (swab).

1 Many types of false nails are available – curved, wide or slim-fitting. If possible, check they are the right shape before you buy by holding them against your nails.

3 If the false nails are brittle and inflexible, dip them in warm water or warmed olive oil and dry thoroughly. Apply a very small dab of glue to the curved underside.

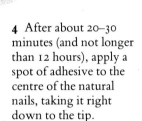

2 Smooth down any rough edges on the natural nails with an emery board, then file the false nails to the required shape, filing them down if too long and pointed.

4 After about 20–30 minutes (and not longer than 12 hours), apply a spot of adhesive to the centre of the natural nails, taking it right down to the tip.

5 One by one, position the false nails carefully over the natural nails and press them down firmly for a few seconds to allow the adhesive to grip properly.

6 To remove, apply a drop of nail adhesive remover under the nail tip (from the capsule provided or on a cotton bud) and lift the false nail off gently with a rocking movement.

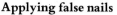

skin travels with it and tears. If this happens, trim the cuticle to prevent further tearing and apply a cuticle cream. It is a good idea to do this promptly to lessen the chances of an infection.

Nail biting is such a common habit that there is no point being prostrated with guilt about it. However, it does unfortunately make it hard to have attractive hands. Those who bite their nails, rather than just picking at them, may find a nail biting deterrent in the form of a bitter-tasting solution some use. Nail biters generally neglect their hands so it often helps to set up a definite hand care regime, including a manicure of whatever nails there are. Becoming aware of them in this way sometimes makes it easier to give up idly nibbling or picking at them all the time. While the nails are growing, avoid aggressive colours that will draw attention to them. A pale peach or pink or a transparent matte polish is best.

If you feel your nails are too unsightly, you could always try false nails (see above), which can give morale a real boost on a special occasion.

Manicure

Everyone can improve the condition of their hands by a regular home manicure, preferably once a week. The first priority is to keep the nails clean and, using a fine emery board, well shaped. Cutting with scissors can jar and split the nail; steel files are too abrasive and inflexible. File weak, split nails across into a square shape to encourage the skin to cling to the sides, so ensuring more protection.

Step-by-step manicure

For the basic manicure you will need: cotton wool balls, an orange stick, an emery board, a bowl of warm water with a little mild soap and baby oil added, nourishing cream or special cuticle cream, cuticle remover – gel, cream or lotion – a soft leather buffer, hand cream and a soft towel. Work in a good light and remove old polish before beginning the manicure.

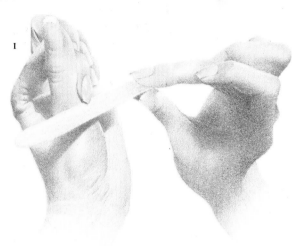

3 Apply cuticle remover all round the nail, rubbing in cream or gel with the thumb, applying lotion with the applicator provided.

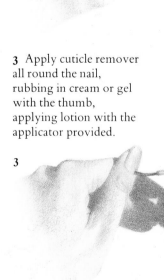

Removing nail polish

Soak a piece of cotton wool in oily nail polish remover. Hold it between the index and middle fingers (to avoid smudging intact polish), press it on to the nail for a second, to allow the remover to soak in, then wipe off the polish with one or two strokes.

1 With a fine emery board, shape the nail into a gentle oval, filing from each side towards the centre in one direction only – filing back and forth leads to rough edges. Do not file too much away from the side, as this can cause hang nails and damage the nail itself.

2 Rub nourishing cream or cuticle cream into the cuticle area and round the sides of the nail with small circular movements of the thumb. Soak the fingers in a bowl of warm soapy water for at least three minutes to soften the cuticles, then dry gently on a soft towel. Treat one hand at a time in this and the three following stages to ensure that the cuticles remain soft.

4 Wrap the blunt end of an orange stick in cotton wool and use it to push the cuticle gently down all round the nail. With a neat circular movement, remove any bits of cuticle still remaining on the nail surface. Roll the orange stick down the nail to push the cuticle gently down to the base.

5 Wrap the pointed end of the orange stick in cotton wool and gently clean out the nail tip. Do not poke the stick into the nail too violently as this can damage the tip and the base. Repeat the soaking and cuticle removing with the other hand. If necessary, neaten off the nails with the emery board.

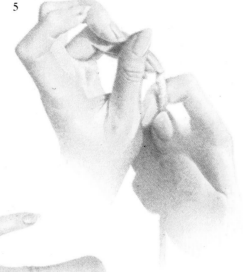

5

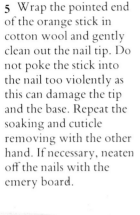

6

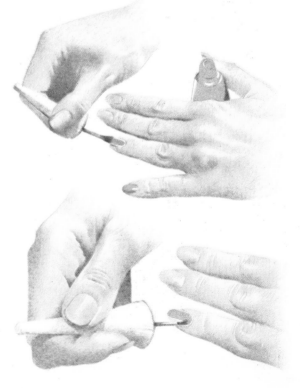

To promote a healthy shine, gently buff the nails from the tips to the cuticles with a soft leather buffer. Buffing also stimulates the blood, so strengthening the nails and promoting their growth.

7

Vigorously rub a small nut of hand cream into each hand. Pay particular attention to the fingers and rub the cream in as if trying to remove a tight ring from each one. This improves the circulation and increases the blood supply to the base of the nail. Remove all traces of cream from the nails with a dampened pad of cotton wool.

Applying nail polish
Rest your hand on a cushion with a towel folded over it. To prevent the pigment in the polish from discolouring the nail, it is essential to apply a base coat. Holding the bottle between the thumb and forefinger, start on the little finger with a broad sweep down the centre of the nail from the cuticle to the tip. Then, with two firm strokes, brush down either side of the nail. Remove any surplus with the brush. Continue with the other nails, dipping the brush into the bottle for each one. Let the base coat dry a little, then apply to the other hand.

Apply the first coat of polish in the same way. It may look streaky, but the second coat gives a denser, finished effect. At first, it is hard to judge how much polish to have on the brush: too little will dry quickly, leaving a rough, dragged surface, but too much will smudge on the skin. Wipe off smudges with a cotton bud dipped in polish remover.

Apply a top coat of colourless polish, and allow to dry for as long as possible (up to an hour) before using the hands. For faster drying use a spray-dry aerosol or briefly dip the nails into iced water.

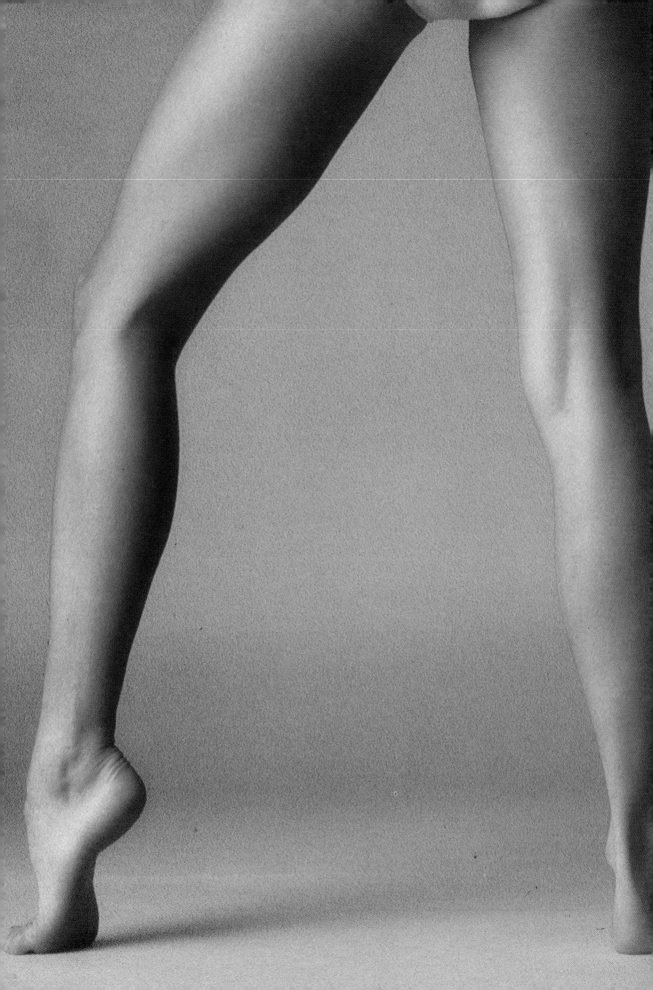

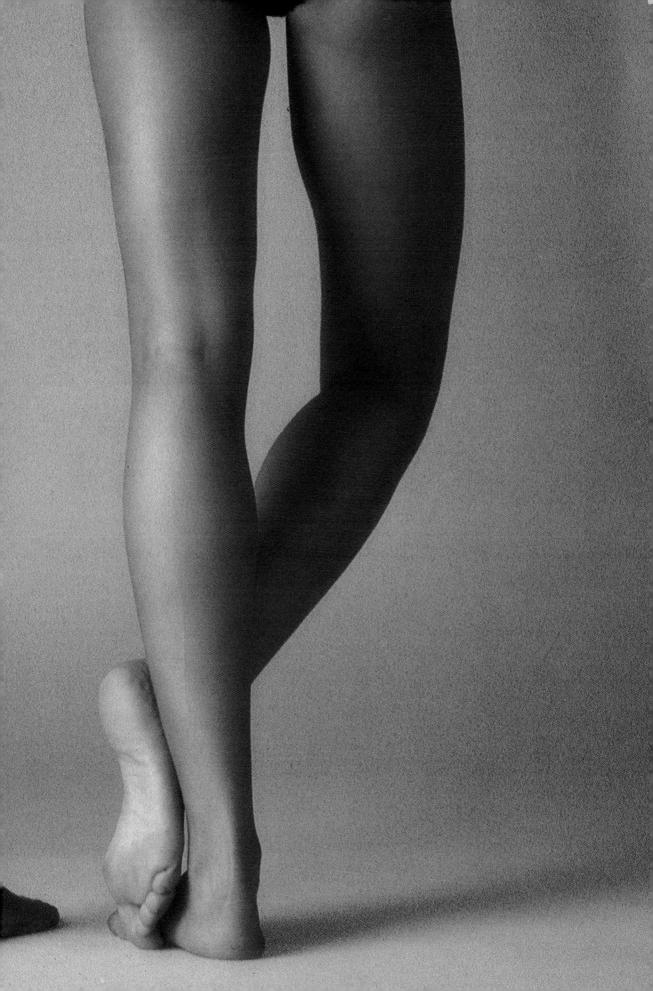

Legs and Feet

One of fashion's major themes through the twentieth century has been the increasing exposure of women's legs. Ankle, calf, knee and thigh have all had their turn in the limelight. The fact that so few of us possess legs that measure up to the ideal – long, slim, gently rounded – is unfortunate but perfectly natural. The basic function of the human leg for thousands of years was to help us survive through flight and escape. Muscle, bone and tendon have all evolved for strength and power and their appearance inevitably reflects their history.

Structure

The muscles of the legs are among the largest and most powerful in the body. At the back of the thigh are the hamstrings, so called because they end in strong tendons (strings) that form on either side of the knee. These muscles flex the knee joint and push the foot off the ground in running – hence they played a crucial role historically in our ability to survive through running from danger.

At the front of the thigh is the quadriceps femoris muscle group, of which the rectus femoris is the most centrally placed. This powerful group of muscles is responsible for extending the knee joint, enabling us to stand, as well as giving power to the action of kicking.

The shape of the calf comes from the gastrocnemius muscle, which ends at the heel bone in the long and extremely strong Achilles tendon. This raises the heel in walking and running and helps to point the toes. In negro races the muscle tends to be higher on the leg bone (tibia) and slimmer (but still powerful) than in Caucasians.

The two major bones in the leg, the thigh bone (femur) and tibia, meet behind the kneecap (patella) to form the flat knee joint. A lengthy spell of kneeling down can lead to swelling of the bursa (the cushion of fluid that acts as the knee joint's shock absorber) and the collection of fluid (housemaid's knee). Because of the weight the knee has to carry, even a minor injury like a knock may take months to become pain-free.

Some women who have large pelvises develop knock knees (see page 67). If this condition is detected in childhood it may be possible to correct the shape of the legs – it is worth consulting an

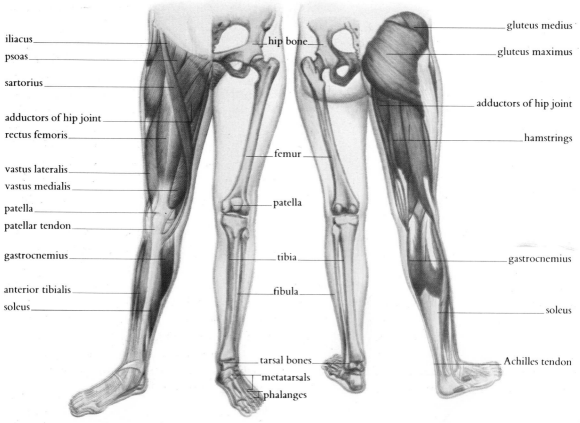

iliacus
psoas
sartorius
adductors of hip joint
rectus femoris
vastus lateralis
vastus medialis
patella
patellar tendon
gastrocnemius
anterior tibialis
soleus

hip bone
femur
patella
tibia
fibula
tarsal bones
metatarsals
phalanges

gluteus medius
gluteus maximus
adductors of hip joint
hamstrings
gastrocnemius
soleus
Achilles tendon

orthopaedic specialist for an opinion because after adolescence no treatment can remedy the condition. The same is true of the opposite to knock knees, bow legs. Fortunately the latter are now extremely rare: the main cause used to be rickets in childhood, a complaint almost unheard of today in the developed countries. It is quite untrue that horse riding or playing the cello can make a person bow-legged.

Women's legs have a naturally smoother, more rounded appearance than men's because they carry more subcutaneous fat. A pad of fat on the inside of the upper thigh in particular is a female characteristic (a useful one too since it acts as a cushion during sexual intercourse). Because of the tendency for fat to accumulate in this area on women it is very hard to shift it. Exercises will make the muscles less flabby (see pages 138–139) but the only real cure for fat here, as elsewhere, is to diet. (Sometimes people in the beauty business call fat on the thighs cellulite; see page 69 for a discussion of this term.)

Making legs look better

There is a limit to the extent to which any part of the human body can be improved and the limit is reached very quickly with the legs. Genetic factors determine their length, overall shape, thickness of ankle and many more subtle characteristics. No amount of diet or exercise will change these essentials any more than they will change the colour of your hair or eyes. For legs that fall a long way short of the ideal, camouflage may be the only practical answer. Clever dressing and make-up can do a great deal to disguise the legs' defects. Dark stockings make legs look slimmer and so does dark make-up applied to the outsides of calves and ankles. Light-coloured stockings or thick tights give a plumper look. Length of skirt can also be important and it is sensible to avoid a skirt that ends in mid calf if your legs are heavy.

Short of window dressing, the only way to improve the appearance of legs that are neither fat nor flabby is to keep the skin looking good. Dark hairs show up sharply on pale skin and many women choose to remove them from their legs (see pages 46–47 for a survey of methods of depilation and advice about which to use).

Apply a moisturizer to the skin on the legs as often as possible because the area is usually very dry. This is partly as a result of exposure to sun and wind most of the year round but also because the legs tend to be undernourished – by the time the blood reaches them it has already lost most of the oxygen it carried when it began its journey from the heart. It is particularly important to use a moisturizing cream or lotion after shaving the legs: soapy lather has a defatting effect and the soak in the bath that may accompany shaving will dry the skin out still further.

The tiny broken veins that some women develop on their legs are part of their genetic inheritance, like broken veins on the face. They tend to show up more the older one gets. Putting the legs near a source of direct heat (such as a radiator or fire) makes the veins more prominent and wearing tight garters can exacerbate them too. If the veins are a source of embarrassment, they can be disguised with make-up or dark-toned stockings, but it is impossible either to prevent them developing or to cure them.

Aching legs

Legs ache for three main reasons: cold (which makes the blood vessels contract), overwork or disuse. Many of the women who complain that their legs ache by the end of the day have spent long periods standing or walking in ill-fitting or unsuitable shoes. If the shoes are too big, for example, the wearer has to bunch the toes up in an attempt to keep the shoes on. This forces the muscles in the calf to flex unnaturally and eventually makes the legs ache. Very high heels also make the calf muscles overwork. The best way for these women to avoid aching legs is to wear properly fitting shoes with heels less than 6.25 cm (2½ in) high.

If the legs feel stiff after a long time spent sitting down, try doing a few simple foot exercises every now and then to flex the muscles in the calves. Lifting the feet off the ground and rotating them from the ankle improves blood circulation and makes the legs more comfortable. Another excellent way of flexing unused leg muscles is to point the toes first downwards and then draw them up hard towards the knee (see pages 144–145 for more exercises for the lower leg).

Sluggish circulation of blood through the legs should not on its own make them ache and neither should varicose veins. However, if leg ache is associated with swollen ankles, as it often is for women with varicose veins, the following position should alleviate both the discomfort and the swelling. Lie down flat with your feet propped up against a wall at as steep an angle as possible. This encourages the blood to flow freely back to the heart and as a bonus increases blood supply to the brain, which should leave you feeling lively and refreshed.

A gentle massage is another way to relax tired, aching muscles and the legs are among the easiest parts of the body to massage yourself. The quick routine described here is easy to fit in even on a busy evening. Damp the hands with oil or lotion and begin the massage at the ankle, moving the hands firmly up both sides of the leg towards the knee. Then return the hands lightly to the foot, running them down the shin bone. Finally massage the knee gently with a circular movement. For more discussion of massage techniques see pages 172–175.

Those who suffer from recurrent leg ache may find it helps to wear support hose made of strong elastic fibre. These apply mild pressure at the heels, mid calves and lower thighs, thereby helping the pumping action of the leg muscles during walking. There are many types of support hose available: some are thick enough to disguise varicose veins, while others look almost identical to ordinary tights or stockings.

Feet

Most people are born with perfect feet but four out of five develop foot trouble later in life. The two overwhelming causes of foot problems are badly fitting shoes or tights and neglect of proper foot care. Follow the step-by-step pedicure on page 93 and remember: it is almost invariably easier to prevent a foot problem than it is to cure it or to learn to live with it.

We rarely become conscious of the numerous muscles, bones and ligaments in our feet until something goes wrong. One common accident – stumbling so that the outer edge of the foot turns sharply inwards – will make us acutely aware of the ligaments on the outside of the foot near the ankle. When these are torn, the foot becomes extremely sore, swollen and painful to tread on – a condition known as a sprained ankle. Treatment is to rest the foot completely for three or four days, preferably firmly bandaged and raised on a stool.

The other part of the foot that is particularly vulnerable to everyday stresses and strains is the joint of the big toe. As the drawing on the opposite page shows, this joint transmits the whole weight of the body on to the front of the foot if we wear high-heeled shoes, forcing it to work very hard, often in cramped conditions. The result may be a bunion, for which surgery offers the only real cure (see Common leg and foot complaints, below).

Shoes and stockings

The first essential for a shoe is that it should fit the foot properly. It should be wide enough to allow the toes to lie naturally (rather than being forced inwards) and at least 1 cm ($\frac{1}{2}$ in) longer than the foot, to allow the toes to move freely. The shoe should fit snugly at the heel and instep so that it is not necessary to bunch the toes to keep the shoe from slipping. It is essential to try the shoes out before buying. Stand up in them and wear them to walk around inside the shop. A shoe that feels fine while you are sitting down may be far from comfortable in action. Remember that feet swell in hot weather, so try to avoid shopping for summer sandals on a cold day.

The second essential in choosing a shoe has already been mentioned: heel height. Heels over 6.25 cm ($2\frac{1}{2}$ in) high subject both feet and legs to such strain that to wear them for long periods of standing or walking is simply asking for trouble. Shoes with low heels distribute body weight far more evenly over the foot and avoid over-straining any one part of it. If you normally wear high heels through the day, try to change into a flatter pair whenever the chance arises – in the lunch break, perhaps, or as soon as you get home. Varying the height of the heels you wear from day to day also helps your feet to feel less tired.

The evils of unsuitable shoes are fairly widely known but it is less generally appreciated that nylon tights can be just as harmful. Nylon does not stretch, as old-fashioned silk stockings do, to accommodate different shapes of foot or to adjust to foot movements. By the end of the day it can constrict swollen tired feet with a grip like steel. Nylons can cause just as many bunions and other foot complaints as badly fitting shoes.

Walking barefoot (see below) is one of the best ways to exercise the feet. Wearing wooden-soled exercise sandals is the next best thing and far more practical than bare feet outside the warmth and shelter of the home. Traditional exercise sandals are carefully balanced to give the muscles in the feet and legs the right kind of stimulus. The gripping/relaxing toe movements they encourage help the calf muscles to contract efficiently, improving the circulation of the blood through the legs and helping pump it back up to the heart.

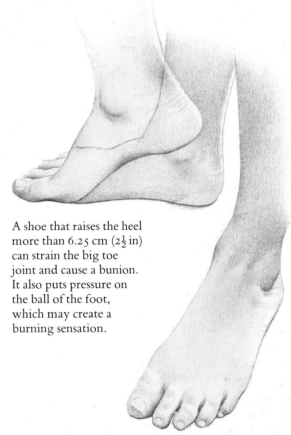

A shoe that raises the heel more than 6.25 cm (2½ in) can strain the big toe joint and cause a bunion. It also puts pressure on the ball of the foot, which may create a burning sensation.

Tired feet, swollen ankles

It is quite common for women who spend much of the day on their feet to experience some swelling of the feet and ankles by evening, particularly in warm weather. This is nothing to worry about, provided that the swelling goes down overnight. Swelling of the ankles during pregnancy, however, may be a danger sign: it is one of the symptoms of pre-eclampsia and should be reported to a doctor at your next ante-natal visit.

All of the following exercises should help to alleviate the discomfort of tired feet:

1 Wrap the feet in cold wet towels for speedy relief and put them on a stool.
2 Take off shoes and stockings and walk around barefoot for as long as you can.
3 Alternately curl the toes tightly for the count of ten and then stretch them out, repeating five or six times. Finally wriggle the toes to the count of ten.

The next set of exercises tones up the foot muscles so that they tire less quickly. Try to practise them every day.

4 Stand with feet together and slowly rise up on to tiptoes and down again (policemen often do this exercise to strengthen their feet and calf muscles).
5 Stand with bare feet on a thick book such as a telephone directory, toes jutting out over the edge. Try to curl the toes down over the edge of the book to grip it as hard as possible. This tones up the muscles in the sole of the foot.

Common leg and foot complaints

● Athlete's foot

This is a fungal infection that attacks the toe nails and the spaces between the toes, making the skin feel sore and peel. It is difficult to clear an infection focused in the toe nails simply by the use of cream or powder since the spaces between the toes will continually be reinfected. Treatment with an oral anti-fungal agent may be needed for several months. Although athlete's foot is infectious, people with dry skin who sweat little normally resist the fungus.

● Bunions

This is a condition that may affect the bursa of the big toe, a cushion of fluid that normally protects the joint from shock each time the foot meets the ground. Chronic overstrain (often caused by wearing badly fitting shoes or high heels) can inflame and thicken the bursa so that it can no longer act as a shock absorber. The only treatment for this painful condition is surgical: removal of the ends of the two toe joints and the old fibrous bursa, to give a stiff but eventually pain-free toe.

- Chilblains

See page 27

- Cold feet

Because the feet are the very furthest points in the body from the heart it takes them a long time to recover from being chilled. Women tend to wear lighter footwear than men and are particularly likely to complain that their feet feel cold at night. One sensible preventive measure is to wear warmer foot coverings and possibly thermal insoles in cold weather. A hot water bottle, electric blanket or bed socks should cut down the time it takes for the feet to warm up in bed.

- Corns (calluses)

These pads of thick, hard skin on the toes and the soles of the feet are the body's way of protecting a part that takes a lot of friction and pressure. Tight, ill-fitting shoes may give rise to painful corns, on the little toe especially. Wearing a corn plaster may ease the pressure on a troublesome corn but if this does not help it may be wise to have the corn treated by a chiropodist.

- Fallen arches (flat feet)

If the muscles that form the arch of the foot are weak, they are strained by carrying the body's weight and may start aching. The shape of the arch may be improved by special exercises, provided that it is spotted early enough. Wooden exercise sandals also help. An adult with painful flat feet may find it more comfortable to wear shoes built up on the inside to give the fallen arch support. (See also page 164 for a yoga posture that helps to correct flat feet and strengthen the arches.)

- Ingrowing toe nails

Sometimes a toe nail, instead of growing straight outwards, curves over and bites into the flesh at the sides of the toe, causing pain or discomfort. This is more likely to occur when the toe is broad and plump and the toe nail small – the nail may naturally sink into the toe as a result of wearing tight shoes or socks. Since the shape of the toes is genetically determined, it is difficult to prevent the nails from growing inwards, but sensible precautions are never to cut the nails away at the sides, or to cut them too short, and to avoid tight footwear. An ingrowing nail usually has to be removed under local anaesthetic and the operation may have to be repeated later.

- Sweaty feet

It is quite natural for the feet to sweat and a daily wash and change of stockings should be enough to prevent the perspiration becoming a problem. However, some people have excessively sweaty feet. This is in no way abnormal, simply a variation, and the problem can be helped by keeping the feet as clean and dry as possible, changing the socks or stockings twice a day if necessary. Foot powders may help, both to keep the perspiration in check and to deal with the smell that often accompanies this condition. If none of these measures works consult a doctor.

- Varicose veins

These arise as a result of damage to the valves in the superficial veins (commonly in the legs). The effect is to make the blood stagnate in the veins, giving them a contorted, swollen appearance. Swollen ankles and dermatitis of the feet may be associated with the complaint. The most usual cause is a deep vein thrombosis (blood clot), which is most likely to occur during pregnancy, immediately after having a baby or after a surgical operation. The best way to stop varicose veins developing is therefore to take preventive measures against blood clots, including exercise as soon as possible after having a baby or operation and keeping the legs mobile while lying in bed. Sitting with legs crossed does no lasting harm normally, but someone who is predisposed to develop varicose veins should avoid the position because it tends to make circulation of blood through the legs more sluggish. Tight garters worn round the upper leg should also be avoided for the same reason.

Varicose veins tend to run in families, so take special care if others in your family have them. Treatment depends on severity of the condition: support stockings may help in mild cases; more severe cases may be treated by stripping the vein surgically. Injecting the veins is a purely cosmetic treatment.

- Verrucae

A verruca is an ingrowing wart on the foot, caused by a virus. It is infectious, so do not swim in a public swimming pool while you have a verruca. Consult a doctor for treatment: if you try to deal with a verruca on your own you may end up with a permanent and painful scar.

Step-by-step pedicure

You will need: a bowl of warm soapy water, a towel, pumice stone, nail brush, nail clippers, cuticle cream or liquid cuticle remover, cotton bud (swab) or orange stick, cotton wool balls, foot or body lotion; base coat and nail polish – optional. Remove all traces of old polish beforehand (see Manicure page 84).

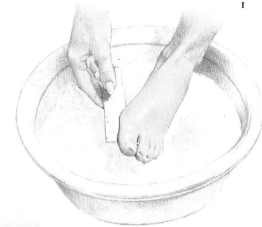

1 Wash each foot in turn in warm soapy water, but do not let them soak as this strips the skin's natural oils, leaving it rough and dry. Gently rub the pumice stone over the soles and heels to remove hard skin. Clean under and around the nails with the nail brush. Dry the feet thoroughly, especially between the toes.

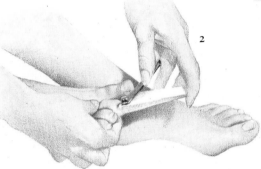

2 Every three or four weeks trim the nails, cutting straight across to discourage ingrowing nails; leave them long enough to cover the tip of the toe. Nail clippers are better than scissors as they have slightly curved ends, which ensure that the nail is cut to the correct shape.

3 Apply a cuticle cream to the base of the nails with the fingers or apply cuticle remover on a cotton bud or an orange stick wrapped in cotton wool. Work round the base and sides of the nails gently, easing the skin back to show the half moon. Never use a sharp or metal instrument to do this as you may split the skin and so cause damage to the base of the nail.

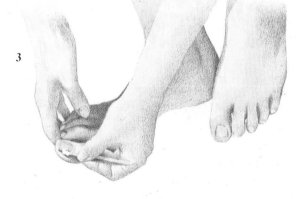

4 Squeeze a little foot or body lotion on to the palm of your hand and work it in all over the foot to leave the skin feeling soft. Massage each toe, then firmly move the hands upwards over the bridge of the feet, from the toes to the ankles, to stimulate the circulation. Continue the massage up to the knee if desired (see also pages 173–175 for further information on massage techniques for the feet and legs).

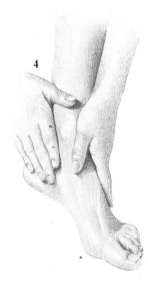

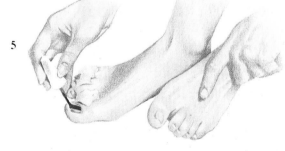

5 Separate the toes with cotton wool. To stop the pigment in the polish discolouring the nail, apply a base coat with one smooth stroke down the centre and two firm strokes on either side. Let it dry and apply polish in the same way, starting with the big toe. Allow to dry for 5–10 minutes. For a longer-lasting finish apply another coat.

A Coordinated Approach

The essential sequel to a knowledge of how the body works is an understanding of how to keep it functioning smoothly. In good health, we assume that our bodies will respond to whatever demands we make of them. But to elicit the best performance and to preserve energy and health, it is important to provide proper maintenance in the form of a well-balanced diet, regular exercise, adequate sleep and periods of relaxation. Only with a combination of all four of these essentials can good health and natural good looks be achieved.

The

While the wisdom of this four-point plan is evident, it is not so simple to choose a regimen that fits your lifestyle and individual needs. A routine that works for one woman may be anathema to the next and only a programme that you enjoy will work for you. Fortunately, the range of methods of relaxation and forms of exercise is sufficiently wide to cater for all tastes and, with exercise, for all levels of stamina and fitness. There are, too, many different approaches to maintaining, losing and gaining weight; simply trying to achieve a well-balanced, nutritious diet can be fraught with complications. Again, familiarity with the fundamental principles of nourishing the body and with its basic needs will enable you to choose the most appealing dietary approach for your purse, palate and figure. Armed with this knowledge, taking care of your body can become a delight instead of a rushed chore or a guilty awareness of neglect.

Essentials

Diet and Nutrition

Food needs

Eating should be both pleasurable and well-balanced – two aims that, far from conflicting, as many people believe, are readily compatible. What is essential first is an understanding of food values and nutritional needs. With this knowledge we can achieve both nourishment and variety in eating because all foods contain a whole range of nutrients in varying amounts. While a particular vitamin or mineral may be present only in small amounts, these contributions from different foods can add up to a significant part of the daily requirement. And so it is misleading to think of foods, as is often the case, in terms of their major nutrients, regarding meat, for instance, solely as 'protein food' or milk as 'calcium food'.

It is more useful to think of foods as having complementary values. Milk, for example, is an excellent source of protein and calcium but contains little vitamin C, while oranges are rich in vitamin C but contain little protein or calcium. So, armed with the facts, the imaginative cook is able to reconcile those warring adjectives 'tempting' and 'wholesome' once and for all.

In nutritional terms, food enables the body to function – it is the engine's fuel. It allows all its components to work smoothly; it renews and repairs parts and, most important of all, it provides energy.

Energy cost of some everyday activities

	kcals/min		kcals/min
Sleeping	0.9	Ironing	1.5–1.9
Sitting	1.1	Polishing	2.0–2.9
Standing	1.2	Vacuuming	3.0–3.9
Walking	3.0–4.0		

The energy provided by food is used up at varying rates according to the activity: clearly the more strenuous the activity, the more energy is used. For calorie consumption rates for different sports, see pages 150–161.

Energy is present in all foods – its value being expressed in calories (strictly kilocalories or kcals) – although the exact energy content of any particular food depends on its nutrient composition. Fat is the richest form of energy in food, while foods low in fat and high in water (which has no energy value at all) have relatively low energy values. Vegetables, for instance, fall into this category.

The body uses food energy for two main purposes. First, to power all the body functions that are essential for life and health, such as breathing, blood circulation, digestion and excretion – this is called the basal metabolic rate (BMR). Second, to provide energy for all the work done by the body – that is, any sort of physical activity, from maintaining body posture to taking part in a sponsored walk. Normally, BMR accounts for about two-thirds of the body's energy needs and work uses up the remaining third except in people who habitually have a high level of activity through their work or recreation. Since both BMR and physical activity can vary enormously from one person to another it is difficult to be precise about the energy requirements of an individual. However, most authorities agree that a healthy adult woman of average height and weight, leading a normal life with a balance of work and recreation, needs about 2000 to 2200 kcals each day.

A healthy person who is neither gaining nor losing weight will use up the same amount of energy as she consumes in the form of food. Although energy intake and output do not match exactly on a day-to-day basis, in the long term they normally balance each other quite accurately. If more 'energy' is eaten than the body can use, the excess is stored as body fat, which usually comprises 25 per cent of the body weight of a slim healthy woman. If energy intake is inadequate, this body store of energy will be used. Maintaining energy balance is an important part of weight control (see pages 112–115).

Liquid needs

Nearly two-thirds of the total body weight is composed of water, so it is hardly surprising that water is the body's prime nutritional need. A healthy person can survive for weeks, even months, without food, but without water death inevitably occurs in a few days. An adequate and regular fluid intake is therefore a fundamental need for good health; any diet that suggests restricting fluid should be viewed sceptically.

Energy value of food

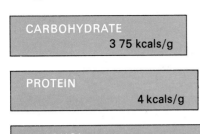

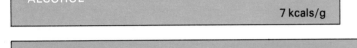

CARBOHYDRATE	3·75 kcals/g
PROTEIN	4 kcals/g
ALCOHOL	7 kcals/g
FAT	9 kcals/g

Most foods contain a mixture of protein, fat and carbohydrate and fall within the middle range of energy values.

The quantity of water required each day is highly variable, ranging from a minimum of 200 ml ($\frac{1}{3}$ pt) to 4 or 5 l (7–9 pt) upwards, although these are extremes and for most people doing everyday occupations in temperate climates 2–3 l (3–5 pt) are sufficient. The body is designed to achieve 'water balance', that is, it is able to maintain a fluid intake large enough to make up for all its fluid losses, as in urine and sweat. Generally, the body does this quite efficiently through the sensation of thirst, signalling the need for more water – although if fluid losses are drastically altered, as in very hot climates or during illness, the slaking of thirst may not be compensation enough. Failure to match losses by intake quickly results in dehydration, the early symptoms of which are merely discomfort and weakness. Further dehydration leads to extreme thirst, weight loss and changes in skin texture and, unless treated, is eventually fatal.

Contrary to popular belief, there are no disadvantages in a generous fluid intake, because water in excess of the body's immediate needs is quickly and efficiently removed by the kidneys and lost via the urine. What is important, however, is the type of fluid intake. Anything other than water could have a profound effect on the rest of the diet. For example, if thirst is satisfied with milk or fruit juice alone, without a corresponding reduction being made in food intake, then almost certainly an excessive amount of calories would be consumed (see pages 120–121). There is therefore a good case for at least part of the daily fluid intake being in the form of plain water, both from the point of view of weight control and of dental health.

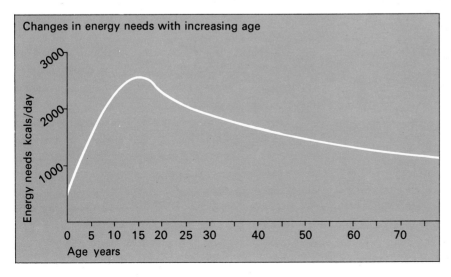

Changes in energy needs with increasing age

Energy needs kcals/day

Age years

Body size affects energy needs: taller and bigger (but not fatter) people tend to need more, while after puberty increasing age diminishes energy needs.

The Major Nutrients

Protein

Needed in the manufacture and repair of tissues, protein is essentially the building material of the body. It manufactures new tissues during growth and pregnancy, renews tissues worn out by everyday wear and tear and repairs those that are diseased or injured; since every tissue – whether muscle, skin, blood or nerve – contains it, protein is a material for which there is a constant demand.

This demand is met by food proteins, which come in many different types, although they are all similar chemically being made up of smaller units called amino acids. There are 20 different amino acids and varying numbers of them can join up into long chains to form an infinite variety of proteins, each specific to a particular tissue. So the amino acid pattern of, say, blood protein differs from that of skin or muscle protein.

Protein content of common foods		
	g/100 g	g/oz
Cheese, hard	26.0	7.4
Peanuts	24.3	6.8
Chicken	20.5	5.8
Beef and other lean meats	20.3	5.8
Liver	20.1	5.7
Cod	17.4	4.9
Eggs	12.3	3.5
Bread	7.8	2.2
Peas	5.8	1.6
Natural yogurt	5.0	1.4
Milk	3.3	0.9

In developed countries we tend to eat too much protein. The excess is used as a source of energy, which is rather uneconomical because protein-rich foods are usually more expensive than energy-giving carbohydrates and fatty foods.

The process of digestion and metabolism of protein is aimed at converting the many types of food protein into the specific type needed by the body at any particular time. To achieve this, first the protein is broken down into its component amino acids, which then circulate in the blood. When they reach the tissue requiring new protein, they are reassembled in the appropriate patterns and proportions for that particular protein. Clearly the 'ideal' food protein would be one that exactly matched the body's needs for amino acids so that the protein requirement of each individual tissue could be met. Alas, no such single food exists.

The nutritional quality of proteins can be judged from their amino acid pattern, and on this basis a mixture of vegetable proteins can be as good as animal proteins. This eliminates the old idea of animal proteins being 'first class' and vegetable proteins 'second class'. In fact, different food proteins are complementary and offset each other's surpluses and deficiencies in amino acid pattern. The way in which the amino acid patterns of bread and cheese complement each other is a good example and the same applies to a number of traditional combinations such as rice and pulses.

Healthy adult women need about 50 g of protein each day. This is more than the minimum requirement, but the extra allows for variation in individual needs and for scope to encourage both the enterprising cook and the discerning palate. Obviously there are many foods able to supply the required amount of protein. Most of a loaf of bread, for instance, could provide a day's quota but that is hardly a tantalizing thought for the gourmet. The best diet is one that is varied, containing proteins from a number of different foods and, contrary to popular belief, the amount of meat and fish included need be only small. Even those committed to the purest forms of vegetarianism need have no trouble meeting their protein requirements (see pages 105, 111).

Carbohydrates

The major function of carbohydrates is to provide energy and in developed countries they usually account for 40 to 50 per cent of the intake. There are two categories of carbohydrates, available and unavailable. The former include sugars and starches, which the body can digest and metabolize. Unavailable carbohydrates, such as celluloses and pectin, cannot be digested but, as roughage, they play an important part in the functioning of the digestive system (see also Fibre on page 100).

Both sugars and starches are important in maintaining the bulk and palatability of the diet.

Starch is a plant product found in cereals such as wheat and rice, cereal products such as bread and also in root vegetables. Sugars, on the other hand, come mostly in the form of refined sugar (sucrose), the white crystalline substance that we add to food and drinks. Only small amounts come from fruits (fructose) and milk (lactose).

Sugar content of common foods		
	g/100 g	g/oz
Boiled sweets and candies	86.9	24.7
Honey	75.4	21.4
Jam	69.0	19.6
Raisins	64.4	18.3
Milk chocolate	56.5	16.0
Fruit cake	43.1	12.2
Sweet pickle	32.6	9.3
Sponge cake	30.9	8.8
Muesli	26.2	7.4
Biscuits, sweet	24.1	6.8
Peaches, canned	22.9	6.5
Ice cream	19.7	5.6
Fruit yogurt	17.9	5.1
Coca-Cola	10.5	3.0
Baked beans	5.2	1.5
White wine, medium	3.4	1.0
Tomato soup	2.6	0.7

Sugars seem to be intrinsically attractive to humans but this universal sweet tooth often leads us to consume much more than energy needs demand.

In chemical terms the simpler carbohydrates – known as monosaccharides – are the sugars. Many monosaccharide molecules linked together form polysaccharides – starch – a more complex structure. The body digests polysaccharides by splitting them into monosaccharides, which are eventually converted into glucose. This is circulated to all parts of the body via the blood and is stored in the liver and muscles, where it helps to maintain blood glucose levels between meals. This ability to convert *all* carbohydrates to glucose means that sugar itself is not essential in the diet, nor does manufactured glucose have any advantage over sucrose as a source of energy for healthy people.

Fats

Although food fats occur in several forms, the most important, and abundant, are the triglycerides, which are made up of chemicals called fatty acids (or glycerides) joined on to glycerol (or glycerine). Each molecule of glycerol can combine with three fatty acid molecules, which may all be the same, or any of 40 different ones. So a large number of different triglycerides are possible and this accounts for the great variety of fats found in nature. Two other types of fat found in foods are phospholipids, such as lecithin, and sterols such as cholesterol. Food fats as a group are often referred to as 'lipids'.

Fat content of common foods		
	g/100 g	g/oz
Vegetable oils	99.9	28.3
Lard	99.0	28.1
Butter	82.0	23.3
Margarine	81.0	23.0
Mayonnaise	78.9	22.4
Peanuts	49.0	13.9
Cheese, hard	33.5	9.5
Pastry	27.8	7.9
Sardines	13.6	3.9
Fruit cake	11.0	3.1
Ice cream	8.2	2.3
Ham	5.1	1.4
Beef, lean	4.6	1.3
Milk	3.8	1.1
Bread	1.7	0.5
Cod	0.7	0.2

Those cutting down on 'visible' fats such as butter can still be left with a more than adequate intake from 'invisible' sources such as peanuts and cheese.

The main function of fats in the diet is as a source of energy and in most developed countries fats provide 35 to 50 per cent of the total energy intake. Although there is no physiological need for this much fat, it does help to reduce the bulk of food that has to be consumed to meet energy requirements. If fat is removed from the diet; it has to be replaced by carbohydrates (or protein), which contain less energy, weight for weight. Fat is also important in maintaining palatability, as anyone who has followed an enforced low-fat diet knows, and in providing the body with two essential fatty acids (EFA).

There is no recommended intake for fats, as the quantity required physiologically is very small. The amount consumed depends largely on national and personal eating habits. However, concern is growing over the possible effects of too much fat in the diet, particularly with problems of overweight and the increase in heart and circulatory diseases. Nearly all nutritional authorities now agree that a general reduction in the total amount of fat consumed is advisable and most also advocate a change in the type of fat – from animal (saturated fats) to unsaturated or polyunsaturated (see page 109).

Fibre

Unavailable carbohydrate includes celluloses and hemicelluloses present in plant tissues, pectins present in fruits, and lignin, which is woody plant tissue. As they cannot be digested these substances, known as roughage or dietary fibre, pass through the digestive system unchanged. Until recently fibre was thought to be of little importance in nutrition but because it is not absorbed, fibre helps to hold water in the waste products in the bowel, which makes the stools soft and bulky and speeds up the passage of food through the digestive system. This is obviously important in the prevention and treatment of constipation and other digestive disorders.

Dietary fibre occurs in all foods of plant origin, the most important sources being wholegrain cereals and flours, starchy roots such as potatoes, pulses such as peas and beans, nuts and fruits. However, the type of fibre present differs from one group of foods to another, fibre in cereals, for example, containing a much higher proportion of hemicelluloses than that in vegetables and fruit (see page 109 for the importance of cereal fibre).

Minerals

● Calcium

Primarily important because it makes bones and teeth hard and strong, calcium is also concerned with normal blood clotting, the transmission of nerve impulses and the digestion of milk in babies. Because it is instrumental in bone formation,

calcium needs are highest in childhood, but even in adult life there is a continual removal and replacement of bone calcium. Individuals differ considerably in the amount they absorb from food, so requirements vary from 500 mg to 800 mg per day for an adult woman. Both pregnant and lactating mothers require much more. Although milk and its products are the richest source, calcium occurs in smaller quantities in many other foods, such as fish eaten with their bones, bread, pulses and nuts.

Foods providing 200 mg calcium		
Cheese, hard	30 g	1 oz
Sardines	60 g	2 oz
Yogurt, low fat	120 g	4 oz
Milk	170 ml	6 floz
Bread, white	230 g	8 oz
Peanuts	340 g	12 oz
Cabbage, cooked	450 g	16 oz

Any serving of food that provides around 200 mg calcium will make a significant contribution to the daily needs.

● Iron

Iron forms part of the red pigment of blood, called haemoglobin, which carries oxygen from the lungs to the tissues and carbon dioxide, the waste product, in the opposite direction. Haemoglobin accounts for about half the total amount of iron in the body, the remainder being stored in various body tissues.

Iron requirements for healthy adult women are between 12 mg and 18 mg per day, and on average intakes reach these levels. But despite the presence of iron in many foods, some women still suffer from anaemia. Often this is caused by increased iron losses, due for example to heavy or prolonged periods, rather than to low iron intakes. In anaemia, haemoglobin levels are reduced, resulting in a general lack of vitality. However, many people have lower than normal haemoglobin levels without any other symptoms of anaemia, and iron supplements in the form of tablets or tonics have little or no effect in these cases. Iron supplements are, however, a cheap and effective way of treating genuine anaemia.

Foods providing 6 mg iron		
Liver	30 g	1 oz
Beef	120 g	4 oz
Eggs	2	–
Apricots	150 g	5 oz
Bread, wholewheat	210 g	7 oz
Peas, cooked	480 g	17 oz

Body stores regulate how much iron is absorbed from food – if they are low, absorption will improve, and vice versa.

● Other essential minerals

Sodium, potassium and chloride are so widely distributed in foods that it is impossible not to get enough. The balance between sodium and potassium is important in maintaining the internal environment of the body, particularly in the body fluids. Individual variations in sodium intake largely depend on the amount of salt (sodium chloride) added to food. Excessive salt intakes have been linked with high blood pressure.

Magnesium and phosphorus both have many essential functions, but again occur widely in foods, and deficiencies are rare. Magnesium deficiency can arise, but only from metabolic conditions that cause large magnesium losses, such as chronic diarrhoea or alcoholism.

Iodine is needed by the body as it forms part of the hormone thyroxine – secreted by the thyroid gland in the neck – which is important in the control of metabolic rate. Iodine intakes are generally adequate except in areas where water, soil, and therefore locally grown food have a low iodine content. Sea food is usually the richest dietary source of iodine.

Fluoride is generally found in water, although in varying content, and also in tea. It is needed to form hard enamel on teeth, thus greatly reducing the likelihood of dental decay, and as such it is particularly important for children.

Vitamins

● Vitamin A

Sometimes known by its chemical name of retinol, vitamin A occurs in food in two different forms – as retinol itself and as carotene, which the body is able to convert to retinol. The former is found in animal fats and the latter in green and yellow vegetables.

Vitamin A has many functions in the body, including maintaining the fine membranes that line all the body tubes, and as part of a pigment in the retina that enables the eyes to see in dim light. An adult woman needs about 750 to 800 µg of retinol a day, but because this vitamin is soluble in fat rather than water, it can be stored in the liver, which means that two or three meals a week that are rich in vitamin A are just as good as a smaller daily intake. In developed countries an excess of vitamin A is a more common problem than vitamin A deficiency, usually as a result of overdosage of concentrated vitamin preparations, such as halibut liver oil. Too much vitamin A is toxic and can even be fatal, so it is vital to follow prescribed doses exactly.

Foods providing 250–300 µg vitamin A – one third of daily needs		
Liver	7 g	$\frac{1}{4}$ oz
Butter	15 g	$\frac{1}{2}$ oz
Carrots, cooked	30 g	1 oz
Margarine	35 g	$1\frac{1}{4}$ oz
Eggs, large	1	
Cheese	75 g	$2\frac{1}{2}$ oz
Milk	415 ml	$\frac{3}{4}$ pt

Generally animal fats, and foods containing animal fats, provide over half the total intake of vitamin A, while vegetables provide around a quarter, mostly from carrots.

● B vitamins

What used to be called the 'vitamin B complex' has been broken down into three major B vitamins – B_1, B_2 and nicotinic acid – and a number of others, some of which are important in human nutrition and some of which are of rather obscure value.

The three major B vitamins play an important part in the metabolic process that releases energy from carbohydrate, so people who eat significantly more carbohydrate will also need more of these vitamins in order to utilize the energy properly. Fortunately, many foods that are rich in carbohydrate – such as cereals and bread – also contain some vitamin B_1, or thiamin as it is sometimes known, and it is also present in pork and its products, milk and vegetables. This fairly wide distribution of thiamin means that a varied diet is the best insurance against a deficiency, which is rare in well-nourished populations. Unlike vitamin A, thiamin is soluble in water and so cannot be stored; any excess to the body's needs is simply excreted in the urine. In an average diet the loss of thiamin during cooking is around 25 per cent – nevertheless intakes are still more than adequate to meet the body's needs.

Vitamin B_2, or riboflavin, is similarly present in a wide variety of commonly eaten foods, such as milk, white meat, liver and kidneys, cereals, eggs and vegetables. As with the other B vitamins, riboflavin is soluble in water and cannot be stored in the body. Some will be lost during cooking and it can also be destroyed by light (bottled milk standing on a doorstep in bright sunlight could lose 10 per cent of its riboflavin content every hour). A lack of riboflavin in the diet can cause lesions on the lips, tongue and skin, but a deficiency of this vitamin is extremely unlikely in any country where dairy products are regularly eaten.

The third major B vitamin concerned with the release of energy from carbohydrate is nicotinic acid, or niacin. Like vitamin A it is found in food in two different forms – as the vitamin itself and as an amino acid called tryptophan, which the body can convert to nicotinic acid. Meat, especially liver, is the most important source of this vitamin, which is less affected by heat and light than the other B vitamins – although there are some losses when chopped or minced foods are cooked in water. A normal varied diet easily provides sufficient nicotinic acid to meet an adult woman's daily needs, and deficiencies are virtually unknown in affluent countries.

Vitamin B_6, or pyridoxin, is involved in the metabolism of amino acids, so the amounts needed are linked to the proportion of protein in the diet. It is present in cereals, meat, milk and fish and there is little evidence of a deficiency ever occurring in humans. Folic acid plays a part in the prevention of anaemia and although it is present in a variety of foods, supplements of it are usually given during pregnancy to offset higher needs. Vitamin B_{12} is also concerned with the prevention

of anaemia and occurs only in foods of animal origin, so deficiencies can arise in people following strict vegetarian diets (see page 111).

Foods providing one third of daily needs of the major B vitamins		
Vitamin B_1: (0.3 mg)		
Nuts	30 g	1 oz
Pork (lean)	50 g	2 oz
Liver or kidney	120 g	4 oz
Bread, white	170 g	6 oz
Vitamin B_2: (0.5 mg)		
Liver	20 g	$\frac{3}{4}$ oz
Cheese	100 g	$3\frac{1}{2}$ oz
Eggs	2	
Milk	380 ml	13 fl oz
Nicotinic acid: (6 mg)		
Nuts	20 g	$\frac{3}{4}$ oz
Liver	60 g	2 oz
Meat, any kind	140 g	5 oz
Bread, white	140 g	5 oz

The most likely dietary sources of the major B vitamins are given here, but they are present in many foods and deficiencies are rare in developed countries.

● Vitamin C

Often known as ascorbic acid, its chemical name, this vitamin has received much publicity in recent years, mostly because of claims that regular large doses could prevent colds. Generally, any excess is lost in urine but there are some indications that taking massive doses (2–3 g per day) can cause kidney stones and affect bone metabolism. It seems probable that much of the benefit attributed to vitamin C is due to a placebo effect.

The normal nutritional function of vitamin C is in the formation and maintenance of the 'cement' substance that in effect sticks the cells of the body together. (The now rare deficiency disease, scurvy, is the result of this connective tissue breaking down.) It is also involved in hormone production and wound healing, but its precise role in these metabolic processes is not yet fully understood. Authorities disagree over how much vitamin C we need. One school of thought believes that body tissues should be 'saturated' with the vitamin, while another considers a lower level of intake quite adequate. Since both levels are well above that at which scurvy occurs, these arguments are of little practical value, and most people's daily intakes fall somewhere in between.

Vitamin C is less widely distributed in foods than, for example, the B vitamins, and fruits and vegetables are the only foods to make significant contributions to the total intake. Even here there is great variation in vitamin C content, as the table shows. Nevertheless moderate sources of vitamin C can be important to the overall diet if they are eaten regularly in sufficient quantity.

Vitamin C is soluble in water and losses during the preparation, cooking and storage of fruits and vegetables can be considerable, possibly resulting in low intakes. Root vegetables can lose up to 50 per cent and green vegetables up to 70 per cent of their original vitamin C content during cooking (see pages 106–107).

*Foods providing 25 mg vitamin C – over half a day's needs		
Blackcurrants	15 g	½ oz
Sprouts	25 g	1 oz
Mustard and cress	30 g	1 oz
Cabbage	40 g	1½ oz
Orange	50 g	2 oz
Grapefruit juice	60 g	2 oz
Melon	80 g	3 oz
Turnip, cooked	100 g	3½ oz
Peas	105 g	4 oz
Lettuce	180 g	6½ oz
Potatoes, cooked	225 g	8 oz
Banana	250 g	9 oz
* raw, unless stated otherwise		

In a standard diet potatoes can often provide up to a third of an average vitamin C intake, although authorities differ on the optimum level required.

● Vitamin D

This vitamin, now sometimes called cholecalciferol, differs from the others in that it can be made in the skin by the action of ultra-violet light, that is, sunlight, and so does not have to be eaten at all. The amount of vitamin D acquired in this way is extremely difficult to estimate, depending on the length of exposure and amount of melanin pigment in the skin. But it is probable that a white-skinned person can, with normal reasonable exposure of the face, arms and legs over the course of a year, meet their needs for vitamin D entirely, while a dark-skinned person who does not expose their skin, perhaps for religious or social reasons, will need an additional food source.

The function of vitamin D is to aid the absorption of calcium (and phosphorus) from food and to ensure that these minerals are used properly in bone formation. This means of course that it is especially important for babies and children, but it is also necessary for adults, as the mineral part of bone is constantly being renewed. A lack of vitamin D causes rickets in children and osteomalacia in adults. Both these diseases are happily much less common in well-nourished populations, but still occur where the diet is low in vitamin D and exposure to sunlight limited.

Vitamin D is a fat-soluble vitamin and is found naturally only in fatty fish, such as herrings, salmon, pilchards and sardines, and in eggs. In some countries it is also added to margarine by law and to baby milks and foods, as both butter and milk products are poor sources. Vitamin D can be stored in the liver, so a weekly serving of a food rich in it is generally adequate for adults if combined with some exposure to the sun.

● Other vitamins

Of other substances thought to have vitamin-like properties only vitamins E and K have much direct relevance to nutrition and health.

Vitamin E, or tocopherols, is certainly essential to man, although its exact function is not clear. Over the years it has been claimed as the miracle cure for almost everything, very largely without supporting scientific evidence. It is found in many foods and a deficiency is unknown in humans.

Vitamin K is vital to the blood-clotting mechanism. It is present in plant foods, but can also be manufactured by bacteria that are normally found in the human intestines, so exact needs are hard to estimate. A deficiency is rare, but occasionally occurs in new-born babies.

A Well-balanced Diet

A diet that is properly balanced not only provides the correct amount of essential nutrients, but matches the needs of the individual as well, both in nutritional requirements and in food preferences and eating habits. It is far from being a strict, monotonous regimen consisting of nothing apart from 'healthy' foods.

Interdependent nutrients

The components of food that are essential for health are part of an integrated system, a bit like a jigsaw, and one missing link can destroy the effectiveness of the whole system.

The body's major need is for energy, and normally we meet this need by eating a mixture of proteins, fats and carbohydrates. However, if insufficient energy is available for any reason, the body will attempt to rectify the situation by burning up food protein instead of using it for essential construction and repair. This does not matter if there is plenty of protein in the diet, but the consequences can be drastic if there is not, especially in children, whose protein needs are relatively high. It also highlights the importance of having adequate amounts of protein in slimming diets (see pages 122–123).

Some nutrients cannot be utilized efficiently without the presence of other, complementary, nutrients. For example, the energy available in carbohydrates cannot be properly released without the B vitamins (see pages 101–102) and the absorption of iron from food is greatly improved by vitamin C, which is why the two nutrients are often combined in iron preparations. This strong interdependence of nutrients means that taking extra amounts of one particular nutrient is more likely to be harmful than beneficial, because it unbalances the diet.

Individual variation

Great efforts have been made to work out exact figures for the nutrient needs of the so-called 'average' person. However, it is now becoming increasingly clear that such figures are accurate only when applied to large groups of people for whom an average figure is probably fairly representative, and that individual needs can vary above and below these averages. In the case of energy requirements, for instance, this variation can be as much as twofold for comparable people. Even when we exclude variables such as work and exercise and simply compare basal metabolic rates (see pages 96–97), there are still large variations. Such differences may affect our lives more than we think – the skinny person who eats enormous quantities without increasing weight probably has high energy requirements, and some overweight people, who are classically portrayed as gluttons, genuinely need less food than average. The moral of all this is that it is impossible to assess a diet purely on the quantities of nutrients it provides – the state of health of the person eating it must also be considered.

General principles

One factor that can be of great help in the matter of staying healthy is the body's ability to adapt, within reasonable limits, to variations in the quality and quantity of the diet, and to short-term changes in the need for food.

The body responds to a shortage of food energy by using what energy it does get more efficiently, and this is one reason why weight losses get slower and slower on long-term slimming diets. In a similar fashion the body reacts to shortages of several nutrients by absorbing a higher proportion of these from food, and by a more economical use of what is available. The same thing happens if the body's requirement for a particular nutrient increases for any reason – for example, more protein, calcium and iron are necessary during pregnancy. Such extra needs are partly met by better absorption and utilization, so that only small changes have to be made in the actual diet in order to achieve good nutrition.

This ability we have to adapt to different diets without detriment to our health makes it possible to outline general principles that are the basis of a well-balanced diet for anyone. The first principle is to eat as wide a variety of foods as possible, because this will ensure that any nutrient deficiencies of one particular food will be cancelled out by the relative excesses of others. Remember that no single food can provide completely adequate nutrition. The second principle is embodied in that old saying 'all things in moderation'. Although we tend to think of many foods in terms of 'good' or 'bad', these labels can be misleading. For example, a 'good' food such as milk if drunk in excessive amounts would effectively become 'bad', while 'bad' foods, such as those containing high levels of sugar or fat, are harmless, or even beneficial, when eaten in small quantities.

The food group system

Nutritional theory can be a rather daunting subject, but fortunately it is possible to combine general principles and theory into a practical system that anyone can use as an easy guide to choosing their everyday diet, and this is known as the food group system.

In this system foods are grouped together according to their nutritional content to form five main groups (see chart). Although these groups are distinct there is considerable overlap, which is an additional insurance against any deficiencies.

The simple measure of eating at least one portion of food from each group, every day, is sufficient to ensure that the basic diet is well-balanced.

Even within a food group there can be considerable variation in nutritional value, and where these differences are relevant they have been noted in the righthand column of the chart. This system is also extremely useful for people who need to exclude a particular food from their diet. For example, vegetarians who exclude meat and fish can see at a glance that the same range of nutrients is provided by groups II and III, so that they can substitute these without any loss of nutritional value.

The sizes of portions indicated are a minimum and the average person will obviously need more food to satisfy her requirements – this can be chosen from any group, according to personal taste, once a daily portion from each has been eaten.

Food groups

Group	Foods	Minimum daily portion for an adult	Main nutrients provided	Points to note
I	Meat of all kinds, poultry, liver and kidneys, white and fatty fish, shellfish, eggs	90 g (3 oz) meat or 2 eggs or 120 g (4 oz) fish	Protein, energy, fat, iron, vitamins B_1, B_2, nicotinic acid	Liver and kidneys are much richer in iron, vitamins B_1, B_2 and a good source of vitamin A. Fatty fish and eggs are also good sources of vitamin D.
II	Milk, cheese, cream and yogurt	300 ml ($\frac{1}{2}$ pt) milk or 60 g (2 oz) cheese	Protein, energy, fat, calcium, vitamins A, B_2	Cream and cream cheese are low in protein and very high in energy.
III	Cereal, bread, flour, breakfast cereals, pasta, rice, peas, beans and pulses, nuts	4 slices bread or 120 g (4 oz) nuts or 230 g (8 oz) cooked pasta	Energy, protein, carbohydrate, calcium, iron, vitamins B_1, B_2, nicotinic acid	Wholegrain cereals also provide roughage. Cereal-based foods made with sugar and fat, such as cakes, pastries and biscuits, have high-energy and low-nutrient content.
IV	Butter, margarine, cooking fats and oils	30 g (1 oz) butter or margarine	Energy, fat, vitamins A and D	Margarine is a richer source of vitamin D than butter. Cooking fats and oils contain few vitamins.
V	Fruit and vegetables of all kinds	1 orange or 120 g (4 oz) cooked green vegetable	Iron, vitamins A, B_1, C	Raw or lightly cooked fruit or vegetables also provide roughage. Citrus fruits, berries, currants and green vegetables are richest in vitamin C.

Eating Habits

Meal patterns

It may be surprising to find that not only *what* you eat, but also *when* and *how* you eat it, can have a marked effect on how your body deals with food and ultimately on fitness and health. Over the last 20 or 30 years there have been slow but steady changes in meal-eating patterns in many developed countries, the trend being away from substantial breakfasts and main meals at midday and towards very light convenient breakfasts, 'snack' lunches and a main meal eaten fairly late in the evening – due in large part to the fact that more and more women go out to work. Such changes may seem fairly trivial but the effects are noticeable. Eating a large meal in the evening encourages more food energy to be converted to fat (because less exercise is taken at this time of day), while small or non-existent breakfasts are known to reduce working efficiency in adults and to affect school performance in children. Snack lunches encourage the consumption of high-energy, low-nutrient foods, simply because they are convenient, rather than nutritious.

Many studies have been made of the differences between people who eat small, more frequent meals ('nibblers') and those who eat fewer, larger meals ('meal-eaters') and it is generally agreed that meal-eaters invariably have more body fat than nibblers. Some slimmers find that a diet designed on a nibbling pattern helps to avoid hunger pangs and there is evidence that it may speed up weight loss. Certainly most digestive systems, and particularly those that suffer disorders such as ulcers or indigestion, prefer a nibbling pattern, and eating 'little and often' is a recognized measure to combat nausea in pregnancy.

Many of the vital body functions follow a definite pattern of changes over a 24-hour cycle, including the metabolism of food. Although this is still an area of research, there is interesting evidence that food energy consumed during the first half of the day is used *less* efficiently than that eaten in the second half, which again explains why a late, large evening meal encourages the accumulation of extra fat in the body, since the excess energy is stored rather than lost as heat.

Of course, the way in which we eat food, and at what times, is, to some extent, governed by the many other demands of our lives, but on health grounds alone there is good reason for regulating eating habits. Small changes, such as beginning the day with a nourishing breakfast and avoiding high-energy, low-nutrient snack foods and drinks, will not result in any immediate improvement in health, but they are a long-term insurance policy from which you will benefit later in life.

Nutrient losses and cooking for health

Although perhaps achieving gastronomic delights, even the most imaginative cook can do little to improve the nutritional value of poor foods. But cooking has such a profound effect on the appearance, taste, texture and palatability of our meals, as well as on their nutritional value, that it is in consequence of incalculable importance to the overall quality of the diet. A meal with high nutrient content has no value whatsoever if rejected as totally inedible.

The major food constituents – protein, fat and carbohydrate – and fat-soluble vitamins A and D are relatively unaffected by cooking. But some loss of nutrients is inevitable, particularly of the water-soluble vitamins (see pages 102–103). As the table shows, a certain amount of these vitamins is lost however food is cooked – especially from vegetables, which are prone to losses of vitamin C – but some methods, including prolonged boiling, will increase such wastage considerably. The figures look frightening, but it is comforting to know that in fact most normal diets still provide adequate amounts of vitamins even after cooking – although it is well worth remembering these commonsense procedures:

- do not finely chop foods and allow to soak for a long time before cooking.
- use a minimal amount of water in boiling.
- do not cook for longer than necessary (pressure cookers and microwave ovens reduce cooking time and the former are particularly good for preserving the nutrient content of vegetables).
- do not keep food hot or warm for a long time before serving.
- try to include raw fruit and vegetables in the diet.

Apart from loss of nutrients, cooking methods can play an important part in other ways in long-term good health and weight control. For example, grilling, baking or poaching rather than

Percentage of vitamins lost during cooking	Vit B₁	Vit B₂	Nicotinic acid	Vit C
Cereals: boiled	40	40	40	–
baked	25	15	5	–
Eggs: boiled	10	5	–	–
fried	20	10	–	–
Fish: poached	10	–	10	–
fried	20	20	20	–
Meat: roast/grilled	20	20	20	20*
stewed	60	30	50	
Milk: boiled	–	10	–	30–70
Vegetables, leaf: boiled	40	40	40	70
Vegetables, root: boiled	25	30	30	40

* for liver only

The figures for nutrient losses are averages; actual losses depend on variable factors such as the volume of water used, cooking time and whether the food is finely chopped or cooked whole – the finer it is chopped, the greater the exposure to oxidation and the greater the loss of nutrients during cooking.

frying can markedly reduce your fat intake, especially with foods such as onions, mushrooms, potatoes and bread, which soak up enormous quantities of fat when fried. Or try cuisine minceur cookery with its emphasis on dishes that are low in calories and cholesterol but high in appeal and palatability.

Adding sugar in cooking may be hazardous to both health and figure. Artificial sweeteners such as saccharin are helpful, but on the whole it is better to try to wean yourself from sweet tastes altogether. In most recipes it is possible to reduce the sugar content by at least half without changing the nature of the dish. If you go about it gradually, you will find that you quickly become accustomed to 'sharper' flavours.

Modern food technology

Today a great many of the foods we eat have been preserved by such methods as canning, drying, freezing or accelerated freeze-drying, and with the help of food technology and additives reach us in an entirely wholesome state. Canning and dehydration tend to result in some loss of nutrients, but very often preservation improves the nutritional quality of a food. For example, when peas are picked in the pod, sent to wholesale markets and then to retail shops, vitamin C losses can be very high, whereas peas that have been frozen within two or three hours of being picked have a much higher vitamin C content when they reach the dinner table. As always, the best safeguard is not to rely entirely on manufactured or processed foods, but to strike a compromise between convenience and freshness.

● Novel protein foods

Much research effort has been expended in the search for new protein-rich foods, with three main aims in mind: the need for new infant foods to prevent malnutrition in developing countries; the need to produce cheaper protein concentrates for animal feeding; and the need to provide a cheap but acceptable alternative to meat.

Protein can be extracted from plankton, algae and leaves, all of which contain too much indigestible matter to be part of the human diet in their natural state. So far none of these has proved successful on a commercial scale. Micro-organisms such as yeasts and bacteria are a more useful source of protein and have produced concentrates suitable for animal feedstuffs, but not yet protein foods of a high enough standard for humans. The most useful sources of man-made protein are oil seeds and legumes, notably the soya bean and the field bean. The protein content of these can be extracted, textured or spun and then flavoured so that it resembles meat. The resulting products are sold under various names, but are collectively known as textured vegetable protein (TVP). Such proteins are now frequently incorporated in manufactured meat products and used for large-scale catering, as in school meal programmes, as well as being increasingly available to domestic consumers.

Since meat provides significant amounts of several nutrients, such as iron and B vitamins, it is reasonable to expect that a meat substitute should also contain these and national and international food agencies are currently very much concerned with establishing consistent high standards for novel protein foods.

Food Problems and Problem Foods

Food is a necessity of life, but it is not entirely problem-free. At one end of the food/man equation are thousands of foods, all containing many different substances, quite apart from essential nutrients. At the other end are millions of individuals each with a unique genetic make-up, which is reflected in their metabolism. So it is hardly surprising that some foods may cause some people problems, either because of something in the food itself, or because of that person's particular physiology.

Food hygiene

Food poisoning attacks rarely reach the news unless they are fatal or affect large numbers of people, yet they occur all too frequently – around 20,000 cases per year in the U.S.A. and 10,000 in the U.K. The symptoms can vary from mild discomfort to serious illness, depending on the type of bacteria involved. These harmful bacteria may be present in the raw food, or introduced during manufacture or preservation, or while the food is being prepared for consumption. The following are some common mistakes that can easily be responsible for food poisoning in the home:

• failing to keep raw and cooked foods separate, during storage or preparation.
• inadequate thawing of frozen foods, so that cooking is incomplete.
• leaving food at warm temperatures, which encourage micro-organisms to multiply.
• allowing food to be contaminated by dirty hands, flies or rodents.

Food allergy

'Allergy' means an abnormal reaction of body tissue after contact with a foreign substance, or 'allergen'. In the case of food allergies, the allergen reaches the tissues via the bloodstream after being absorbed from the digestive system. The resulting allergic reaction is basically an immunological response, which damages cells, releasing histamine and other substances that cause the symptoms of the allergy.

Food allergies are generally more common in children and frequently involve eggs, wheat or cow's milk. For example, coeliac disease has now been identified as an allergy to a wheat protein, gluten. Fortunately many childhood food allergies disappear spontaneously, and until quite recently the subject of food allergy in adults received scant attention. But trends are changing and new interest in the subject has resulted in speculations that food allergy may in fact be responsible for a wide range of diseases – physical and mental.

Allergic reactions range from the trivial to the potentially fatal and may occur within a few minutes of contact with the allergen or not for several hours or even days. Diagnosing a food allergy accurately requires careful and painstaking assessment. The most usual method is to put the patient on an 'exclusion diet', which is designed to cut out potential allergens, such as meat, eggs, milk, and canned, dried or frozen foods. The patient's reactions to this neutral diet are carefully monitored, and if there is no initial allergic response, then the likely food allergens are added to it one at a time until the rogue food is detected. Skin tests with injections of suspect foods to see if they provoke an abnormal reaction are another way of diagnosing food allergies.

If you suspect that you are allergic to a particular food, you can certainly make preliminary investigations yourself by excluding it from your diet and keeping a careful record of your food intake and reactions. However, if the symptoms are at all severe it is wise to consult a doctor, since the cause may not be a food allergy or may require special medical treatment or dietary advice.

Common food allergens and their effects		
Allergen	System affected	Allergic reaction
Gluten Milk	digestive	e.g. coeliac disease, diarrhoea
Gluten	skin	e.g. eczema
Milk	respiratory	e.g. asthma
Chocolate	central nervous	e.g. migraine, behavioural problems

Food allergens affect other body systems apart from the digestion, which may complicate diagnosis whether by skin tests or by an 'exclusion diet'.

Diet and migraine

Migraine appears to be caused by certain changes in the arteries carrying blood inside and outside the skull, but what exactly produces these changes is not clear. They may possibly be due to a build-up of histamine-like substances, which can occur after an emotional upset, or perhaps as part of an allergic reaction to a food. It is not uncommon for sufferers to find that their migraine attacks appear after eating one, or several, specific foods. Chocolate, cheese and alcoholic drinks, especially sherry and red wine, are often implicated and are known to contain substances that can affect the arteries in the head. Food is by no means the only cause of migraines, but it is useful to keep a daily record of what you eat, as this may help to identify the cause. Mild attacks can be helped by the stimulant properties of caffeine in coffee.

Drugs and nutrition

Drugs are substances that alter the body chemistry in some way and are generally taken to relieve symptoms or to encourage natural body processes. The dividing line between the effects of drugs and nutrients is small and the body metabolizes both in exactly the same way – breaking them down into smaller chemical units, which can be used or eliminated. Not surprisingly, there is considerable interaction between food and drug metabolism. For example, cheese generally contains a substance called tyramine, which is known to increase blood pressure. This is normally destroyed quickly by enzymes called monoamine oxidases (MAO); however, a certain group of drugs used for treating depression prevents MAO from destroying the tyramine, with the result that blood pressure rises, causing headache, nausea and dizziness and possibly other dangerous side-effects. Patients using these drugs are therefore instructed to avoid foods containing tyramine. This is a rather extreme example, but if your doctor is prescribing drugs for you, always tell him if you are on a special diet, and follow any dietary instructions relating to the course meticulously.

Digestive problems and dietary fibre

The popular idea that a daily bowel movement is essential for health is misleading. In fact it is perfectly normal and healthy to defaecate only every two or three days. Genuine constipation affects sedentary people, those taking drugs and often pregnant women as well. The effects tend to be exaggerated and it does not cause serious illness (although it can be a symptom of one), but it does cause headaches, abdominal discomfort and a general lack of well-being. Including fibre in the diet (see page 100), taking adequate daily exercise and drinking plenty of water are helpful. Purgatives are necessary only in extreme cases.

Cereal fibre is now thought to be more effective than that from other plants in the prevention and treatment of digestive disorders, such as dyspepsia and diverticulosis (a disorder of the large bowel). This has resulted in an enormous upsurge of interest in bran, which is the outer coating of wheat grains containing the fibre. Since wholewheat flour and bread contain all the bran portion of wheat, as do bran-containing or wholegrain breakfast cereals, pasta and baked goods, increasing fibre intake is relatively simple.

Saturated fats and cholesterol

A high intake of fat in the diet is known to be harmful in several ways – it causes overweight and therefore a predisposition to heart disease, and, more specifically, it can be responsible for atherosclerosis, the gradual thickening of the arteries.

Animal fats contain a high proportion of saturated fatty acids (recognizable because they are mostly solid at room temperature – butter, for example). In chemical terms, these contain more hydrogen than unsaturated fats (mono- or poly-), which predominate in vegetable oils and are liquid at room temperature. Saturated fats (and also sugar) increase fat levels in the blood, whereas it is thought that unsaturated fats (and particularly polyunsaturated ones) tend not to do this because they are chemically different from body fat and follow different metabolic paths.

Cholesterol (see page 99) has recently been strongly linked with atherosclerosis, but as many dietary factors other than cholesterol can alter blood cholesterol levels, it may in fact be less important than previously thought. A diet that is low in saturated fat will also be low in cholesterol, and vice versa.

Healthfoods, Wholefoods and Vegetarianism

Natural and organically grown foods

The term 'natural' is hard to define, since nearly all foods have been natural at some stage, but it is generally taken to mean food that has been grown without the aid of pesticides, herbicides or fungicides, has not been 'processed' or preserved and that does not contain additives. However, it is a description commonly misused by food manufacturers and advertisers, who, for example, on the one hand claim that butter is natural (although it has been processed from milk, blended, and salt added), and on the other that margarine has been made from natural ingredients, despite the fact that they have been altered chemically and physically. It is right that the consumer should have a choice, but for those who cannot afford or do not wish to buy 'natural' foods it is still perfectly possible to have a healthy and nutritionally balanced diet without them.

'Organically' grown foods are highly valued by those who believe that the use of animal or plant manure produces nutritionally superior food crops and that other fertilizers are detrimental. While there is no doubt that organic material is a valuable aid to agriculture, there is no evidence that organically grown foods have greater nutritional value or even that they taste any better. Like 'natural' foods, they are expensive because of low yield and high production costs. In recent years, too, there has been a disturbing number of instances of dishonest labelling.

Wholefoods

As the name implies, these are foods that have not been put through any refining process, which inevitably removes some part of the nutritional content. Wholegrain cereals have long been prized by healthfood enthusiasts as a source of roughage and their claims are now supported by an ever-increasing weight of scientific evidence as to the value of dietary fibre (see pages 100, 109). The vitamin and mineral content of such cereals is marginally higher than that of refined cereals, but less may be absorbed owing to the presence of other substances, so in practice the additional amounts are hardly significant. Foods such as brown sugar are often misleadingly regarded as wholefoods, although this has already undergone nearly as much refining as white sugar. If the concept of wholefoods were taken to a logical extreme, all fruit and vegetables should be eaten with their peel and skins.

Vitamin pills, herbal and 'magic' remedies

Many healthfood advocates believe that it is impossible to get enough of all the essential nutrients from a 'modern' diet, despite clear evidence to the contrary. There is also a widespread idea that chemically manufactured, or 'synthetic', vitamins are of little nutritional value and that only 'natural' vitamins obtained from food sources are useful, despite the fact that these have also been extracted and purified. In fact there is no difference between the two, either in chemical structure or in the way in which the body uses them. It is likely that vitamin pills and tonics have a placebo effect, so their efficiency is exceedingly hard to prove one way or the other.

There is currently an enormous range of herbal remedies and pills of simple inorganic salts on the market, which between them have probably claimed to cure just about every ailment known to mankind. There are various arguments against the self-administration of these so-called cures, the main one being that they may delay, or even prevent, a person taking proper medical advice. Other points to bear in mind are that common substances such as salt, sand and plaster of Paris are marketed under unusual names and at vastly inflated prices; the over-zealous use of herbal remedies can give rise to medical problems; and drug-active substances are found only at very low levels in plants, so extraction and concentration is necessary before they are of use pharmaceutically.

Perhaps the least helpful of all healthfoods are those that have become associated with magical health-giving properties. Included in the group are honey, cider vinegar, yogurt, molasses, garlic, ginseng and buckwheat. Usually such foods are promoted on the premise that because they conferred special health attributes on one population, they will do the same for another. Yogurt is a good example here – it was reputed to be responsible for the longevity of Bulgarian peasants and so was marketed in Western Europe and America as promoting long life. Honey has been attributed magical properties for centuries, despite the fact that it is only sugar (glucose and fructose) and water. Cider vinegar has been claimed to melt away unwanted body fat (with the aid of a diet) and the newest recruit, ginseng, is currently gaining ground as the elixir of life. However, apart from undoubted placebo effects, nutritionally such foods do nothing for health that cannot be attained by a well-balanced diet.

Vegetarian diets

A vegetarian diet is usually thought of as one that excludes the flesh of animals, but in fact there is a range of vegetarian regimens:
- an ovo-lacto-vegetarian diet excludes meat and fish, but allows dairy products and eggs.
- a lacto-vegetarian diet excludes meat, fish and eggs, but allows dairy products.
- a pure vegetarian diet excludes *all* animal products, including dairy products and animal fats, and foods containing them. Vegans, as they are called, also reject leather and wool.

The nutritional quality of a vegetarian diet obviously depends on the degree of variety allowed. Thus it is much easier for an ovo-lacto-vegetarian to get adequate nutrition than it is for a vegan. Nevertheless, as studies of diets and the state of health of vegetarians confirm, it is perfectly possible for all types of vegetarians to obtain the nutrients they require.

The most obvious consequence is that protein must be derived from foods other than meat and fish. If milk, cheese and eggs are allowed, then this is fairly easy – if not, cereals, nuts, peas, beans, pulses and other vegetables become the major protein sources. To these can be added a range of soya bean products, including soya flour, soya milk and meats – analogues made from soya protein (textured vegetable protein, or TVP, see page 107).

Milk is by far the best source of calcium and excluding it may result in a calcium deficiency, especially among children and pregnant and lactating mothers, whose needs are high. But green vegetables, peas and beans all contain significant amounts, and in some countries cereal foods such as bread and flour are fortified with extra calcium to ensure a reasonable intake.

Vitamin D occurs in relatively few foods (eggs, liver, margarine and fatty fish) and if all these are eliminated from the diet, there may be a problem.

Vegetarian protein sources		
	Protein content	
	g/100g	g/oz
Soya flour, low fat	45.3	12.9
Cheese, hard	26.0	7.4
Peanuts	24.3	6.8
Peanut butter	22.6	6.4
Textured vegetable protein	17.0	4.8
Almonds	16.9	4.8
Cheese, cottage	13.6	3.9
Oatmeal, dry	12.4	3.5
Eggs	12.3	3.5
Brazil nuts	12.0	3.4
Walnuts	10.6	3.0
Bread, wholewheat	8.8	2.5
white	7.8	2.2
Lentils, boiled	7.6	2.2
Cob or hazel nuts	7.6	2.2
Butter beans, boiled	7.1	2.0
Baked beans	5.1	1.4
Peas, boiled	5.0	1.4
Spaghetti or macaroni, boiled	4.2	1.2
Sweetcorn, kernels	4.1	1.2
Soya milk	3.4	1.0
Milk	3.3	0.9
Rice, boiled	2.2	0.6
Chestnuts	2.0	0.6
Potatoes, boiled	1.4	0.4

Even if dairy products and eggs are excluded from the diet, a mixture of cereal and vegetable proteins can be just as valuable in quality as proteins that are derived from animal foods.

Average exposure to sunlight normally satisfies requirements, but in its absence the use of a vitamin preparation is sensible.

Similarly, meat and milk provide vitamin B_2 (riboflavin); without these the vitamin has to be obtained from green leafy vegetables, peas, beans and wholegrain cereals and bread. In vegan diets vitamin B_{12} will certainly be insufficient and may possibly result in a form of anaemia and even nerve damage. An acceptable synthetic form of vitamin B_{12} can be taken regularly by vegans to avoid the possibility of a deficiency.

A Rational Approach to Slimming

We tend to think of malnutrition in terms of lack of food, but strictly speaking it should apply to overeating too, for this is potentially just as serious. Overweight is primarily a disease of affluence, indeed in poor countries being fat is regarded as a sign of wealth, even to the point of being deliberately sought after. The current fashion in developed countries, however, is for slimness and people go to great lengths in pursuit of this ideal.

Being overweight means that the body has accumulated more fat (stored energy) than normal. If this extra fat becomes excessive – and it can double the body weight – the condition is known as obesity and poses a serious risk to health. Obesity always starts as a mild degree of overweight, so it makes sense to take action early. Prevention is, of course, far easier than cure, and the best means of prevention is a long-term policy of weight control, adjusted to your individual needs. In order to evolve such a policy and to be able to evaluate the many different types of slimming diets and 'cures' on offer, it is first important to be aware of and understand both the causes and effects of overweight.

The problem of overweight

It is hard to give exact figures about the incidence of overweight because investigators often use different standards in their assessments. However, usually 10 per cent or more above the ideal-weight range (see table) is considered to be overweight, while 20 per cent or more above ideal indicates obesity. On this basis there seems little doubt that around half the adult population of North America and Britain, for instance, are overweight, and that a sizeable proportion of these are obese. For both men and women, the incidence of overweight tends to increase with age, but at most ages more women are overweight than men.

The causes

Genetics, environment, metabolism, lifestyle and psychology are all involved in the complex problems of overweight and obesity. The respective role played by each of these factors almost certainly varies from one individual to another. However, in *all* cases it is true that in order to accumulate excess fat the energy consumed as

Percentage incidence of overweight among women		
Age group	10%+	20%+
U.S.A. and Canada		
20–29	23	12
30–39	41	25
40–49	59	40
50–59	67	46
60–69	68	45
London, U.K.		
15–29	16	8
30–49	33	17
50–65	50	32

Studies of overweight tend to be localized, but available figures suggest that in developed countries half of all women are overweight and about a third are obese.

food must exceed the energy that the body uses up. This does not mean that all fat people are gluttons – some people do undoubtedly overeat, but others just seem to need less food than average and are unable to burn off excesses.

The energy balance equation		
ACCUMULATION OF BODY FAT =	FOOD ENERGY INTAKE	– ENERGY USED BY BODY

When energy intake is higher than energy output, for whatever reasons, excess fat is stored. Conversely when energy intake is less than output, body fat is burnt up – which is the fundamental prerequisite of any successful slimming diet.

The part played by genetics is hard to assess because it is impossible to separate the effects of heredity from environmental factors. Children of overweight parents are certainly more likely to become overweight than children of slim parents, but it is difficult to judge whether this is because they have inherited a tendency to accumulate fat or simply learnt bad eating habits. Lifestyle is important too, because it determines the level of social eating and drinking and the amount of physical activity undertaken. Boredom, anxiety or depression are also reasons for overeating, as they cause some people to turn to food for consolation. The resultant weight gain may then worsen the psychological outlook, leading to further 'comfort eating'.

The effects

A mild degree of overweight has little effect, other than the inconvenience of one's clothes no longer fitting and perhaps a general feeling of being unfit. The more serious effects start to appear at a weight of 10 per cent or more above the ideal. It is now well-accepted that at this level of overweight you stand a much greater chance of suffering from high blood pressure, heart disease, diabetes, back trouble, respiratory infections and even from an increased number of accidents. These varied health risks inevitably express themselves in higher mortality rates for over-weight people – although obesity is rarely designated as the cause of death.

For most people, however, appearance and self-confidence are probably more compelling reasons than health alone for avoiding, or getting rid of, excess weight. Marked obesity is as much a psychological as a physiological strain, the effects of which can severely hamper efforts to lose weight and stay slim, however pronounced the desire may seem to be.

Your ideal weight

If you are honest with yourself it is a simple enough matter to detect overweight. A regular weight check is an obvious measure and clothes are quick to indicate the presence of excess fat in the middle regions. It is much harder, however, to decide what your ideal weight *should* be and therefore how much you need to lose. If you have only recently gained weight, then obviously it makes sense to aim for what you were before. But if you have suffered from overweight for a longer period, you will probably need some additional guidance. Such help comes in the form of weight tables, which indicate the ideal weight, or weight range, for people of different heights. The only disadvantage of these tables is that they are based on life-expectancy statistics compiled by in-surance companies and so indicate the best weight for survival rather than the weight that is best for healthy living and a good figure. Nevertheless, ideal-weight tables are the most useful guide currently available, if used sensibly.

You will probably find that some tables give ideal weights for different body frame sizes, but as there is no accurate way of deciding what frame size you are this can be misleading. When slimming, do not feel compelled to aim for an exact weight, as it is very much up to you to decide what weight you can maintain with reasonable ease, and at which you are happy with your shape and appearance. If you have a lot of excess weight to lose, you will probably find it more encouraging to set an intermediate target to achieve, and then to assess the next target weight when you have reached it.

Weight guide for women			
Height without shoes		Ideal-weight range (without clothes)	
cm	ft in	kg	lb
147	4 10	42–51	92–112
150	4 11	43–53	95–116
152	5 0	44–54	97–119
155	5 1	45–55	100–122
157	5 2	47–57	103–126
160	5 3	48–59	106–130
162	5 4	50–62	110–135
165	5 5	51–63	114–139
167	5 6	53–65	117–144
170	5 7	56–67	121–148
172	5 8	57–69	125–152
175	5 9	58–71	128–157
177	5 10	60–73	132–161
180	5 11	62–74	136–165
182	6 0	63–75	139–170

These guides cover most body frame sizes; if you are within the range shown for your height you will be near your personal ideal weight.

Diet versus exercise

To reduce the amount of energy stored in the body as fat we have to eat less energy, in the form of food, than the body uses up. Any slimming regime that claims to be able to reduce weight without doing this should be regarded cautiously, because it is either misleading or dangerous.

Losing weight can be achieved in three ways – by cutting down the amount of food consumed, by increasing the body's energy needs by extra activity, or, of course, by a combination of both approaches, in which case neither remedy needs to be quite so drastic.

For an overweight woman whose normal energy needs are 2000 kcals per day, even a fairly generous diet of 1500 kcals per day creates an energy deficit of 500 kcals per day, or 3500 kcals per week, which is equivalent, in energy terms, to 450 g (1 lb) of body fat. Her weight loss a week would therefore be around 450 g (1 lb), but probably more as she would also lose some fluid with the fat – and this on a generous diet. To achieve the same sort of weight loss by extra exercise alone would require an enormous physical effort – as much as an hour or more a day of sustained activity such as squash, or up to an hour and a half of something less strenuous such as swimming or tennis. Obviously this is beyond the capabilities of all but the super-fit, and in any case would be too time-consuming for most people.

Dieting is by far the most popular way of losing weight, because it gives the best results for the least time and inconvenience. Nevertheless, exercise can be an extremely useful part of a slimming campaign, as long as you are prepared to stick to a regular regime over a slightly longer period. For example, half an hour's brisk walk every day would use an additional 150–175 kcals per day, or over 1000 kcals per week. In three to four weeks this would add up to the energy equivalent of 450 g (1 lb) of fat, which may not seem much until you think that in the course of a whole year it would be equivalent to about 6.5 kg (14 lb), providing, of course, that you do not step up your food intake meanwhile.

The pattern of weight loss
If you are about to embark on a serious slimming campaign it is most important to understand the physiology of weight loss, the possible side-effects and to have realistic expectations of how much weight you are likely to lose and how quickly.

The first week on a diet can be a shock to the body, and it is quite common for women to experience losses of as much as 3 kg (7 lb) or more, even on fairly generous diets. But by no means all of this is fat – much of it is carbohydrate (stored in the form of glycogen in the liver and muscles). When energy intake falls below the body's needs, glycogen is the first reserve of energy called on. Quite a lot of water is associated with it, which also accounts for a significant part of the weight loss. After this initial large and encouraging drop, the weekly loss normally settles to about 0.5–1 kg (1–2 lb), although obviously it will vary depending on the degree of overweight, previous level of food intake, strictness of the diet and amount of physical activity. In practice weight losses are often less than estimated, because the slimmer has difficulty in following the diet accurately; they may also be irregular, as a result of fluid retention just before menstruation (see opposite) and the loss of fluid afterwards.

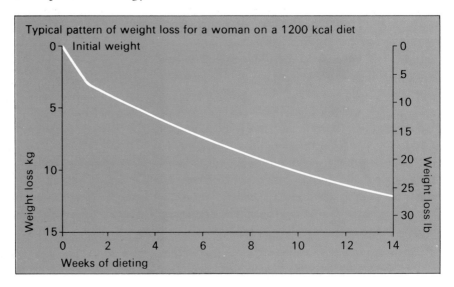

Weight loss during the first week of a diet is often dramatic, but then settles down to a more gradual rate.

After several months of successful slimming, it is a common experience to reach a 'plateau' – partly because the body has adapted to its enforced low-energy intake by becoming more economical, but also because even the most dedicated slimmer can tire of dieting and have simply failed to follow the diet to the letter. The problem is usually resolved by changing to a stricter diet, or else by having a short period of weight maintenance before restarting the diet. This latter course is especially helpful for very overweight slimmers, who may have to diet for up to a year in order to reach a reasonable weight.

When slimming, it is important to remember that the weight rarely, if ever, comes off evenly from all parts of the body – a fact that may cause unnecessary distress if figure proportions seem to change drastically. Perversely, the areas less prone to weight gains lose fat first, while the more vulnerable areas are the last to go. So a woman with a small bust that never increases very much when she puts on weight is likely to find that it appears to shrink alarmingly when she first starts to lose. Fortunately, as slimming progresses weight also comes off other areas and body proportions return to normal. Similarly, a woman with heavy hips and thighs will probably find that these slim down only as the last bit of excess weight is shed.

Changes in fluid balance and in glycogen stores can alter body weight by as much as 1 or 2 kg (2-4 lb) in the course of a single day, while premenstrual fluid retention may cause increases of up to 3 kg (7 lb) or even, in rare cases, double that. For these reasons it is misleading, and probably discouraging, to weigh yourself every day – once a week is generally sufficient. The morning is best, preferably after going to the lavatory and before breakfast. Always use the same scales, and if for any reason you choose some other time of day, try to wear clothes of similar weight on each occasion.

Choosing the right diet

Because weight problems can be caused by an infinite variety of factors and are different for each individual, it is hardly reasonable to expect a single diet to be the solution for every overweight person. Furthermore, we all have our own food preferences, eating habits and lifestyle, so what might be an ideal and convenient slimming diet for one woman could be impossibly rigid for another.

Every year, literally thousands of diets are published. The critical factor that determines whether or not you succeed on any one of them is how accurately you can adhere to the limitations it imposes. Here are some points to bear in mind:

• is it too strict? You cannot expect to work or run a home on much less than 1000 kcals a day. Most slimmers lose well on up to 1500 kcals.

• is it flexible? This is essential in a good diet, as few people lead lives so well-organized that they can stick rigidly to day-by-day menus for any great length of time.

• are the permitted foods acceptable to you? Do not choose a diet that suggests eating a lot of something you do not like or rarely eat.

• does it allow small indulgences? Many people find it easier to have a small daily allowance of, say, sweets or drinks, rather than stretching their willpower to the limits by excluding them completely.

• will it fit in with family catering? This is an obvious requirement for many female slimmers.

• is it well-balanced nutritionally? You can check this with the food group chart on page 105.

• is it too expensive? Any diet that demands smoked salmon and best steak will quickly ruin most family budgets.

Weight maintenance

Many people who diet lose weight successfully, but then in the following months gradually slip back to their former state. A good slimming diet therefore has to fulfil a number of functions – it must obviously promote a steady weight loss, but in addition it must re-educate eating habits, so that even when there is no longer a need to diet actively, there is no return to the old patterns of eating that caused overweight in the first place.

Evolving a method of weight maintenance that suits you is an essential part of any slimming campaign. When you have reached a weight (and shape) with which you are satisfied, step up food intake a little at a time, until you reach a normal diet at which you can maintain your weight. As body weight fluctuates for natural reasons, it is sensible to aim to keep your weight below an upper limit that allows for daily and monthly changes, rather than trying to stick to a specific weight. Some women find that dieting one or two days a week helps in weight control, while others prefer to eat fairly freely, resorting to a diet only when their weight level has exceeded their uppermost limit.

Slimming aids

There is a vast array of aids for slimmers, ranging from the extremely expensive to the relatively cheap and from the ineffectual to the positively helpful. It is impossible to be comprehensive, but this guide should help you to assess the different types in relation to your weight problem, and to consider the merits and shortcomings inherent in all of them.

● Appetite suppressants

The most effective appetite suppressants are available only from doctors or hospitals. These are *not* a substitute for a diet, but simply help you to overcome hunger and stick to your diet. They do not affect metabolic rate or weight loss and often cause unpleasant side-effects, such as headaches and drowsiness. Most doctors use them only as a last resort when there has been repeated failure to lose weight by other means.

Many other products claiming to be appetite suppressants can be bought freely over the counter. However, there is little evidence that any of these claims can be justified scientifically, and any beneficial results that may occur are probably due to a placebo effect, that is, the products work simply because the consumer believes they will. Their high cost is certainly unjustified.

● Behavioural psychotherapy

This type of treatment aims primarily to correct the faulty attitudes to food and eating that created the weight problem in the first place, although you should also lose weight as an indirect result of therapy. Its effectiveness is hard to assess and probably depends on the individual patient and psychotherapist. But it is expensive and so best left until other methods of weight reduction have failed (see also pages 248–251).

● Bulking agents

These include substances such as methylcellulose, gum guar and bran fibre, which, if taken before meals, are purported to swell up and fill the stomach, so reducing the amount of food eaten at the meal. In fact scientific tests have shown that this happens only when dangerously large amounts of bulking agents are taken and not with the relatively small doses usually recommended. Most brands also include a diet with their instructions, which would of course produce a weight loss, if followed properly and conscientiously, even without the bulking agent.

● Dental splinting

In cases of apparently incurable compulsive eating, it is possible to wire the jaws together so that only liquids, or liquidized food, can be taken. Weight losses are usually excellent while the splint is in place, but considerable re-education is needed if the reduced weight is to be maintained after its removal. In the few cases where this procedure has been tried, long-term weight maintenance has not always been satisfactory.

● Exercise

From the slimmer's point of view there are two types of exercise. The first involves actively moving the body around from one place to another, thus using up energy. The second is the 'keep fit' exercise, which basically tones up muscles in a specific area, but uses little extra energy. The first type, if done regularly, will help to promote weight loss, while the second will improve the figure. Ideally most slimmers need some of both and it is sometimes possible to combine them in a single activity such as swimming. Do not make the mistake of embarking on a course of isometrics or yoga in the belief that you will lose weight, although it will help your figure, and probably your mental outlook.

Exercise machines fall into similar categories – cycles and rowing machines help to increase energy output, while passive exercise machines concentrate on toning up specific muscles. For further information on the relative merits of different types of exercise machine, see pages 166–167.

● Health farms or clinics

These establishments generally offer a fairly strict diet combined with exercise for weight reduction, plus various other treatments such as sauna baths and massage to promote a feeling of relaxation, well-being and good health. It is expensive, of course, but providing you do not expect miracles, a visit to a health farm can be an extremely pleasant way of taking a holiday *and* improving your health and looks (see pages 238–241).

● Hypnosis and acupuncture

Both have been used to treat overweight, although little is known about their success or otherwise. If you are tempted to try either, do make sure that the person consulted is properly qualified and belongs to the appropriate professional body, and be prepared for it to be expensive (see pages 232 and 236 for further details of these forms of treatment).

● Localized slimming aids

From machines that massage, vibrate or pummel, to soaps and herbal lotions, the one thing that localized slimming aids have in common is their ineffectiveness. There is no scientific evidence for the sort of claims these products make. The only really successful way to remove fat from the body is by dieting and/or vigorous exercise, and even this can lose it only generally, not from specific areas. Cures for 'cellulite' or 'lumpy fat' are similarly useless.

● Meal replacements

The idea of presenting the slimmer with a nutritionally complete meal, perhaps in the form of biscuits or a milk-based drink, is quite good in theory. It cuts out the possibility of choosing the wrong foods, cooking them the wrong way and eating too much, and for slimmers who need a quick, convenient meal such products do have a limited usefulness. The drawbacks are that they do little to re-educate eating habits, are often very sweet and quickly become boring if used more than occasionally.

● Slimming groups

Groups and clubs are highly popular with slimmers and on the whole play an informative and helpful role. They vary enormously in cost, size and organization and in the type and range of diets they offer. Being part of a group of people, all with the same problem of overweight, is valuable in sorting out difficulties that you may feel are unique to you but which in reality are shared, and the competitive element also gives you the incentive to succeed. If you are thinking of joining a club, it is a good idea to go along to a meeting as a visitor first, to make sure that you like the group and that they have a diet to suit you, before parting with any money.

● Special foods

There is now an increasing number of special slimmers' foods on the market – the range including soft drinks, low-fat spreads, mayonnaise dressings, sauces, soups, bread, crispbread and artificial sweeteners. The aim is to provide a saving in calories as compared with similar normal foods, which is usually achieved by adding a calorie-free 'filler', such as water or air, or flavour substitute such as saccharin. Inevitably low calorie foods are more expensive, and it is largely a matter of personal preference whether you pay the extra or choose to cut out, or eat less of, the normal food. It is always worth checking the calorie saving made by a low calorie food – it may not be large. For those on low carbohydrate diets there are also some starch-reduced products. Take care not to confuse special slimming foods (sometimes called 'dietetic' foods) with 'diabetic' foods, which may be sugar-free but contain a substance called sorbitol instead and are no lower in calories or carbohydrates.

● Surgery

Generally surgery is used only as a last resort when severe obesity threatens a patient's health (see also page 228). Two main types of operation are possible: an apronectomy, in which excess fat is cut away from the abdominal wall, or an intestinal bypass operation, which involves shortening the small intestine so that less food can be absorbed. The latter invariably causes quite a large weight loss, but the side-effects on the digestive system can be quite unpleasant. For cosmetic surgery operations to remove excess fat from the thighs, hips and buttocks and from the upper arms, see pages 228–229.

● Sweating

Taking a sauna or Turkish bath is relaxing and invigorating, and so beneficial to health and beauty. But the only thing a sauna removes from the body is water, in the form of sweat (see entry under Slimming treatments page 247). No fat is lost, so it cannot be counted as a method of slimming. The same is true of the plastic garments designed to make the body sweat; the fluid lost through sweat is quickly replaced by the body.

Calorie Controlled Diet

Slimming by controlling calorie intake is probably the most successful and popular type of diet. It involves keeping the intake below a fixed limit by adding up the calorie content of every item of food and drink consumed. You can either follow a set menu that has been worked out by someone else, in which every meal has a given calorific value, or with a little extra effort you can design your own and count the calories yourself.

You will need a reliable calorie chart, kitchen scales, a measuring jug, a notebook and a pencil. Everything you eat or drink must be weighed or measured and its calorific value calculated and recorded in the notebook. If you have planned the meals carefully, your daily or weekly calorie intake should correspond to the level you have set yourself – usually somewhere between 1000 and 1500 kcals a day. For a calorie chart of basic foods and drinks, see pages 120–121.

Mistakes to avoid

There are a number of pitfalls for the unwary. It is easy to forget the calories contained in the milk added to tea or coffee, or the butter you spread on bread, or even the bits and pieces you nibble while you are preparing a meal. These items may seem small, but their total calorie content can make the difference between success and failure on the diet. Do not be tempted to guess the weight of food, because this can result in considerable errors in calorie intake. Do not forget to record your food intake and then try to add up the day's calories in your head – this is the most common mistake made by calorie-counters and it is almost impossible to recall everything that you have eaten and drunk with complete accuracy.

The nutritional value of what you eat is still important. Aim to get about half your calories from valuable foods such as milk, cheese, meat, fish, eggs and vegetables – a diet composed entirely of jam doughnuts will not do much for your general health. But if your previous attempts at dieting have failed because you have been unable to resist certain foods it may be a good idea to include them within reason in your daily intake. The likelihood is that you will probably find that you no longer crave your pet indulgence as soon as it becomes a permissible part of your daily diet.

Planning ahead

One of the advantages of calorie counting is that you can allow for special occasions such as parties or meals out without ruining your entire diet campaign. If you have a busy social life you may find it helpful to aim for an average weekly calorie intake – this will allow you to eat a fairly generous diet on one or two days and be stricter on others. A weekly allowance of about 10,000 kcals should provide an average intake low enough to ensure a steady weight loss. You do need to plan carefully, however, to avoid consuming your entire weekly allowance in the first three or four days.

People who are not as well organized may find it simpler to plan only a day or so ahead. When you know you are going to a function at which it will be impossible to avoid exceeding your calorie allowance, cut down your food intake beforehand, and on the great day try to select the less calorific foods and drinks available. You will have to compromise between abandoning all control over calories and appearing antisocial by refusing everything that is offered.

The pros and cons

No diet is perfect for every slimmer. Before embarking on any regime you should consider whether it is right for your own requirements and style of life.

The advantages of a calorie controlled diet:
- its great flexibility suits most individual needs.
- no food need automatically be excluded.
- you can still enjoy eating out.
- it fits in with family catering and any pattern of meals.
- you are not involved in extra expense.
- it teaches you about energy values as you go along.
- the transition to a normal diet for weight maintenance is straightforward and painless.

The disadvantages:
- weighing and recording food can be inconvenient and a chore.
- it is easy to make mistakes in calculating calorie intake.
- if you like a rigid diet regime you may find it gives you too much choice.
- it puts the onus on you to select a nutritionally balanced diet.

Low Carbohydrate Diet

Reducing the amount of carbohydrate you eat is really just another way of cutting down calorie intake. Foods that contain starch or sugar are strictly limited, while you can eat more or less as much as you want of the carbohydrate-free foods such as meat and fish. The nutritional value of your diet is not affected, while its fat content should be automatically reduced. For instance, if you eat less bread you will tend to eat less butter.

How it works

Instead of counting calories you add up the carbohydrate values of what you consume. Since many of the foods you will be eating contain little or no carbohydrate, the procedure is slightly simpler. You need a chart of carbohydrate values (see pages 120–121) and a notebook and pencil to keep a daily record of what you eat. These values are usually expressed in units, 1 unit being equivalent to 5 g of carbohydrate. Ideally each meal you eat should contain a carbohydrate-free food – meat, fish, eggs, cheese and many vegetables – but all other foods must be noted down and the carbohydrate units recorded. Most low carbohydrate diets suggest a daily limit on carbohydrate intake of 10–12 units (50–60 g), which usually results in steady weight losses but does not affect the palatability of the overall diet. The calorie intake of such a diet is usually between 1200 and 1500 kcals per day.

By far the most common error on a low carbohydrate diet is to eat an excess of the carbohydrate-free foods, especially those that are rich in fat and thus high in calories, such as cheese, cream and fatty meat. The extra calories can easily increase weight or slow down weight loss.

Although some leafy vegetables are free of carbohydrate, many vegetables and fruits do contain small but significant amounts, so check on your chart before eating them. In chemical terms alcohol is not strictly a carbohydrate but since it is metabolized in the same way and provides energy, if your diet includes alcohol, allow for it in your carbohydrate count. At 5 or 6 units, a glass of wine cannot be more than an occasional treat.

If you are ever tempted to have all the allowed carbohydrate units in one go – as a slice of cake or a packet of potato crisps – remember that you will have to live on entirely carbohydrate-free foods for the rest of the day, which can be difficult, unless you possess superhuman willpower. Most people find the diet more acceptable if the allowance is spread out evenly during the day.

It is important not to cut out *all* carbohydrate from your diet, since this can result in a condition called ketosis, when the end products of the breakdown of fats accumulate. This will not happen on a normal low carbohydrate diet providing 10–12 units (50–60 g) of carbohydrate.

A low carbohydrate diet can also be expensive but this depends on the foods that you choose. Smoked salmon and fillet steak will obviously be more costly than chicken and eggs.

Sociable eating

Eating out in a restaurant should present fewer problems than a dinner party. Providing you remember which foods are free of, or contain very few, carbohydrates, you need not worry too much about portion sizes (unlike calorie-counting). But, like alcohol, most soft drinks have a surprisingly high carbohydrate value and more than one will almost certainly take you over your allowance. Low calorie soft drinks are generally also low in carbohydrate, so these can be a help. You can try to budget your carbohydrate allowance over several days, although this is less successful than when calorie counting. If your life is socially demanding, a calorie controlled diet will probably suit you better.

The pros and cons

The advantages:
- it is simpler to follow and involves less calculating than a calorie controlled diet.
- it ensures a diet of high nutritional value.
- it lays the foundation for good eating habits.
- it is ideal if you have a lot of weight to lose.
- it is suitable for every member of the family.

The disadvantages:
- it is probably not suitable if you crave sweet foods, alcoholic drinks, etc.
- it is less flexible towards individual likes or social occasions than a calorie controlled diet.
- some slimmers, especially those with only a little weight to lose, find it too generous.
- it still puts a limit on high fat foods such as cheese, even though they are carbohydrate-free.

Calories and Carbohydrate Units

	kcals /100g	/oz	c* units /100g	/oz
Cereals and cereal products				
Biscuits, chocolate, full-coated	524	149	13½	4
Biscuits, digestive, plain	471	134	13	3½
Bran, wheat	206	59	5½	1½
Bread, white	233	66	10	3
Bread, wholewheat	216	61	8½	2½
Cornflakes	368	105	17	5
Cream crackers	440	125	13½	4
Doughnuts	349	99	9½	2½
Eclairs	376	107	7½	2
Flour, plain	350	99	16	4½
Flour, wholewheat (100%)	318	90	13½	4
Fruit cake, rich	332	94	11½	3
Gingerbread	373	106	12½	3½
Ginger nuts	456	130	16	4½
Ice cream, dairy	167	47	5	1½
Jelly, packet, made with water	59	17	3	1
Macaroni, boiled	117	33	5	1½
Muesli	368	105	13	3½
Pastry, shortcrust, cooked	527	150	11	3
Rice, boiled	123	35	6	1½
Rice Krispies	372	106	17½	5
Shortbread	504	143	13	3½
Shredded Wheat	324	92	13½	4
Spaghetti, boiled	117	33	5	1½
Sponge cake, without fat	301	85	11	3
Milk and milk products				
Cheese, Cheddar type	406	115	0	0
Cheese, cottage	96	27	0	0
Cheese, cream	439	125	0	0
Cream, double (heavy)	447	127	0	0
Cream, single (light)	212	60	0	0
Milk, cows', fresh, skimmed	33	9	1	½
Milk, cows', fresh, whole	65	18	1	½
Milk, evaporated, whole, unsweetened	158	45	2½	½
Milk, goats'	71	20	1	½
Yogurt, fruit	95	27	3½	1
Yogurt, natural	52	15	1	½
Eggs				
Egg, boiled	147	42	0	0
Egg, fried	232	66	0	0
Egg, whole, raw	147	42	0	0
Fats and oils				
Butter, salted	740	210	0	0
Compound cooking fat	894	254	0	0
Low fat spread	366	104	0	0
Margarine, all types	730	207	0	0
Olive oil	930	264	0	0
Vegetable oils	899	255	0	0

* carbohydrate units

	kcals /100g	/oz	c* units /100g	/oz
Meat and meat products				
Bacon, grilled back	405	115	0	0
Beef, corned, canned	217	62	0	0
Beef, minced, stewed	229	65	0	0
Chicken, roast, meat only	148	42	0	0
Gammon rashers (hamsteak), grilled, lean	172	49	0	0
Ham, canned	120	34	0	0
Kidney, lamb's, fried	155	44	0	0
Lamb chops, loin, grilled, lean	191	54	0	0
Lamb, leg, roast, lean	290	83	0	0
Liver, lamb's, fried	232	66	0	0
Liver sausage	310	88	1	½
Pork chops, loin, grilled, lean	226	64	0	0
Pork, leg, roast, lean	185	53	0	0
Sausages, beef, grilled	265	75	3	1
Sausages, pork, grilled	318	90	2½	½
Sirloin, roast, lean	192	55	0	0
Stewing steak, cooked, lean and fat	223	63	0	0
Tongue, canned	213	60	0	0
Turkey, roast, meat only	140	40	0	0
Veal, roast	230	65	0	0
Fish and fish products				
Clams, raw	81	23	0	0
Cod, baked	96	27	0	0
Cod, fried in batter	199	57	1½	½
Haddock, smoked, steamed	101	29	0	0
Herring, grilled	199	57	0	0
Kipper, grilled, baked in oven	205	58	0	0
Lemon sole, steamed	91	26	0	0
Lobster, boiled	119	34	0	0
Oysters, raw	51	14	0	0
Plaice, fried in crumbs	228	65	1½	½
Prawns, boiled	107	30	0	0
Salmon, canned	155	44	0	0
Salmon, smoked	142	40	0	0
Salmon, steamed, poached	197	56	0	0
Sardines, canned in tomato sauce	177	50	0	0
Scampi, fried	316	90	6	1½
Striped bass, oven fried	196	56	1	½
Swordfish, canned	102	29	0	0
Tuna, canned in oil	289	82	0	0
Vegetables				
Beans, broad, boiled	48	14	1½	½
Beans, runner (string), boiled	19	5	0	0
Beetroot (beets), boiled	44	12	2	½
Brussels sprouts, boiled	18	5	0	0
Cabbage, winter, boiled	15	4	0	0
Carrots, old, boiled	19	5	1	½
Cauliflower, boiled	9	3	0	0

	kcals /100g	/oz	c* units /100g	/oz
Celery, raw	8	2	0	0
Cucumber, raw	10	3	0	0
Lettuce, raw	12	3	0	0
Mushrooms, raw	13	4	0	0
Onions, boiled	13	4	0	0
Peas, frozen, boiled	41	12	1	½
Peppers, green, raw	15	4	4	1
Potatoes, boiled	80	23	3½	1
Potatoes, chips	253	72	7½	2
Potato crisps	533	151	10	3
Potatoes, roast	157	46	5½	1½
Spinach, boiled	30	9	0	0
Sweetcorn, kernels, canned	76	22	3	1
Tomatoes, raw	14	4	0	0
Fruit				
Apples, cooking, raw	37	11	2	½
Apples, eating	46	13	2½	½
Apricots, fresh	28	8	1½	½
Avocado pears	223	63	0	0
Bananas, raw	79	22	4	1
Cherries, eating, raw	47	13	2½	½
Currants, black, stewed without sugar	24	7	1	½
Currants, dried	243	70	12½	3½
Dates, dried	248	70	12½	3½
Figs, green, raw	41	12	2	½
Fruit salad, canned	95	27	5	1½
Grapefruit, raw	22	6	1	½
Grapes, black or white, raw	61	17	3	1
Lemons, juice, fresh	7	2	0	0
Mandarin oranges, canned	56	16	3	1
Melons, yellow, honeydew	21	6	1	½
Olives in brine	103	29	0	0
Oranges, raw	35	10	1½	½
Peaches, fresh	37	11	2	½
Pears, eating	41	12	2	½
Pineapple, canned	77	22	4	1
Prunes, dried, raw	161	46	8	2½
Raisins, dried	246	70	13	3½
Raspberries, raw	25	7	1	½
Rhubarb, stewed without sugar	6	2	0	0
Strawberries, raw	26	7	1	½
Sultanas, dried	250	71	13	3½
Tangerines, raw	34	10	1½	½
Nuts				
Almonds	565	160	1	½
Brazil nuts	619	176	1	½
Chestnuts	170	48	7½	2
Cob or hazel nuts	380	108	1½	½
Coconut, desiccated	604	172	1½	½
Peanut butter, smooth	623	177	2½	½
Peanuts, roasted and salted	570	162	1½	½
Walnuts	525	149	1	½

	kcals /100g	/oz	c* units /100g	/oz
Sugar and preserves				
Jam	261	74	14	4
Honey	288	82	15½	4½
Marmalade	261	74	14	4
Molasses	232	66	12	3½
Sugar, demerara and white	394	112	21	6
Syrup, golden	298	85	16	4½
Treacle, black	257	73	13½	4
Confectionery				
Boiled sweets, candies	327	93	17½	5
Chocolate, milk	529	150	12	3½
Peppermints	392	111	20½	6
Toffees, mixed	430	122	14	4
Beverages				
Coca-Cola	39	11	2	½
Cocoa powder	312	89	2½	½
Coffee, infusion of grounds	2	1	0	0
Drinking chocolate	366	104	15½	4½
Grapefruit juice, canned, unsweetened	31	9	1½	½
Lemonade, bottled	21	6	1	½
Orange drink, undiluted	107	30	5½	1½
Orange juice, canned, unsweetened	33	9	1½	½
Pineapple juice, canned	53	15	2½	½
Tea, infusion without milk	1	0	0	0
Tomato juice, canned	16	5	1	½
Alcoholic beverages				
Cider, dry	36	10	2	½
Draught beer	32	9	2	½
Lager, bottled	29	8	1½	½
Red wine	68	19	4	1
Sherry, dry	116	33	4½	1½
Sherry, sweet	136	39	5	1½
Spirits, 70% proof	222	63	7	2
Vermouth, dry	118	34	5	1½
Vermouth, sweet	151	43	6	1½
White wine, dry	66	19	4	1
White wine, sweet	94	27	5	1½
Sauces and pickles				
French dressing	658	187	0	0
Mayonnaise dressings	311	88	3	1
Pickle, sweet	134	38	7	2
Tomato ketchup	98	28	5	1½
Soups				
Chicken noodle, dried, as served	20	6	1	½
Clam chowder, canned, ready to serve	30	9	1	½
Oxtail, canned, ready to serve	44	12	1	½
Tomato, cream of, canned, ready to serve	55	16	1	½
Vegetable, canned, ready to serve	37	11	1½	½

Protein and Fat in Slimming Diets

On an ordinary, non-slimming diet, we derive 10 to 15 per cent of our energy from protein, about 40 per cent from fat and 40–50 per cent from carbohydrate. Of these three, protein is the most important, since the proportions of fat and carbohydrate can be varied significantly, without detriment to the health.

Slimming creates special demands in the body, which are largely met by the protein content of the diet. In order to ensure good health the protein intake must be maintained, even though the total food intake has been reduced. Do not forget that the foods rich in protein are also valuable sources of vitamins and minerals. Moreover, protein helps to create the sensation of satiety and to make the diet palatable. On a strict diet (one providing fewer than 1000 kcals a day) there is always the danger that protein may be burnt to provide energy, instead of being used to build, renew and repair body tissues. Thus not only body fat, but also body protein is lost.

High protein diets

A diet low in carbohydrate can be thought of as a high protein diet, in that more than 20 per cent of the total calorie intake comes in the form of protein, compared with the 10 to 15 per cent on a normal (non-slimming) diet.

However, slimming diets in which protein constitutes 50 per cent, or even more, of the calorie intake have also been advocated, and it has been claimed that such diets produce far greater weight losses than those allowing the same calorie intake but lower amounts of protein. These diets rely heavily on protein-rich foods that are low in fat such as chicken and fish; they often specifically exclude all carbohydrates and severely limit other foods and fluids. Thorough investigations have shown, however, that the apparently high weight loss they achieve is caused by changes in the body's water retention and not by fat loss. Thus in the long term this weight loss still depends on the total number of calories consumed and not on whether they have come from protein, fat or carbohydrate. In spite of this, high protein diets still appear, often making miraculous claims.

High protein diets have many drawbacks. They are often badly balanced because of the small range of foods allowed. Those that restrict fluid intake not only give a false impression of weight loss, but may be dangerous. Diets requiring high consumption of protein can be expensive and they do little to re-educate eating habits to a pattern that encourages long-term weight control. If you enjoy protein foods, opt for a low carbohydrate diet – it will let you eat them reasonably freely and in a sensible way.

Protein sparing diets

In recent years attention has focused on the ways of speeding up weight loss, either by using very low calorie diets or by complete starvation (see page 125). There is no doubt that if the slimmer can follow such a regime accurately, good weight losses can be achieved, but there are several snags, the main one being that on an energy intake as low as 300–400 kcals, or on starvation, the body is forced to burn protein instead of using it to construct body tissues. This may result in a lower metabolic rate, so that energy needs are less and weight loss becomes even harder.

To obviate this problem, diets have been developed that are low in calories (300–700 kcals per day) but high in protein to minimize body protein losses. In some of them the protein is 'pre-digested' – supplied in the form of separate amino acids – with added vitamins and minerals; in others it comes from everyday foods, with a little carbohydrate to prevent ketosis (the accumulation of the end products of the breakdown of fats). Preliminary results suggest these diets may indeed prevent losses of body protein, a finding contrary to accepted nutritional theories, and one that has been challenged by several leading authorities. There is scope for considerably more research.

This limited type of diet is suitable only for severely obese people who can be kept under close medical supervision, since, followed continuously over a long period, it could have serious effects on the metabolism and nutrition.

Low protein diets

In most affluent countries the average protein intake is well above the minimum necessary for good health and can often be two or even three times as much as the body requires. Once the body has satisfied its need for protein, any excess is burnt for energy or else converted into body fat, with the result that even protein foods can contribute to a weight problem. Much of our protein comes from animal sources and is thus associated with animal fats and their attendant nutritional disadvantages. Moreover, animal proteins are expensive, both in terms of the energy used to produce them and of the money needed to purchase them. There is clearly a need for a slimming diet that avoids these shortcomings while still ensuring a good weight loss.

How low a protein intake is compatible with good health and a palatable diet? The table below shows that minimum protein needs are considerably lower than the recommended levels, which in turn are lower than our actual intakes.

Protein needs and consumption		
	U.K. g/day	U.S.A. g/day
Minimum protein requirement	38	38
Recommended protein allowance	55	46
Average protein intake	71	92

The average woman in developed countries today eats far more protein – most of it derived from animal sources – than she needs to maintain good health.

Even a diet that is low in protein should contain at least 38 g per day; people with special needs, such as children or expectant mothers, require more. Any diet that is low in protein and in fat will have to be high in carbohydrate. Since other nutritional dangers are associated with carbohydrate in the form of sugar, the diet must rely on starches from cereals, root vegetables and pulses. These also provide valuable protein, so that only small amounts of animal protein are necessary, and the final form of the diet is not unlike a vegetarian one. The inclusion of unrefined cereals such as wholemeal bread and flour is said to be beneficial, because the extra roughage creates bulk that helps to reduce food intake, although this claim is not entirely proven. To be really effective this diet must be calorie counted and kept within the usual range of daily allowances.

While there is no doubt that the low fat, high fibre content of this form of diet has several advantages, the low protein intake itself does not seem to offer any specific nutritional benefit. It is possible that in the future we shall all consume this type of diet, since our limited energy resources will demand greater efficiency in food production. At the present time, however, many people, including some nutritionists, still value a relatively high protein intake as necessary for a palatable and satisfying diet.

Low fat diets

Although most calorie controlled diets are moderately low in fats, low carbohydrate diets have a higher fat content. In both types of diet, however, the fats in foods can cause problems. Slimmers following calorie controlled diets often underestimate the calorific value of foods by neglecting their 'invisible' fat content (see page 99). On low carbohydrate diets overenthusiastic consumption of high fat foods that are carbohydrate-free can significantly increase the total calorie intake. Fats are the richest source of energy and if they are reduced a larger volume of food must be eaten to get the same intake of calories.

A low fat diet has recently been designed to work on similar lines to a low carbohydrate one, except that instead of counting carbohydrate units, you count fat units. Each fat unit represents 10 g of fat, and you are allowed 10 units per day, which automatically cuts the daily calorie intake to 1000–1500 kcals. Foods that contain no fat are allowed without limit – these include vegetables, fruit and cereal foods such as bread, pasta, rice and even breakfast cereals. Although this diet is not yet widely used, when followed properly it seems to produce good weight losses, while still providing sound nutritional value. Being low in fats and generous with cereals, vegetables and fruit, it is now fully backed by medical opinion.

Like every diet, it has its shortcomings. Sweet foods and drinks must still be limited, since although they contain little or no fat, they increase the total calorie intake if consumed in too great a quantity. The same applies to alcohol. But a low fat diet does offer a genuine and effective alternative to calorie counting or low carbohydrate diets and can easily be adapted for weight maintenance afterwards simply by increasing the daily allowance of fat units.

Crash Diets and Fasting

The typical crash diet is strict, with a daily calorie intake of well below 1000 kcals – often as little as 500 kcals. The menu is set inflexibly and the limited range of foods allowed does not reflect normal eating patterns. These diets are usually designed to be followed over a period of one or two weeks at the most.

Crash diets make extravagant claims about how much weight you can lose. Do not take these claims too literally, since losses can be variable, although as long as your calorie intake is reduced you should certainly lose some weight.

The initial weight loss is likely to be impressive, owing to the reduction of carbohydrate stores (glycogen) and associated water, as well as some fat and body protein. It may be as high as 3–5 kg (7–11 lb) in the first week, but less than half of this will be fat, which is what you are aiming to lose.

Subsequent weeks' results will seem disappointing in comparison, but the second week of a crash diet can produce as high a fat loss as the first. Reductions in protein and glycogen are negligible and much less water is lost. So if you can follow a crash diet to the letter for two weeks you could lose up to 7 kg (15 lb).

Results are rarely as good as this in practice, however. Do not underestimate the difficulty of following an abnormal diet for more than a few days. You may find the limited range of foods intolerably boring especially if friends and family are eating a normal diet around you. If you decide that you are not proof against all temptations, you will probably do better on a less rigid diet.

Fluid intake

If your crash diet restricts fluids, you will appear to lose more weight, but this is because you are losing water, not fat. There are many calorie-free fluids that can be drunk unlimitedly without spoiling your diet. Restricting fluid intake does not improve health and can be detrimental.

Nutritional value

A diet that restricts the total calorie intake to below 1000 kcals a day is only just adequate. Very strict diets – around 500 kcals a day – cannot provide all the required nutrients for an adult woman. As a result, losses occur from the body tissues, particularly of protein, which is one reason why no crash diet should be continued for longer than two weeks. Taking multi-vitamin and mineral preparations can help a little, but they are no substitute for a well-balanced diet. Make sure you are in good health when you start a crash diet since it may make you feel tired and irritable and will certainly exacerbate a cold or infection.

Weight maintenance

A return to a normal eating pattern will cause a weight increase, as body stores of glycogen are replaced. This can be depressing if you have made a great effort to shed excess weight. Moreover, it is common for a person coming off a crash diet to go on an eating binge and this, of course, will replace some of the lost fat as well as the glycogen. It is best to step up your food intake gradually to allow your body time to re-adapt itself.

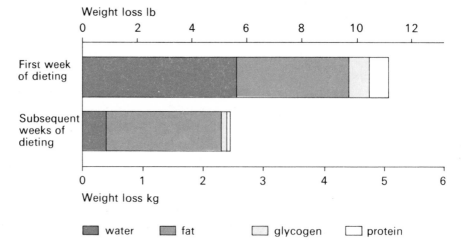

Composition of weight loss on a crash diet

On a diet of about 400 kcals a day roughly half the initial weight reduction is attributable to loss of water.

A crash diet does very little to re-educate bad eating habits, apart from giving you an incentive to keep your new slim figure. By allowing you a limited, and often bizarre, range of foods, in quantities that cannot provide balanced nutrition, it does not encourage a permanent change towards better eating. This makes weight maintenance a particular problem and as a result some people alternate between periods of uncontrolled eating and crash dieting, with their weight fluctuating by several kilos. This is both physiologically and psychologically undesirable.

Nevertheless, crash diets do provide a chance to get rid of a few excess kilos in a relatively brief time and can be a useful aid as far as short-term weight reduction is concerned.

Occasional fasting

Once in a while a single day of fasting can be undertaken by a healthy, well-nourished person without any risk to health or life, providing that adequate amounts of calorie-free or low calorie fluids are drunk. It can be used either for weight reduction or simply for weight maintenance.

As you will probably feel tired and hungry on your day of fasting, select a time when the demands on your life are light. This will depend on your circumstances – a working woman might find a weekend easier, while a housewife may prefer a day when the rest of the family are at school and work. Do not fast for more than one, or at most two, days a week. If you find fasting imposes too great a strain on your willpower, you will probably be happier with a rather less drastic approach to dieting.

Fasting for more than a day or two should never be undertaken unless under strict medical supervision and then only by people who are in good general health.

Intermittent fasting

This has been recommended for people who are very overweight, as an aid to speeding up and maintaining a good rate of weight loss. Patients usually undergo a fast of between seven and 15 days, under hospital supervision, and are then put on a low calorie diet of 500–1000 kcals per day with occasional one- or two-day fasts, on an out-patient basis. Although a lot of weight is lost during the original fast, success is not maintained in the out-patient phase, and in the long term (over a year or more) results are very poor. Indeed, one study showed that those who had undergone intermittent fasting did worse in terms of permanent weight loss than those who had a continuous low calorie diet. There seems therefore little to be gained from intermittent fasting.

Total starvation

Only safe when done under hospital supervision, total starvation offers severely obese people a chance to lose between 0.2 and 0.4 kg (7–14 oz) per day and 1.4–2.8 kg (3–6 lb) per week. The initial weight loss is slightly faster owing to losses of glycogen and water, with slower subsequent losses. Towards the end of a long period of dieting, the rate of loss may decelerate further, as the body attempts to adapt itself to starvation.

There are various potentially dangerous side-effects. Hunger is no longer experienced after the first day or two, and ketosis (the accumulation of the end products from the breakdown of fats) can make some patients euphoric. More seriously, prolonged starvation can disturb kidney function, causing large losses of vital minerals such as potassium, which may affect the heart. Oedema (fluid retention), hair loss and polyneuritis (inflammation of nerves) can also occur. The consumption of small amounts of protein-containing foods, such as lean meat or milk, reduces the side-effects without significantly affecting the rate of weight loss, although even this does not completely prevent the loss of much-needed body protein.

The ultimate success of total starvation depends on the behaviour of the patients after they are discharged from hospital. They are usually put on a low calorie diet before going home to give them time to become accustomed to it, but even so there is frequently a quite rapid weight gain. The proportion of patients who manage to maintain their weight at the new lower level is low and many regain all their lost weight. As a result, medical and nutritional opinion now favours the use of low calorie diets of around 800 kcals per day, sacrificing some speed of weight loss for lower risk to the patient and better long-term maintenance of the reduced weight.

Eating to Gain Weight

A severely underweight woman is one who is more than 10 per cent below the ideal-weight range for her height (see the table on page 113). Many underweight people are apparently in excellent health, although others have decreased body fat and perhaps some wasting of the muscles. Their resistance to infection may be low and they tend to feel the cold because the layer of subcutaneous fat that normally insulates the body is much reduced. The underweight woman – unlike the anorectic (see opposite) – often feels that she looks bony and lacks the necessary curves to look really good.

The causes of underweight

Underweight may be a temporary condition, a result of illness, injury or a period of stress. Food intake has failed to match the energy needs of the body and the stores of body fat have become depleted. This situation usually rectifies itself. As the patient recovers from her illness or stress the appetite improves, food intake increases and she gains weight. The body can aid recovery by using food very economically.

Some people, however, are permanently underweight and although they eat enough to satisfy their energy needs they never succeed in reaching the ideal-weight range for their height. We are probably all familiar with the woman who seems to eat everything, but remains as slim as a rake. There are a number of likely reasons for this. Her food intake may not be as large as it appears, or she may maintain a high level of activity, being constantly on the move and fidgeting while apparently sitting still. She may even have an inherently high metabolic rate so that she burns up energy fast; some people get rid of excess calories after a meal by a temporary increase in the metabolic rate – this is known as the thermic effect. For such people, providing they remain in good health, there seems little point in trying to override the body's system of weight control, even if it does seem to be fixed at a lower level than is considered ideal. After all, ideal weights are worked out statistically and are not necessarily right for each individual.

Overeating to gain weight

This is by no means as easy as it sounds. Experiments on young healthy people who are at or below their ideal weight have shown that overeating does not necessarily cause a big weight gain. Even when eating two or three times their normal energy needs, these people gain only a little weight, probably 'burning off' much of the excess food energy as heat instead of storing it as body fat. This process may involve brown adipose tissue, a special kind of fat tissue present in the body in small amounts and currently the subject of much research. Once food intake returns to a normal level, any weight increase is likely to be quickly lost.

Despite this discouraging outlook, if you are still prepared to try to gain weight by eating more, there are a few guidelines to observe.

● The nutritional balance and quality of the diet should be maintained. The food group system remains a good general guide (see page 105).

● Do not eat more only of the foods that are thought of as 'fattening'. Extra meat, milk and bread are as valuable in energy and better for you.

● Do not be tempted to buy products claiming to promote weight gain in specific parts of the body; there is no scientific evidence that this is possible, any more than the slimming of localized areas.

● Exercise may improve body shape by building up muscles, but it can also increase energy output, so do not get too enthusiastic.

If you fail to make or maintain a significant weight gain, do not be too disappointed. You are probably at the optimum weight for your body and you may do more harm than good by attempting to change things.

Feeding the convalescent

During illness and in the initial stages of recovery it is important to keep up the intake of fluids and to tempt the appetite with favourite foods. Almost any food is better than none and it does no harm to indulge the whims of the patient, as long as they are not too outlandish.

As recovery continues the patient should have food of high nutritional value. Milk is ideal here. In the absence of specific medical instructions, try to include a protein-rich food in each meal, with daily servings of cereal food, vegetables and fruit. Avoid rich and heavily seasoned dishes and serve small portions, as attractively as you can.

Anorexia nervosa

This term describes self-imposed starvation, maintained over long periods and resulting in dramatic weight loss and other side-effects. Sufferers are almost always teenage girls and young women, particularly from the upper social classes and often highly intelligent. Perhaps as many as 1 per cent of girls between the ages of 16 and 18 suffer from anorexia, although they may recover before medical intervention is required. It also occurs in young men, but relatively rarely.

Anorectics go to great lengths to avoid eating food, claiming that they find it repulsive, and even mislead people into thinking they have eaten, while actually throwing the food away. At later stages of the disease, sufferers may make themselves vomit after eating or else take large doses of purgatives. Body weight may fall as low as 30 kg (66 lb) and periods usually stop once the weight drops below 45 kg (99 lb). The body may become covered with fine downy hair (lanugo) and as subcutaneous fat is lost the individual muscles can be seen. Mental and physical activity are not reduced, indeed hyperactivity is a common feature, although usually denied by the sufferer. When the loss of body weight becomes severe, resistance to infection is low and what would normally be a minor illness can become serious and even, occasionally, fatal.

The causes

The rejection of food and subsequent reduction in weight are the outward expression of psychological problems. It has been suggested that the large weight losses and subsequent emaciation are an attempt to deny adult sexuality and to revert to a pre-pubertal state. Certainly sexual experiences can precipitate anorexia, although other stresses may have the same effect. There is sometimes an abnormal relationship with either one or both parents – particularly where the mother is very dominating. In such cases the rejection of food may be symbolic of the rejection of parental love.

Treatment

Methods of treatment are aimed at returning the body weight to normal and maintaining it there. Treatment usually falls into two main categories – psychiatric and medical therapy. The former (see pages 248–251) attempts to resolve the underlying problems, while the latter concentrates on feeding the patient again with the aid of sedative and appetite-stimulating drugs. Often a combination of these two approaches is used.

Nowadays the psychiatric therapy is often designed to include the immediate family of the patient. Parents of anorectics may need reassurance, and information to help them understand the condition and how it may have arisen. Self-help for anorexia sufferers is also now available, in groups rather like Alcoholics Anonymous. These can be extremely helpful and supportive during the period of recovery.

When anorexia has become severe the patient is usually admitted to hospital where she can be kept under the close supervison of skilled and patient nursing and medical staff to ensure that she does eat. Sometimes 'privileges', such as extra visitors or being allowed out of bed, are used as an added incentive for weight gain. This has to be combined with psychiatric treatment to help both the sufferer and her family come to terms with the problem.

Although some girls who suffer a degree of anorexia recover spontaneously – often when a particularly stressful period of life has ended – few who have lost a great deal of weight recover without some form of medical help. As many as 50 per cent make an only partial recovery.

Prevention

Since those closest to the potential sufferer are, in a sense, often involved themselves, prevention is not always easy. The warning signs of anorexia are the rejection of food and loss of weight, although if food is being hidden or vomited the former may not be immediately obvious. Exhorting the person to eat is not usually helpful – the situation must be handled with tact and sympathy, and if weight loss continues should be referred to the family doctor. The earlier medical help is sought, the better the chances of avoiding severe weight loss and making a good recovery, without the need for hospital admission, which in itself can create extra stress.

Above all, it is important to remember that the rejection of food in anorexia nervosa is a symptom of the illness and not a cause.

Exercise

To many women, the idea of sport or exercise has long been anathema, conjuring up unhappy memories of winter afternoons on the hockey pitch or of being goaded on to seemingly impossible feats by a stentorian-voiced gym mistress. Why, then, should women take up exercise? Why is it that more and more women are in fact spending their leisure time on the squash court, in the gymnasium, in the swimming pool? Probably the foremost reason is an urge to improve the figure, coupled with the realization that exercise can be enjoyable as well as highly beneficial.

Exercise is the perfect partner of a good diet, whether it be a weight-reducing one or just a healthy, balanced eating plan. Not only does it burn off calories, but it makes the muscles firmer, redistributes the bodyweight and improves posture. So the figure-conscious woman has every reason to be interested. However, it is not just the figure that benefits: regular sessions – at least three times a week – of any vigorous exercise or sporting activity, the more varied the better, will make you physically fit. Not only will you look and feel healthier and sleep better, but you will find that you are more energetic and alert and less prone to tension and tiredness.

What is fitness?

Fitness means that your muscles are strong and can sustain effort; that your joints are flexible; that your weight is about right for your height (see page 113); and that you have an efficient cardio-vascular respiratory system. This last component of fitness is the most important and simply means the ability of the heart and lungs to keep the muscles supplied with blood and to get rid of the waste products.

If you go pink and breathless when you take vigorous exercise, do not worry. It is good for your heart and lungs to have a real work-out. You should be concerned only if you remain pink and breathless long afterwards or have bouts of breathlessness some time later.

Exercises that improve the efficiency of the heart and lungs are termed aerobic – with the aid of oxygen. Swimming, jogging, cycling and tennis all come into this category. In order not to place too much strain on the heart and lungs, it is important to take plenty of short rests during a bout of energetic exercise.

If you take up any form of exercise when you are unfit, no matter what your age, go carefully and slowly at first. If you are over 35 and at all worried about your health, have a check-up with your doctor, who will take your blood pressure and probably reassure you that physical activity will do you good. Even if you do have a health problem, the chances are that some form of mild exercise will help. If you drink and/or smoke to any extent, exercise may be more of a strain, so consider which you really care about.

Choice of exercise

Clearly, age and health play a large part in the choice of activity, but the next consideration is enjoyment. You will exercise regularly only if you enjoy it. This does not mean, however, that you have to restrict yourself to the things you know you are reasonably good at: with so many forms of exercise to choose from, why not sample something new? Exercise does not have to be hearty and exhausting to be effective, nor do you have to 'win'. Try working some form of exercise into your daily life: walk the dog briskly, cycle to work, climb the stairs rather than take the lift.

What it costs

Although the home exercise programme on pages 134–146 involves little or no equipment, no sport is entirely without expense. As a beginner, try to borrow or hire equipment in case you find you do not like it. Clothing in natural fibres is far more comfortable than the non-absorbent manmade fibres. The right shoes are essential.

Getting down to it

Never exercise on a full stomach – eat only lightly and no less than an hour beforehand to give the food a chance to settle. Spend a few minutes loosening up before launching into action, so that you come to the exercise itself ready and relaxed, less likely to pull a muscle. The daily minimum programme on pages 134–135 acts as a general warming-up sequence for the home exercise programme. Limber up for other forms of activity by running on the spot for a minute; then bend your knees, stretch up on your toes, drop from the waist and let your arms and trunk hang loose a few times. Do the same to unwind at the end of a session of exercise.

Whatever form of exercise you decide to take up, be prepared to put some energy and time into it and to keep at it. By doing so, you will reach a standard where you can really enjoy it and will reap the rewards of a better figure, a more supple body and improved general fitness.

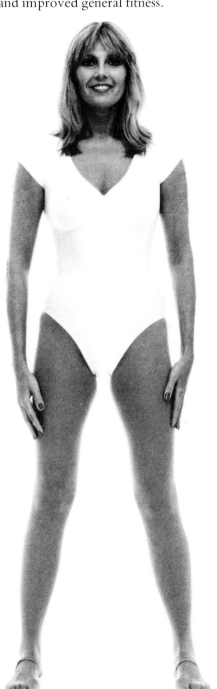

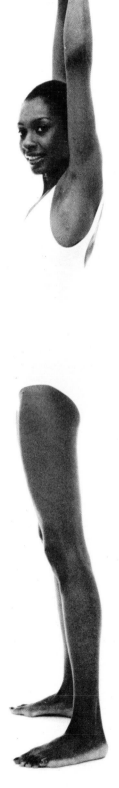

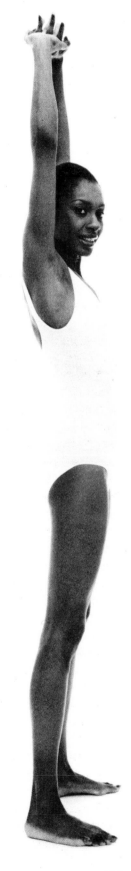

Posture

The mere mention of the word 'posture' may be thoroughly off-putting to many women, evoking, as it often does, unpleasant memories of school gym classes; yet these same women may be worried about their protruding bottom or tummy, round shoulders, poking head or aches in their neck or back. Many of these defects are in fact postural, caused by the way in which the spinal bones are held or not held by the muscles. This can be changed by awareness and practice; it is possible to transform your shape instantly and even appear to grow a little – comforting if you are worried about your apparent dumpiness.

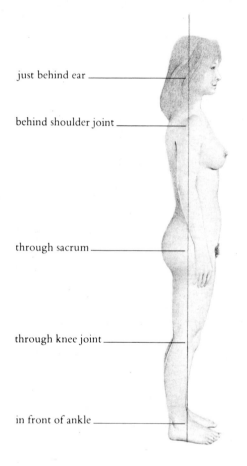

just behind ear

behind shoulder joint

through sacrum

through knee joint

in front of ankle

When you are standing correctly, in good posture, the line of gravity should pass through the points shown above.

The modern approach to posture is different from the old-fashioned militaristic style. The correct position is one in which the fewest possible muscles are being used to hold the body and head up, while, at the same time, the weight is carried through the bones without causing any undue pressure on them or on the ligaments that hold them together. The body is balanced evenly over the feet and the space between them; the wider the feet are apart, the greater the stability, and the narrower the base, the more likelihood there is of falling over.

Every object has a centre of gravity, or point of perfect balance, around which its weight is evenly distributed. In human beings, this is reckoned to be a point just inside the upper part of the pelvis (the second sacral vertebra). The line of gravity is a vertical line that passes through this point. The pelvis is balanced evenly, being tilted neither too far down nor up, or carried too far forwards or backwards.

The more evenly the weight of the body is carried around the line of gravity, the less the muscles have to work. The head weighs about 5 kg (10–12 lb), the arms and hands about 10 kg (20–24 lb) and as weight gradually accumulates downwards – chest, back, hips and so on – the muscles have to work harder to control the bulk. The spinal bones (vertebrae) are graduated in size, being larger lower down the spine to carry the increasing weight.

When the body is upright and still, the spinal column is curved forwards in the neck region (seven bones), backwards in the upper back (twelve bones), forwards in the lower back (five bones) and then is supported by the pelvis, which curves backwards and to which the legs are attached at the hip joints. There should be no sideways curve at all in the whole column. Between each bone there is a pad of gristle, the intervertebral disc, which can be squashed in any direction and so allows movement as well as the various movements already taking place at the spinal joints.

This is the best arrangement for balancing and carrying body weight easily. However, people who habitually wear very high heels tip their weight forwards so that the line of gravity tends to fall outside the base and the spine has to sway backwards to compensate. Equally, if a heavy load is frequently carried in one hand, the spinal column may become crooked so that the back muscles have to work hard on the other side of the spine to keep the body upright. For those with a habitual tendency to slump forwards, the back muscles have to carry the strain and may even become distorted. Any distortion results in strain on the spinal ligaments as well as the muscles and may, if persistent, cause damage to them and to the discs between the vertebrae and even in time to the spinal bones themselves.

Achieving good posture

Take off your shoes and stand with your feet slightly apart; feel that your nose, chin, breast-bone, navel and the front of your pelvis are in a straight line and that this line would fall exactly between your feet. Adjust yourself as necessary by feeling what is happening within you.

Sway slightly backwards and forwards on your feet and then place your weight just in front of your ankles. In this way your weight will be evenly spread back on to your heels and forwards on to your toes, rather like a three-legged stool. Feel that your knees are slightly bent so that you can wiggle your kneecaps up and down freely – they are not fixed.

Adjust the way you carry your pelvis. Try the four possible positions – pushed forwards and pushed backwards, tilted downwards and tilted upwards. Now balance it in the comfortable mid-point. Your pelvis moves easily on the hip joints and the joints of the lower back, so you can readily feel what is happening and register the perfect position for you.

Stretch upwards through all your spinal joints to the top of your head, with your nose and eyes facing straight forwards and your chin at a right angle to your neck. At the same time let your arms drop gently downwards so that your middle fingers hang at the outside of your thighs. If you find they tend to lie further forwards, pull your shoulder blades slightly downwards, backwards and together to correct this. Do all this carefully, feeling each adjustment pleasantly.

You will feel your chest rise into a comely position as you stretch upwards. Keep breathing easily, feeling your lower ribs rise upwards and sideways as you breathe in and fall down again as you breathe out.

Swing your arms loosely forwards and backwards and feel other adjustments taking place in your spine and leg joints to keep you from falling.

Positions of the pelvis

If the pelvis is pushed forwards (a), the spine has to sway backwards so that balance is not lost. If it is pushed backwards (b), weight falls on the heels instead of the centre of the foot. The pelvis may also be tilted up in front (c) by the abdominal muscles so that the lumbar curve flattens and its muscles relax. Alternatively, it may be tilted down in front (d) relaxing the abdominal muscles and causing the buttocks to protrude by tension in the low back muscles.

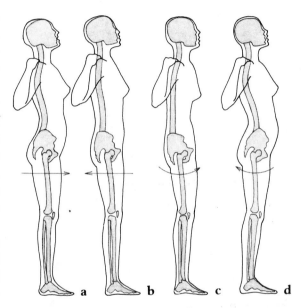

a   **b**   **c**   **d**

Each time you move from the fundamental stance where the body is correctly aligned with the line of gravity, other muscles all over your body spring into action to do the necessary work. This is called 'dynamic posture' – ready for movement – because the spine and other joints move to adjust your weight.

Walk round the room with the same upheld posture, head high and arms gently swinging with the opposite hand and foot forwards and back. Try to walk like this as often as you can every day, with bare feet and without a handbag or shopping, which would curtail the lovely free feeling. Never try to retain the corrected posture rigidly. It will be continually altering as you move and your balance shifts.

Sitting at rest

When sitting, the same rules apply whenever possible. If you are sitting having a rest, remember that is what you are trying to do. Many women sit sideways on the front of a chair, cross their thighs and perhaps curl one leg around the other, fold their arms across their front and hardly use the back of the chair at all.

Instead, choose a chair that supports your back, the whole of your thighs and allows both feet to rest evenly on the floor. Place your bottom right back in the seat and try not to cross your legs as this may impede the upward flow of blood. Stretch upwards against the back of the chair; support your heavy head on the back and your arms on the arms of the chair.

You will feel peaceful, you will look peaceful and you will really have a rest. How much more pleasant it is to chat to someone in this position than to someone rolled up in a bundle perched precariously on the edge of a chair.

Sitting at work
Your work will be mainly in front of you, whether writing, typing, sewing or bathing a baby – even ironing, much food preparation and working on a car engine can all be done sitting down – so the tendency is to bend the head downwards. The weight of the head curves the whole body forwards, which causes great strain on the neck and back. To prevent this, bring your hands forwards to your work instead, while keeping the back upright. Remember that the shoulder joints are the loosest joints in the body, so it is easy for the arms to move forwards, sideways, upwards and even backwards with only minimal accommodatory movement from the back. It is a good idea to practise these movements as a separate exercise (see pages 142–143) to get used to loose arm movements in all directions.

If it is absolutely necessary to bend forwards to work, try to do so with a straight back and head held high, moving from the hips. In this way, the large buttock muscles will be used to lower the weight forwards and the spinal muscles will not be strained. Make a habit of stretching up tall in your chair and pushing your hands high above your head after you have finished a job.

Now that you know how to adjust your weight anywhere in your body whenever you feel it is getting out of alignment and straining your joints, your general health should benefit considerably and you will look and feel better.

The Alexander Principle
When fatigue and constant hoarseness began to threaten the career of Matthias Alexander, the Australian actor and reciter determined to cure himself. By studying in detail exactly how his body produced sound and the way in which the muscles worked, he managed to cure his voice, and went on to devote the rest of his life to teaching the method he developed – the Alexander principle. He came to London in 1904 and started by teaching actors such as Henry Irving and Lily Langtry and later went to America to make his theories more widely known. His work was taken up with enthusiasm by many doctors and influential celebrities, including Aldous Huxley and George Bernard Shaw, who found that their potential was more fully realized by the greater awareness of the interplay between body and mind that Alexander taught them. His teachings are widely used, not only in hospitals for the relief of back pain and other disorders, but also as part of the curriculum in several drama and music colleges. Sports centres, too, often include study of his methods. It is important to realize, however, that the Alexander principle cannot be self-taught but requires a certain amount of instruction from a specialist teacher.

The Alexander principle is a coordinated approach to the health of both body and mind. It maintains that most of us function inefficiently both physically and mentally because we develop tension habits in our muscles. This manifests itself in the form of back problems, rheumatic disorders and the whole range of tension and stress problems – asthma, hypertension, tension headaches, anxiety states and general fatigue can all be caused by this misuse. It is apparent, too, in the majority of people who cope well in normal circumstances but find that their bodies let them down when they want to give of their best, whether it be in a major crisis, competitive sport, making love or music. The Alexander principle teaches an intimate awareness of body use. If we know what our bodies are doing and why, we can employ them to better advantage.

The most important area of body misuse, according to Alexander, is centred round the head, neck and upper back, through which the most important blood vessels and nerves pass; it is here that the misuse of the body manifests itself most clearly. Faulty breathing patterns, for instance, throw the muscles of the lower neck and upper ribs into excessive spasm, while the eating and speaking mechanisms need good vertebral posture. Misuse often produces a hump on the back, created by wrongly distributed muscle tension. Re-education starts by developing an awareness of these abuses and subsequently at the most subtle level teaches the release of faulty tension patterns all over the body, which leads to a better postural balance.

Any movement requires a complicated inter-action of the messages sent by the brain and the nerves and muscles and even a simple act, such as sitting down, can involve misuse of the body – practically everybody upon sitting down throws the head back and stiffens and shortens the neck. Even when we are aware of this, it is impossible to alter the pattern immediately simply by being given a new set of directions.

The head and neck area must be gradually brought into correct alignment by gentle ma-nipulation on the part of the teacher as well as by verbal direction. These directions are not instruc-tions to be carried out by conscious effort, but are intended as a guide that the mind gradually absorbs, so that the body slowly reprogrammes itself into a more efficient use. Eventually a balance should be achieved so that no part of the body has to work harder than any other.

End-gaining

Too many people, according to the Alexander principle, aim purely for final goals without any thought of how they are going to be achieved. This can cause the muscles to tense up before even starting. With the Alexander principle you learn how to use the body at every stage of an action, thereby increasing its efficiency and reaching the ultimate goal as a logical conclusion of all the preceding actions. Much interest has been focused on this 'end-gaining' theory. Many sportsmen, dancers, even writers and musicians, have found that by following the Alexander principle they have released their talents to further heights as they become relieved from the inhibitions of the instinctive constraints put on them by an overstriving mind and body. This release from

Misuse of the muscles of the neck and back

Bending the head forwards to work instead of bending from the hips and keeping the spine straight is a common fault, particularly among sedentary office workers. The ribcage and lower back tend to slump downwards and a hump forms where the neck joins the back. This encourages misuse of the neck muscles so that when the head is lifted to look straight ahead, the forward curve of the neck is exaggerated (a). This forward curve of the neck and backward curve of the upper back may become so ingrained that the distortion is maintained when standing, forcing the lower back to curve forwards to compensate (b). Good use involves a minimal backward curve of the upper back and forward curve of the lower back (c).

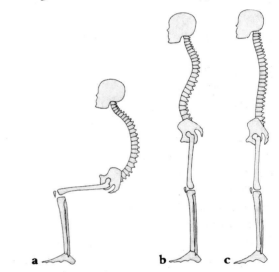

a   b   c

the obsession with the ultimate outcome of our actions can help everyone to enjoy a more relaxed way of life. When the body is freed of unnecessary tension, the mind will be freed also.

The Alexander principle is as much a mental exercise as a physical one and does not require a vigorous, exhausting routine. It can be helpful at a simple level, showing how to use muscles as they were designed to be used and therefore allowing them to work at their best, or it can be developed into a comprehensive awareness of body use in every situation, including rest. Many people resort to alcohol, tranquillizers, collapsing at the weekend or even self-induced hypnosis to relax. Alexander maintains that all these methods offer only temporary respite. A balanced resting state is an important part of the principle and offers as much relief as correct use during activity.

Daily Minimum Programme

Practised every day, these exercises will strengthen all the muscles of the body and will promote and maintain a supple figure. If you want to firm one particular area, supplement this programme with exercises from the following pages. Initially, repeat each sequence eight times; build up to between 30 and 40 repetitions, increasing your speed. Repeat the facial exercises only as often as is comfortable. Make the movements look attractive: move smoothly and stretch toes and fingers. Always try to breathe evenly. If you are under medical supervision or suffer from a weak back, consult your doctor before starting; never persist with an exercise that causes pain.

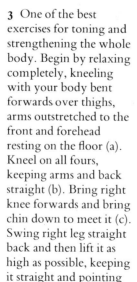

1 Standing with feet apart, bend from hips (a), and swing arms through legs, keeping arms straight but bending knees a little (b). Repeat.

Bend forwards in the same way, but place your hands, palms facing downwards, just in front of your feet (c). Bounce up until standing nearly straight (d) and down again.

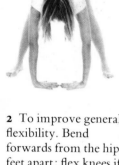

2 To improve general flexibility. Bend forwards from the hips, feet apart; flex knees if you are a beginner or have a weak back. Keeping arms straight, place hands on floor, palms down and fingers facing each other (a). Swing hips to the right and bend right knee sideways as far as possible, keeping feet and hands flat on floor and left leg straight (b). Swing over to the left, bending left knee, and repeat the movement to right and left.

As you become more flexible, bend right elbow as you swing to the right until your forearm lies on the floor at a right angle to your feet (c). Repeat to left.

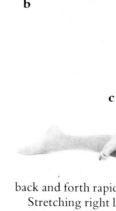

3 One of the best exercises for toning and strengthening the whole body. Begin by relaxing completely, kneeling with your body bent forwards over thighs, arms outstretched to the front and forehead resting on the floor (a). Kneel on all fours, keeping arms and back straight (b). Bring right knee forwards and bring chin down to meet it (c). Swing right leg straight back and then lift it as high as possible, keeping it straight and pointing the toes (d). Swing it

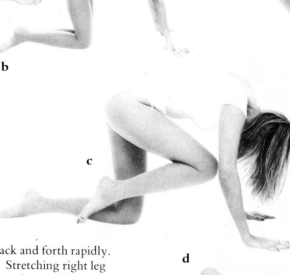

back and forth rapidly.

Stretching right leg straight out to the back, rapidly raise and lower it without letting it touch the ground.

4 To firm the buttocks. Stand with feet together, knees flexed so that your back is straight, and hands on hips to feel the action of your muscles. Roll your pelvis back and out (a) and then forwards and up (b), swinging back and forth in a smooth U-shaped movement, keeping stomach and buttock muscles taut.

5 These half sit-ups help to firm the abdominal muscles. Lie facing upwards, knees bent and feet apart, hands clasped behind head (a). Lift head as high as possible, keeping shoulders and spine on floor (b). Repeat.

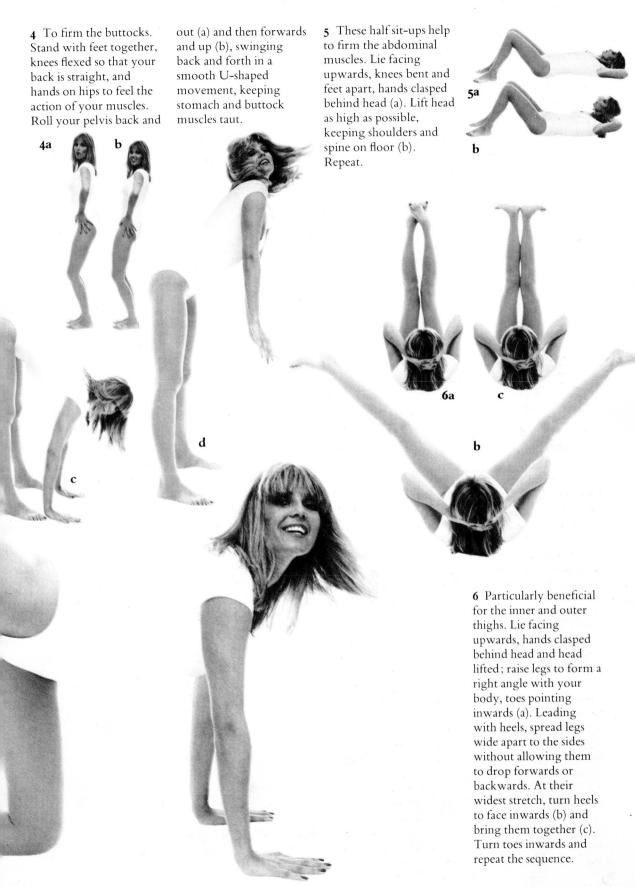

6 Particularly beneficial for the inner and outer thighs. Lie facing upwards, hands clasped behind head and head lifted; raise legs to form a right angle with your body, toes pointing inwards (a). Leading with heels, spread legs wide apart to the sides without allowing them to drop forwards or backwards. At their widest stretch, turn heels to face inwards (b) and bring them together (c). Turn toes inwards and repeat the sequence.

Abdomen and Waist

Right To tone waist muscles. Stand with feet apart, knees slightly bent and arms stretched out in front of you (a). Swing arms sharply to the right, keeping them level with shoulders; move from the waist upwards only, feeling hips, legs and feet locked firm (b). Pause, and twist swiftly to the left. Swing from left to right several times, pausing at the furthest point of each twist.

Repeat the swinging movement, bending right knee as arms swing to the right, left knee as arms swing to the left (c), allowing your body to turn further; twist from the hips.

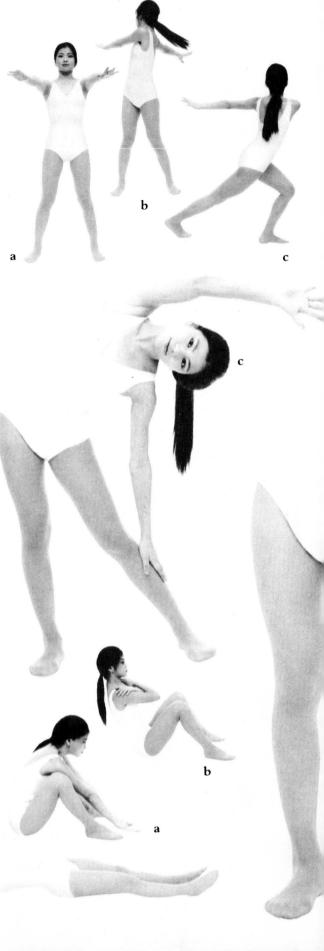

Above Stand with feet apart, knees slightly bent and arms at sides. Bend to the left from waist, running left hand down left leg and bending right elbow to bring right hand up right side (a). Do not lean forwards. Take left hand down as far as possible (b) and bring right arm up and over head, fingers pointing to the left (c). Do not allow right arm to touch head. Bring left arm up parallel to the right, so both arms are stretched horizontally to the left (d). Hold for as long as you can, then slowly straighten up by reversing the sequence; repeat to the right.

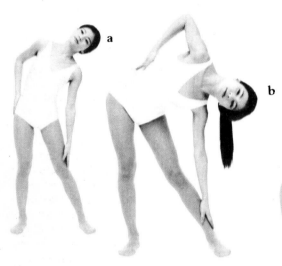

Right For a flat stomach. Lie facing upwards, arms above head. Stretch fingers and toes away from each other and press spine into floor. Clench abdominal muscles for a few seconds and release; repeat.

Right Lie face up, feet apart, legs bent up and arms above head. Sit up, swinging arms over between feet (a). Cross arms, hands on shoulders, and lie back (b). Repeat.

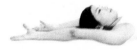

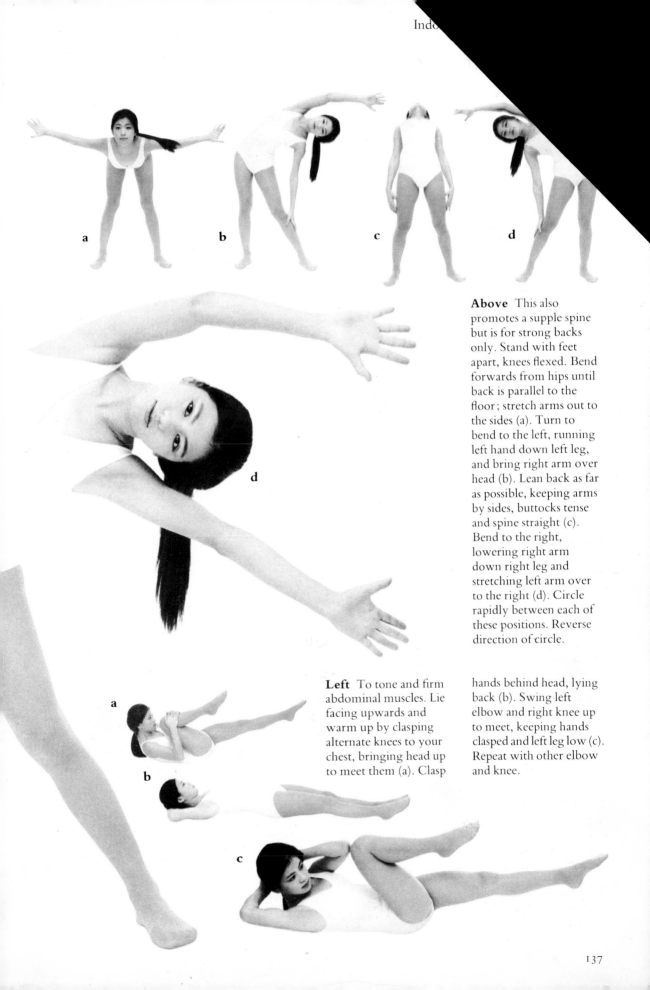

a   b   c   d

d

Above This also promotes a supple spine but is for strong backs only. Stand with feet apart, knees flexed. Bend forwards from hips until back is parallel to the floor; stretch arms out to the sides (a). Turn to bend to the left, running left hand down left leg, and bring right arm over head (b). Lean back as far as possible, keeping arms by sides, buttocks tense and spine straight (c). Bend to the right, lowering right arm down right leg and stretching left arm over to the right (d). Circle rapidly between each of these positions. Reverse direction of circle.

Left To tone and firm abdominal muscles. Lie facing upwards and warm up by clasping alternate knees to your chest, bringing head up to meet them (a). Clasp hands behind head, lying back (b). Swing left elbow and right knee up to meet, keeping hands clasped and left leg low (c). Repeat with other elbow and knee.

a

b

c

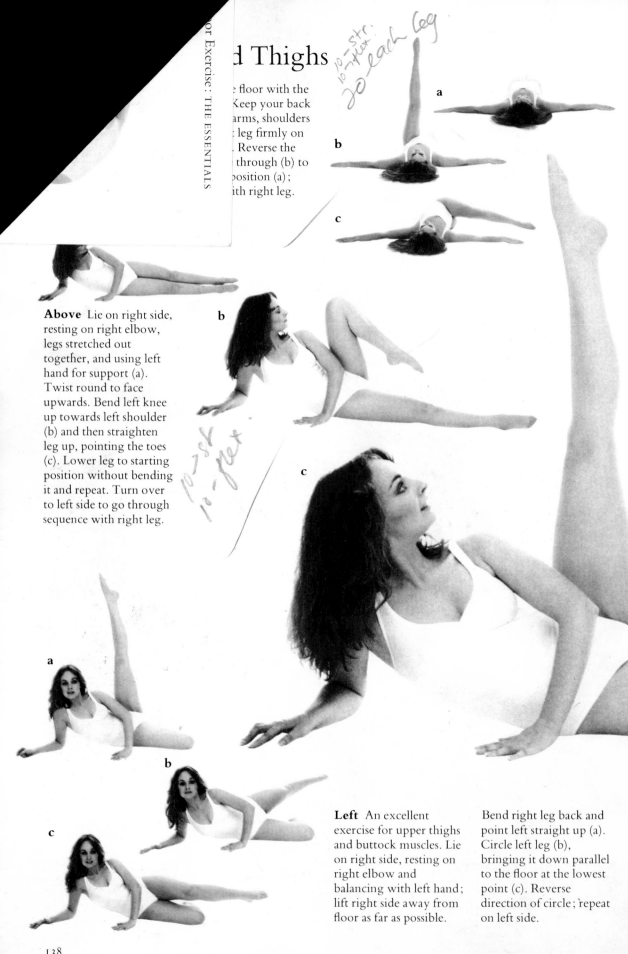

d Thighs

10-str.
10-flet.
20-each leg

e floor with the
Keep your back
arms, shoulders
leg firmly on
Reverse the
through (b) to
position (a);
ith right leg.

a

b

c

Above Lie on right side, resting on right elbow, legs stretched out together, and using left hand for support (a). Twist round to face upwards. Bend left knee up towards left shoulder (b) and then straighten leg up, pointing the toes (c). Lower leg to starting position without bending it and repeat. Turn over to left side to go through sequence with right leg.

b

c

10-st.
10-flet.

a

b

c

Left An excellent exercise for upper thighs and buttock muscles. Lie on right side, resting on right elbow and balancing with left hand; lift right side away from floor as far as possible.

Bend right leg back and point left straight up (a). Circle left leg (b), bringing it down parallel to the floor at the lowest point (c). Reverse direction of circle; repeat on left side.

Right Especially good for stretching and strengthening the muscles of upper hips and thighs. Lie on your back with arms outstretched and legs vertical, toes pointing up (a). Keeping arms firmly on the floor, lower right leg to the right until it is lying on the floor; hold head straight and try to keep left leg vertical (b). Follow with left leg so that both legs are stretched out to the right (c). Raise left leg back to position (b) and then right leg to bring you into starting position (a). Repeat sequence to left.

Below Tones and firms the inner and outer thighs. Crouch down, on tiptoes, feet together, hands on the floor on either side of feet; lean forwards over thighs (a). Twist knees to right, and bounce up and down on tiptoes (b); repeat to left (c). Keep upper half of body facing forwards as legs turn, using hands for balance. Stretch right leg out to the side, keeping left one bent and hands central (d). Walk hands to the right, turning from hips (e) and gently reach towards right knee with forehead (f). Repeat on left side.

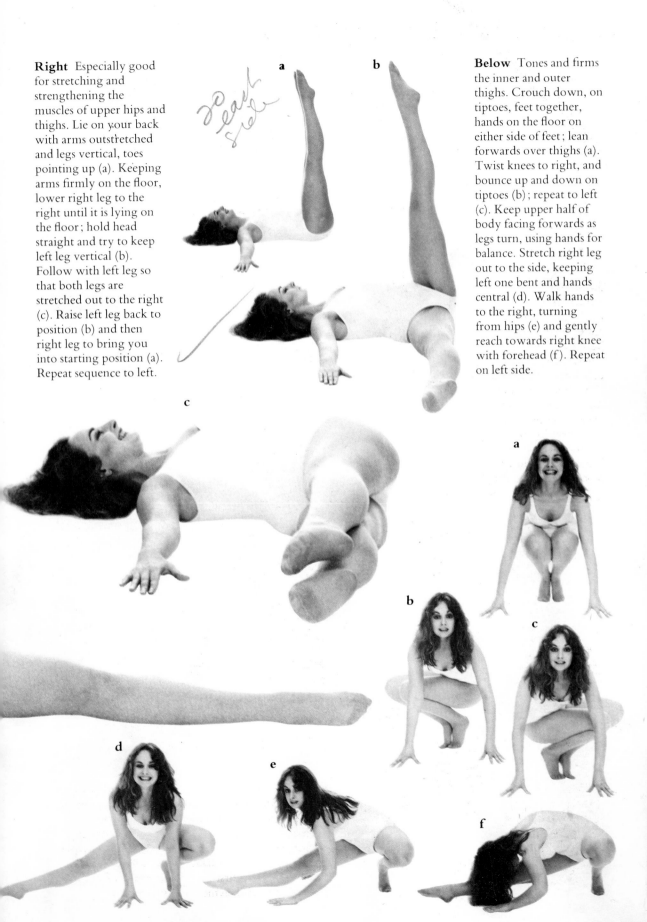

Back

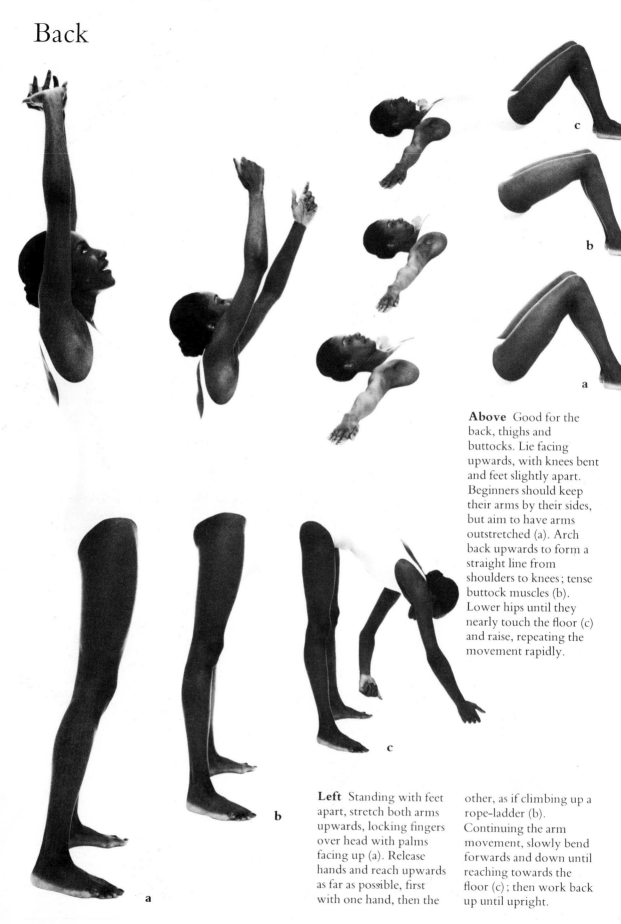

Above Good for the back, thighs and buttocks. Lie facing upwards, with knees bent and feet slightly apart. Beginners should keep their arms by their sides, but aim to have arms outstretched (a). Arch back upwards to form a straight line from shoulders to knees; tense buttock muscles (b). Lower hips until they nearly touch the floor (c) and raise, repeating the movement rapidly.

Left Standing with feet apart, stretch both arms upwards, locking fingers over head with palms facing up (a). Release hands and reach upwards as far as possible, first with one hand, then the other, as if climbing up a rope-ladder (b). Continuing the arm movement, slowly bend forwards and down until reaching towards the floor (c); then work back up until upright.

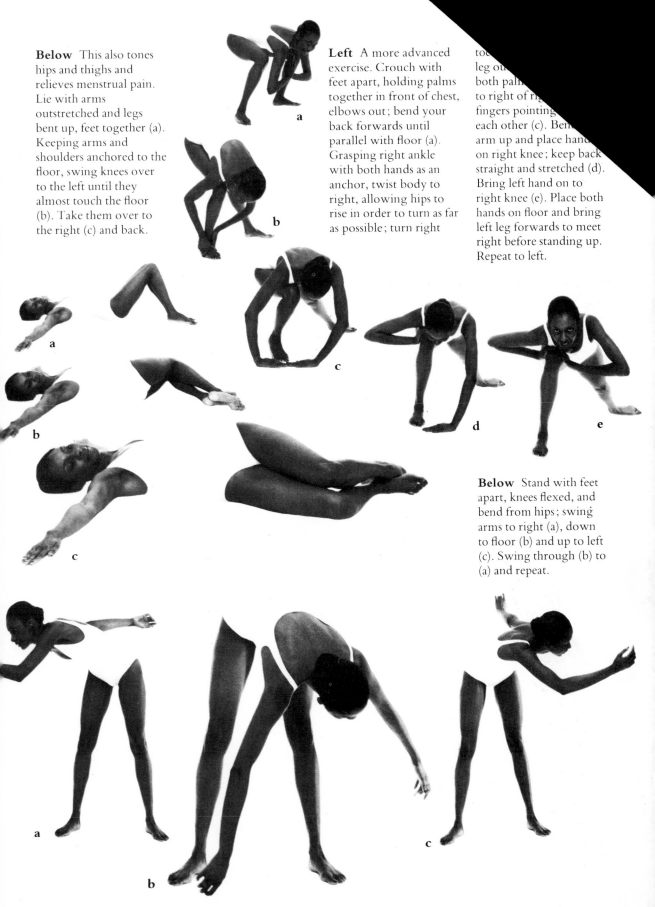

Below This also tones hips and thighs and relieves menstrual pain. Lie with arms outstretched and legs bent up, feet together (a). Keeping arms and shoulders anchored to the floor, swing knees over to the left until they almost touch the floor (b). Take them over to the right (c) and back.

Left A more advanced exercise. Crouch with feet apart, holding palms together in front of chest, elbows out; bend your back forwards until parallel with floor (a). Grasping right ankle with both hands as an anchor, twist body to right, allowing hips to rise in order to turn as far as possible; turn right toe... leg ou... both palm... to right of r... fingers pointing... each other (c). Be... arm up and place hand... on right knee; keep back straight and stretched (d). Bring left hand on to right knee (e). Place both hands on floor and bring left leg forwards to meet right before standing up. Repeat to left.

Below Stand with feet apart, knees flexed, and bend from hips; swing arms to right (a), down to floor (b) and up to left (c). Swing through (b) to (a) and repeat.

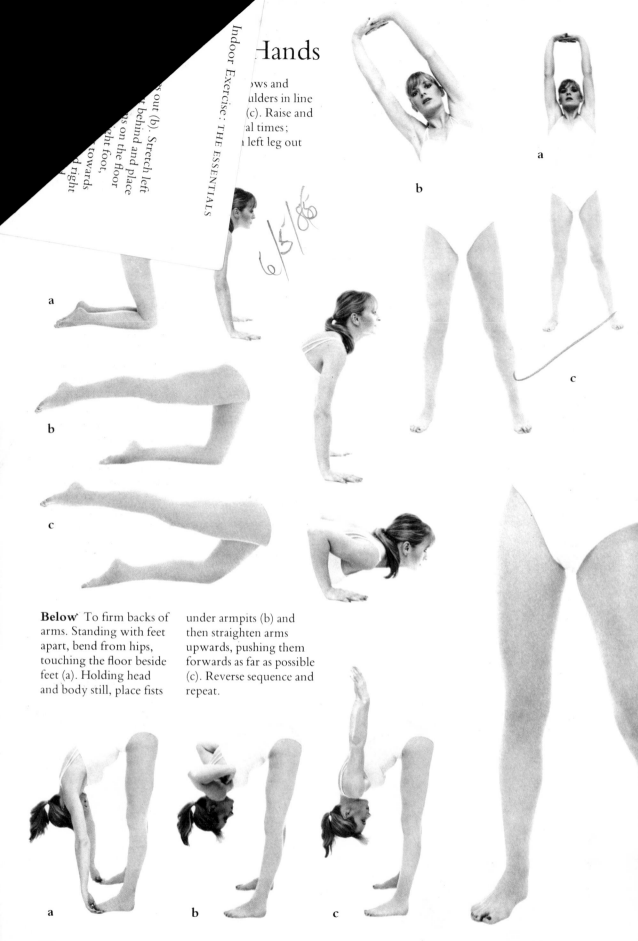

Hands

...ows and
...ulders in line
... (c). Raise and
...al times;
... left leg out

...s out (b). Stretch left
...r behind and place
...s on the floor
...ght foot,
...towards
...d right

6/5/80

a

b

c

a

b

c

a

b

c

Below To firm backs of
arms. Standing with feet
apart, bend from hips,
touching the floor beside
feet (a). Holding head
and body still, place fists
under armpits (b) and
then straighten arms
upwards, pushing them
forwards as far as possible
(c). Reverse sequence and
repeat.

a

b

c

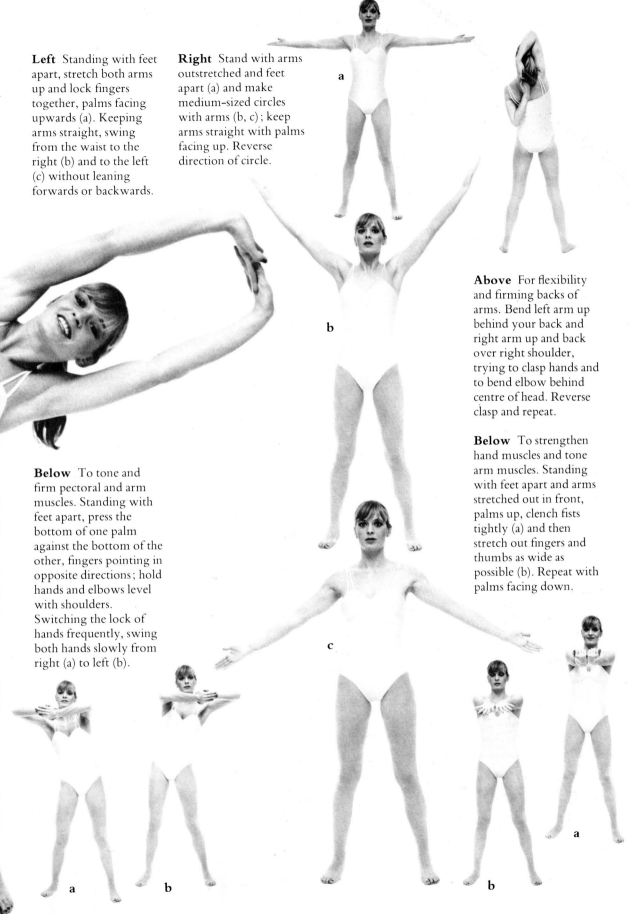

Left Standing with feet apart, stretch both arms up and lock fingers together, palms facing upwards (a). Keeping arms straight, swing from the waist to the right (b) and to the left (c) without leaning forwards or backwards.

Right Stand with arms outstretched and feet apart (a) and make medium-sized circles with arms (b, c); keep arms straight with palms facing up. Reverse direction of circle.

Above For flexibility and firming backs of arms. Bend left arm up behind your back and right arm up and back over right shoulder, trying to clasp hands and to bend elbow behind centre of head. Reverse clasp and repeat.

Below To strengthen hand muscles and tone arm muscles. Standing with feet apart and arms stretched out in front, palms up, clench fists tightly (a) and then stretch out fingers and thumbs as wide as possible (b). Repeat with palms facing down.

Below To tone and firm pectoral and arm muscles. Standing with feet apart, press the bottom of one palm against the bottom of the other, fingers pointing in opposite directions; hold hands and elbows level with shoulders. Switching the lock of hands frequently, swing both hands slowly from right (a) to left (b).

Legs and Feet

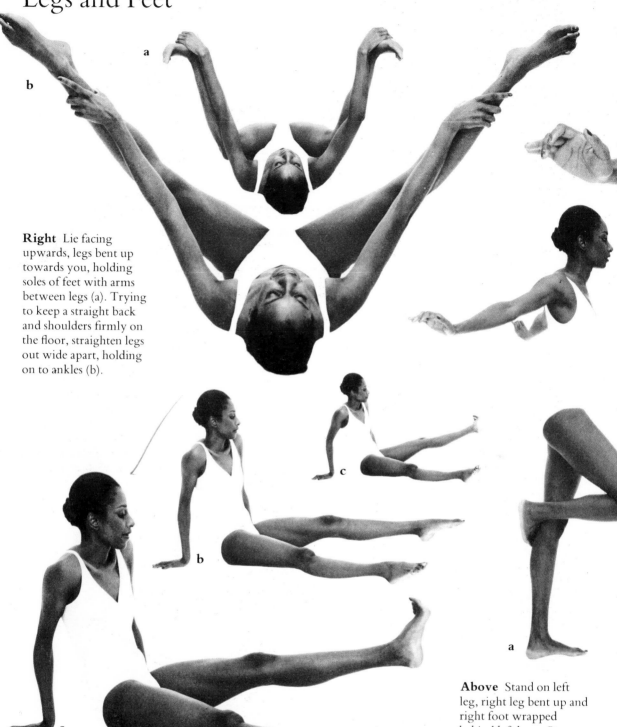

Right Lie facing upwards, legs bent up towards you, holding soles of feet with arms between legs (a). Trying to keep a straight back and shoulders firmly on the floor, straighten legs out wide apart, holding on to ankles (b).

Above Helps to stretch and strengthen all the muscles of the leg, particularly the calf and ankle. Sit with legs straight out, hands on the floor behind you. Lift left leg a little off the ground and flex left toes towards (a) and then away from you. Keeping left foot up, swing leg in towards centre (b), pointing toes inwards, and to the left, pointing toes out (c). Swing from side to side. Repeat sequence with right foot.

Above Stand on left leg, right leg bent up and right foot wrapped behind left knee. Stare at a fixed point and hold, arms outstretched for balance; keep back straight and head up (a). When you feel stable, rise up on to ball of left foot (b) and down again. Repeat several times and then switch to right leg.

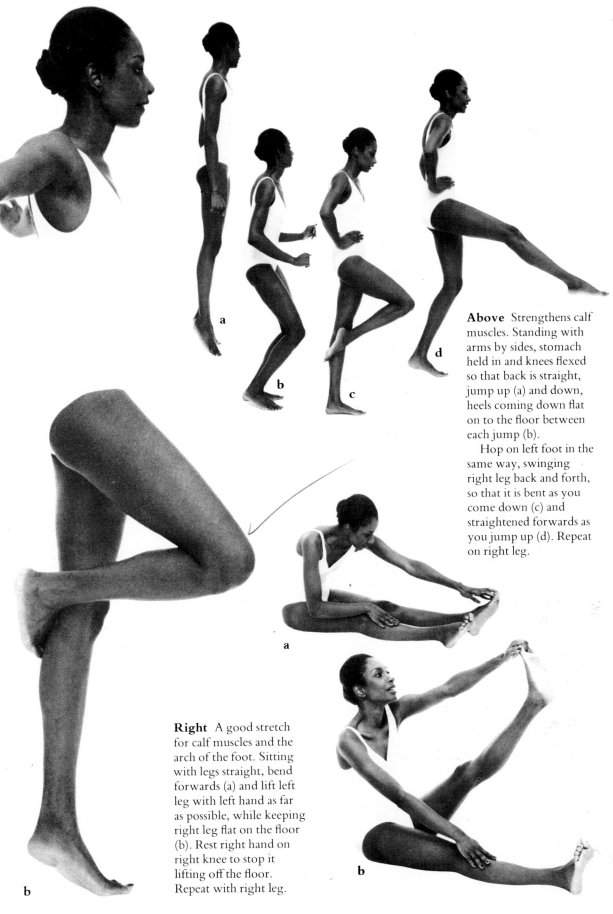

Above Strengthens calf muscles. Standing with arms by sides, stomach held in and knees flexed so that back is straight, jump up (a) and down, heels coming down flat on to the floor between each jump (b).

Hop on left foot in the same way, swinging right leg back and forth, so that it is bent as you come down (c) and straightened forwards as you jump up (d). Repeat on right leg.

Right A good stretch for calf muscles and the arch of the foot. Sitting with legs straight, bend forwards (a) and lift left leg with left hand as far as possible, while keeping right leg flat on the floor (b). Rest right hand on right knee to stop it lifting off the floor. Repeat with right leg.

Face, Neck and Shoulders

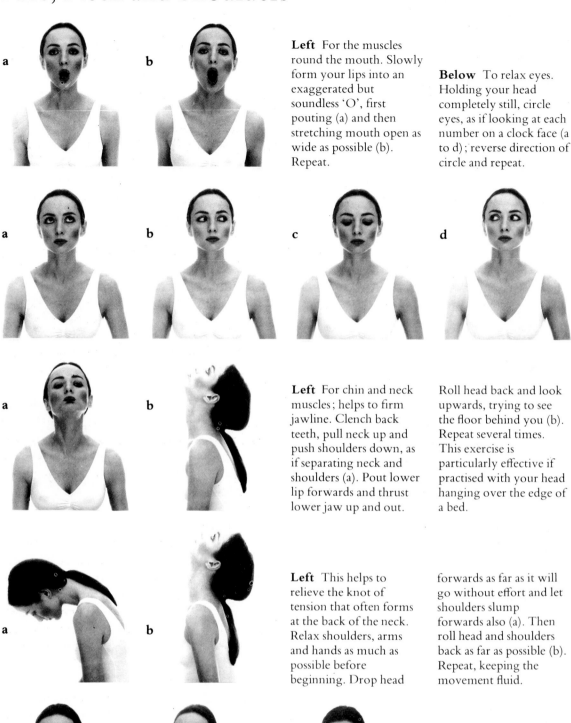

Left For the muscles round the mouth. Slowly form your lips into an exaggerated but soundless 'O', first pouting (a) and then stretching mouth open as wide as possible (b). Repeat.

Below To relax eyes. Holding your head completely still, circle eyes, as if looking at each number on a clock face (a to d); reverse direction of circle and repeat.

Left For chin and neck muscles; helps to firm jawline. Clench back teeth, pull neck up and push shoulders down, as if separating neck and shoulders (a). Pout lower lip forwards and thrust lower jaw up and out.

Roll head back and look upwards, trying to see the floor behind you (b). Repeat several times. This exercise is particularly effective if practised with your head hanging over the edge of a bed.

Left This helps to relieve the knot of tension that often forms at the back of the neck. Relax shoulders, arms and hands as much as possible before beginning. Drop head

forwards as far as it will go without effort and let shoulders slump forwards also (a). Then roll head and shoulders back as far as possible (b). Repeat, keeping the movement fluid.

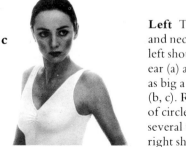

Left To relax shoulder and neck muscles. Raise left shoulder up towards ear (a) and then roll it in as big a circle as possible (b, c). Reverse direction of circle and repeat several times. Switch to right shoulder.

Ante- and Post-natal Exercises

Carrying the baby

During pregnancy the ligaments and joints of the body loosen so that extra room can be made in the pelvis to accommodate the baby. This is therefore a good time to start encouraging your body to be more flexible and to create new habits of regular exercise, correct posture, relaxation and good breathing.

While you are carrying the baby, your spine, abdominal muscles and pelvic floor (see pages 68–69) need to be strong enough to support the growing weight. Strong and supple leg muscles encourage good circulation, which helps prevent tiredness, cramp and varicose veins. Posture is also important when so much extra weight is concentrated in one area and maintaining the correct tilt of the pelvis is particularly beneficial (see pages 130–131). Good breathing and adequate relaxation help the whole body to function efficiently.

Having the baby

The abdominal muscles should be strong to help with delivery and the pelvic floor needs to be in good shape to cope with stretching as the baby passes through it. Suppleness in the hip joints, legs and feet helps you to move into useful positions for labour and birth, such as stooping or squatting. Good breathing and the ability to relax allow you to maintain control and to be as comfortable as possible during the labour, so helping both you and the baby in the delivery.

After the baby

After all the changes and hard work the body has been through during pregnancy, delivery and immediately after the birth, restoring it through exercise is essential if later problems, particularly with the pelvic floor, are to be avoided. The ability to relax and breathe well is helpful in coping with the anxieties and strains of parenthood. Looking after a small child involves hard physical work: if you are fit, you are less likely to tire easily, so you can enjoy and make the best of your baby's first years.

Babies spend a lot of time on the floor. If you can squat and sit on the floor comfortably, both of you will enjoy playing more and you will be maintaining suppleness in your hip, knee and ankle joints at the same time.

Ante-natal exercises

This gentle programme can be part of your relaxation time every day. If possible, try the exercises lying on your back to begin with, so that the trunk is fully supported. Place a cushion or two under your head if it makes you more comfortable. Gradually progress to doing the exercises sitting, first with the back supported and then without additional support, but proceed cautiously. Always be gentle with yourself.

If you find the ante-natal programme is not enough, you may safely add in as much of the post-natal programme as you feel is beneficial; but try not to strain or hold the breath.

Strengthening the pelvic floor

To strengthen the muscles of the pelvic floor during pregnancy and after the birth, try this exercise. Lift, tighten and squeeze the pelvic floor for a count of four, breathing normally, and then release. Practise this lying on the floor at first, but after a while you can do this exercise in any position, as often as possible; it can also be combined with pelvic tilts (see page 149). Do the pelvic floor exercise to keep the area strong and healthy, to encourage full enjoyment of sex and to help prevent incontinence and other problems later in life.

Dos and Don'ts

• Do not hold the breath, but relax, release and breathe well with the exercises. This will prepare you for breathing during labour. Take a deep breath before and after each exercise.

• Do not strain or overdo exercising. A little regular practice is the ideal. The exercises should be pleasant once initial stiffness has been overcome and should make you feel better; what the body enjoys it will ask you to repeat.

• Do not lie on your back and try to lift both legs up. This is far too strenuous and quite unnecessary. Instead follow the gentle but very effective exercises outlined in this programme.

• Do not do exercises that cause you to overarch and squeeze the small of the back.

• Turn on to your side to lie down or sit up.

• In late pregnancy lying on your back may become uncomfortable so avoid it.

• Repeat each exercise four times only.

Ante-natal Exercises

Right For spine, hips, knees and feet. Sitting with legs crossed, on a cushion if it is easier, breathe in and straighten spine, lifting front ribs. Breathe normally, keeping a straight spine, or rest if this is hard.

If this exercise is hard at first, rest your back against a wall for support. Progress to sitting with legs straight out together and then apart. Try to sit cross-legged often, even on a sofa. Stand up slowly after the exercise.

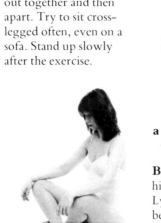

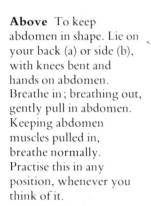

a

b

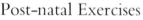

Above To keep abdomen in shape. Lie on your back (a) or side (b), with knees bent and hands on abdomen. Breathe in; breathing out, gently pull in abdomen. Keeping abdomen muscles pulled in, breathe normally. Practise this in any position, whenever you think of it.

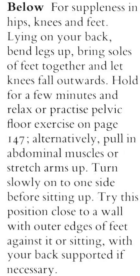

Below For suppleness in hips, knees and feet. Lying on your back, bend legs up, bring soles of feet together and let knees fall outwards. Hold for a few minutes and relax or practise pelvic floor exercise on page 147; alternatively, pull in abdominal muscles or stretch arms up. Turn slowly on to one side before sitting up. Try this position close to a wall with outer edges of feet against it or sitting, with your back supported if necessary.

Left For spine and abdomen. Stand with good posture, feet a little apart and arms at sides. Keeping feet firm, gently twist to the left (a) and to the right (b). Check your posture. Avoid this exercise if it hurts your lower back.

a

b

Below Improves posture. Lie on your back on the floor, arms stretched over head; breathe in and really stretch, pressing lower back and knees into floor. Breathe out and stop stretching. If this causes discomfort in lower back, place a cushion or two under thighs. If still uncomfortable, bend legs up with soles of feet flat on floor and stretch arms and trunk only. This exercise can also be practised sitting cross-legged with your back against a wall.

Post-natal Exercises

Right For abdomen and spine. Lie facing up, legs bent up to chest and hands clasped round knees (a). Breathe in, keeping head on floor. Breathing out, squeeze stomach down and press knees against chest, lifting head (b).

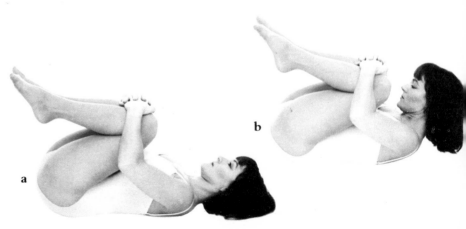

a

b

Below For spine, abdomen, hips and legs. Sit with legs straight, knees facing the ceiling and toes pointing up; sit on a cushion if it is easier. With hands on the floor behind you, shoulders down, try to sit up straight (a); rest. Gradually increase the length of time you hold the position and go on to sit without support of hands (b).

Below Good for lower back, tightens abdominal muscles at sides. Stand with feet apart, arms bent and fingertips resting on shoulders. Lift left hip towards left ribs (a), then right hip towards right ribs (b). Try this lying on your back or on all fours.

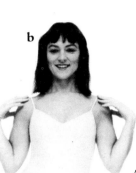

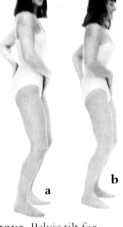

Above Pelvic tilt for improving posture. Standing with feet apart, knees slightly bent, place one hand on abdomen with fingertips on pubic bone, the other on lower back, fingers pointing down (a). Breathe in; breathe out and tilt pelvis, lifting pubic bone forwards and up (b). Hold position for a short while, breathing normally. Later, combine with tightening abdomen, buttocks and pelvic floor. Practise this exercise sitting on a chair or on the floor in any position.

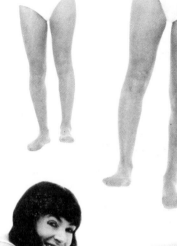

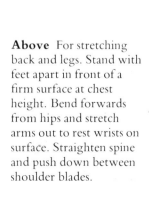

Above For stretching back and legs. Stand with feet apart in front of a firm surface at chest height. Bend forwards from hips and stretch arms out to rest wrists on surface. Straighten spine and push down between shoulder blades.

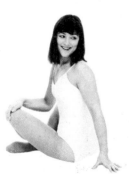

Above For spine and abdomen. Sitting cross-legged, spine straight and left hand on floor, take right hand to left knee and twist to left. Repeat to right.

A–Z of Exercise

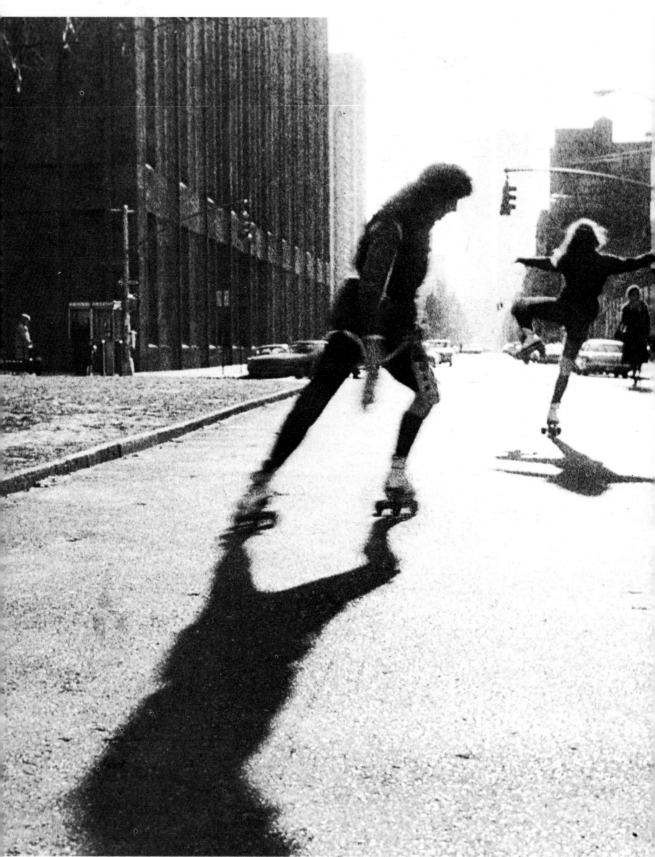

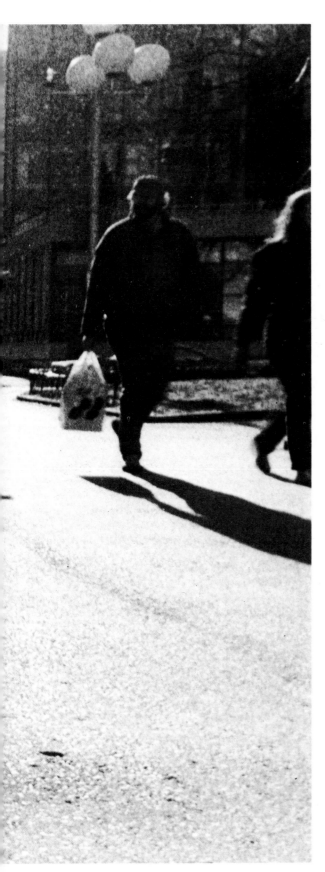

Calorie consumption figures in the following entries denote the approximate number of calories consumed by someone of 65 kg (150 lb) carrying out the sport over a half hour period; consumption varies according to how energetically the exercise is carried out. Asterisked figures are the author's suggestions based on known values of similar sports.

Archery (target)
*Less than 100 calories per half hour

Archery benefits the upper part of the body, i.e. arms, shoulders and chest. You need good eyesight, concentration and coordination, but there is no need to be particularly strong. Men and women compete together, although target distance ranges from 90 m (99 yd) as the greatest for men to 70 m (77 yd) for women. When practised under recognized international rules, archery has an unbroken safety record.

It is a complex skill: knowledge of equipment, the language and the simple mechanics of shooting arrows from a bow will help the aspiring archer, but coaching is the greatest help.

A club will probably be able to rent you the equipment for your first few visits. You need a bow – the modern type is of wood and fibreglass; arrows, made of aluminium alloy; a bracer to protect the arm; a tab or reinforced glove to protect the hand, and a quiver. No special clothing is needed, but for competitions green and white are the preferred colours.

The season runs through the summer, although many clubs organize indoor shooting in winter.

Variations: crossbow archery; field archery.

Athletics
Running 450 per half hour; calorie consumption for other activities varies according to the activity

Activities on the athletics track or field are divided into running, jumping, throwing or a combination of some or all of these. While athletics as a whole makes for complete physical fitness, each activity has its own benefits and appeals to different people and constitutions. If you are interested in athletics but unsure which branch would suit you, visit an athletics club or sports centre where you can try everything and get professional advice about your abilities.

Running: long- or middle-distance running promotes endurance, sprinting and hurdling develop leg strength and all are good for the heart and lungs.

Throwing requires and develops strength in the trunk and in the arms.

Long- and high-jumping develop coordination and flexibility while strengthening the leg muscles.

Weight training, under proper supervision in a gymnasium, is good preparation for all athletics and will help prevent strain and injury.

For warming up and training you will need training shoes and for all outdoor athletics spiked shoes. A singlet, shorts and tracksuit are also desirable.

Badminton

175 calories per half hour

Played vigorously, badminton is fine exercise for the heart and lungs, while it also promotes suppleness throughout the body and builds up powers of endurance. As an overhead game it is especially good for strengthening the back and shoulders and improving posture. Although it is strenuous at a high level, you can enjoy a more social game without overexertion, particularly mixed doubles. Provided you are reasonably fit, you can take up badminton well into middle age.

The beginner must master coordination of racket and shuttle and learn to make all strokes with the wrist, not the armswing as in tennis. The idea is to 'throw' the racket head at the shuttle early in its flight over the high suspended net; a point is won if the opponent on the other side cannot return it before it hits the ground. Play is to 11, 15 or 21 points and a match is usually the best of three games.

The wooden or steel racket weighs a mere 110–140 g (4–5 oz) and the nylon or feather shuttle a fraction of that. A club will often hire out rackets and shuttles. White shorts or skirt and shirt and white rubber-soled shoes are worn. A wooden-framed racket should be stored in a press.

Badminton is an indoor game, played on a wooden-floored court, but it can be played outside on grass providing it is not very windy.

Canoeing

115 calories per half hour

Canoeing improves the efficiency of the heart and lungs and builds up strength in the top half of the body. All canoeists should be able to swim and in rough water or the sea should always wear a lifejacket. All ages can enjoy the fun of canoeing, from young children to the over 70s, but a good standard of fitness is essential because it is a strenuous form of activity.

As canoeing can be dangerous, it is recommended that all aspiring canoeists take an approved course. You will be provided with a canoe, paddle and usually all the clothing, which consists of wetsuit, lifejacket and safety helmet.

You can canoe on lakes, rivers and the sea, but obviously rushing currents call for a greater degree of skill than calm, flat water. Many rivers are graded to international standards of difficulty.

Climbing

A demanding rather than a giving sport, climbing undoubtedly improves certain aspects of fitness, but a high level of physical fitness is an essential prerequisite. You should be supple and agile and have the ability to maintain strength for long periods. You do not need to be bulging with muscles: some of the best climbers are small and neat, or long and lean, but they are always superbly fit.

Climbing is fun, but dangerous. It is not a sport to approach on your own or in an amateurish way and is far more fun in a group. The best way to learn to climb is to join a club with a training scheme. A course in climbing or mountaineering will teach you all the basic techniques and enable you to choose the right equipment such as boots, clothing and ropes. A club will generally provide much of the equipment on loan.

Cricket

120 calories per half hour

Good for general mobility and muscle strength, the sporadic bursts of activity make cricket very demanding, particularly on the heart and lungs. You need to be fit, and if taking up cricket after about 30 you should play some other sport seriously to provide adequate training.

Two teams of 11 players each play on a grass wicket with stumps 20m (22 yd) apart. The batting team aims to make as many runs as possible and the bowling side aims to dismiss the batsmen for as few runs as possible. Although cricket is traditionally a man's game, cricket for women is a flourishing and quite separate sport in its own right, with some variations such as a lighter ball. Equipment, which is generally provided by clubs, consists of bat, leather ball and, for women, white or cream divided skirt and shirt, knee-high socks and white boots with spiked or rubber soles. Pads and gloves are worn by batsmen and wicket-keeper.

Cricket is a summer game, but fitness training goes on all year round.

Croquet

In terms of energy expenditure, croquet is too light to get the lungs and heart working hard or to exercise the muscles to any marked degree, but it is an enjoyable, skilful and serious game if taken beyond the 'teaparty' level. It is leisurely and painstaking, requiring subtlety and guile in the use of tactics, and is one of the few

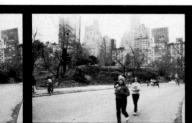
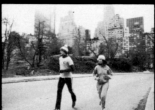
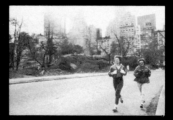
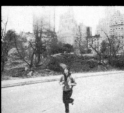

games where men and women can achieve equal prowess.

Play is either between two opponents or two teams of two players. The object is to drive balls, two different coloured ones to each side, through a series of six metal hoops spaced out on a lawn, finishing by striking a wooden post. Players hit the ball with long-handled wooden mallets. The hoops must be negotiated in a certain order and complex rules govern the playing of shots, making croquet an entertaining obstacle race.

Played at home on the lawn, croquet requires no special clothing apart from well-fitting rubber-soled shoes. Club players usually wear white.

Joining a club is the best way for the serious player to improve their game and a club will hire you a mallet to begin with.

Croquet is chiefly a summer game.

Cycling
330 calories per half hour

Cycling is very good exercise for the legs and for the heart and lungs. Although the hunched position of a racing cyclist can encourage shallow breathing, conventional straight handlebars promote good posture and make cycling good for the back.

Age, arthritis, heart or lung conditions, including asthma, are no bar to cycling, providing you have first consulted your doctor.

Which bicycle you choose depends on what you want it for: the modern small-wheel cycles, some folding, are ideal for cycling round town or to shops or office. The conventional 66 cm (26 in) wheeled bicycles are for those who like cycling for its own sake. Racing bicycles are for serious sport and may have up to ten gears.

Racers need special shoes and light absorbent clothing such as shorts and shirt, whereas the more casual cyclist can wear trousers or a skirt and well-fitting shoes. All cyclists should avoid flapping trouser legs, which could catch in the wheels.

Dance
Modern and disco 300 calories per half hour; ballet 200★; ballroom 200★; folk 225★; tap 200★

All forms of dancing are excellent exercise. They aid coordination, flexibility and suppleness, are good for the heart and lungs and, if done energetically, will certainly help you lose weight. Changing into more elegant clothes or a pretty-coloured leotard and exercising to music also has a psychological effect, which is just as important as the physical one.

Ballet: calls for great discipline and control and should be started at an early age. You can return to ballet after a break and still enjoy it. You need leotard, tights and ballet shoes.

Ballroom dancing: few adults are natural dancers, so it is a matter of learning and practising technique. Though formal and controlled, it is a social activity, especially in team dancing. You can begin at any age. Court shoes with a 6–7 cm (2½–3 in) heel are best and soles should be light and flexible; never wear new shoes. For classes, casual clothes such as skirt and shirt are fine.

Folk or country dance: much less formal and much more social than ballroom dancing, folk or country dancing usually takes place in village halls and the atmosphere is high spirited with participants intent on having a good time rather than being stylish. Inexperienced dancers can easily and quickly pick up the steps at any age by participating or by attending special classes. Dress is casual: skirt and shirt, low heels.

Jazz, modern and disco: all these forms depend on the individual's skill at improvisation. Movements are based largely on gymnastics, which makes them good keep-fit exercises. The younger you start the better, because you need to be uninhibited and imaginative, besides very flexible and relaxed.

Tap dancing: can be done solo or as a group, the aim in both instances being to work out a routine of steps. You need flexible ankles and feet, but do not necessarily have to do high kicks, so you can take up tap at any age, provided you build up slowly.

Fencing
150 calories per half hour

Fencing provides all-over flexibility, muscle strength in the legs particularly and is good exercise for the heart and lungs. You can fence in a fast, fierce way and use up a lot of energy or have a more leisurely, gentle bout, which makes fencing suitable for all ages.

It is essentially a game of tactics. Before you can fight in safety you must have professional instruction, which will involve a reasonably long period of training in proper technique before you are ready to engage in freeplay. French is the main language of fencing, although some terms are English and Italian.

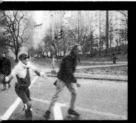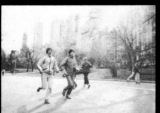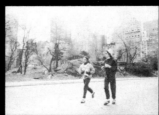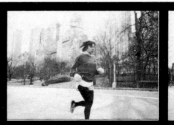

The aim of fencing is to score the prescribed number of hits on your opponent's target area – her trunk – before she can do the same to you. Generally, five hits is the agreed figure.

Fencing clubs usually have a pool of equipment, especially for beginners. You will need a foil – a light sword with its tip protected by a plastic button; a fine wire mesh mask; a padded jacket and strong gloves. Loose tracksuit trousers and rubber-soled shoes are adequate.

Clubs fence throughout the year, in a gym or hall with a wooden floor.

Golf

125 calories per half hour

The main physical benefit derived from golf is from the walking involved, but there is also the twisting movement for the drive, which is good for the waistline; regular energetic playing is necessary, however, for either benefit to be marked. It is possible to enjoy the fresh air, exercise and social side of golf without ever being very proficient or athletic.

Golf can be started at any age. The object of the game is to play your ball into a series of holes using the minimum number of strokes. Individuals can compete against one another or partners play together with either two or four balls, usually scoring hole by hole. Courses are set out with either nine or 18 holes.

A full set of golf clubs comprises 14, but beginners usually start with up to seven. Three types of clubs are used for different strokes – woods, irons and a putter. Beginners should try to buy their clubs secondhand, if possible with the advice of a professional, as a full set of new clubs is expensive. If you are lefthanded, it is worth trying to obtain lefthanded clubs. Special spiked shoes are needed and optional extras include a trolley, a golfing umbrella and a lefthand glove (or righthand if lefthanded) for better grip. The other expense is joining a golf club, most of which are fully subscribed and have a waiting list; a beginner would be better to start on a public course under the instruction of a professional.

Golf can be played all the year round.

Gymnastics

★220 calories per half hour

Good for flexibility and coordination, gymnastics is best started young when fitness is at a peak, but once a basic level of competence has been reached it can be enjoyed well into middle age. Gymnastics calls for great determination and dedication, but the grace and control achieved are proportionately rewarding. The creative aspect and the possibility for self-expression are particularly appealing.

Trampolining helps to develop the qualities of balance, rhythm and endurance needed for gymnastics, and is a sport in itself.

Gymnastics divides into floor and apparatus work. Floor is the more creative, while apparatus calls for strength and endurance. Supervision is essential for gymnastics and trampoline.

The most practical clothing is a leotard, with no tights, shoes or socks.

Hang-gliding

Hang-gliding is exciting and exhilarating – you literally fly like a bird – but the exercise comes from the walking involved to reach the elevated take-off point. With a heavy craft in tow a 100 m (330 ft) hill can seem like a mountain. Anyone reasonably fit can hang-glide but must have proper instruction at a school. It can be a dangerous sport.

The pilot is suspended by a harness from the hang-glider, which looks like a giant canvas kite, and controls movement in the air by moving a triangular control frame. The aim is to use the wind to stay in the air as long as possible.

A school will provide glider and helmet; you need your own warm windproof clothes, even in summer, boots that give ankle support and gloves that will not slip on the control frame.

Hang-gliding goes on all year, subject to weather and prevailing wind conditions.

Hockey

★250 calories per half hour

Good exercise for the heart and lungs, hockey also improves flexibility of the arms and legs and strengthens the body in general.

Each team of 11 players aims to get the hard leather-covered ball into the opponents' goal by hitting and passing it along the field with a curved stick.

The best way to learn and play hockey is to join a club and with good tuition you will soon become proficient enough to enjoy a game.

The size of a hockey stick depends on your weight and

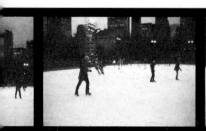
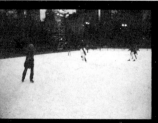
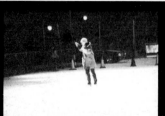
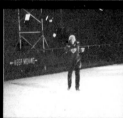

height, but what matters most is that the stick should be comfortable and easy to use. Boots generally have moulded rubber soles and can be used indoors, although hockey is almost always played on outdoor pitches. Women wear knee-socks, shorts or skirt and shirt. The goalkeeper and sometimes other players wear pads and face guards.

Hockey is played through the winter.

Ice-skating

200 calories per half hour

Graceful and exhilarating, skating is good for general mobility, circulation, posture and weight control. Speed skating is the most energetic and beneficial. Skating is probably the best sport for coordination, and the music that accompanies skating at a rink encourages rhythm and self-expression.

Age is no barrier: anyone can get along quite well after only one professional lesson. Dancing and figure skating are for the more proficient skater.

Skates and boots are the only essential equipment and can be hired at a rink. Guards keep the blades sharp when not in use. Boots need to be at least half a size smaller than your shoes and should be worn with tights or thin socks so that they feel like an extension of your foot. Trousers and sweater are acceptable casual wear for skating; frilly dresses look silly unless you are a really good skater. Gloves and hat are useful extras for beginners.

Be wary of skating on frozen ponds and lakes.

Isometrics

Isometric exercises are exercises *without movement*, in which the muscles work against other muscles or against immovable objects. They are good for strengthening all the muscles of the body, but do not provide any exercise for the heart and lungs, nor do they help flexibility of the joints; an isometric programme should therefore be complemented by another form of exercise involving movement, such as running or jogging. Isometrics can be dangerous for the heart as they put it under strain: any isometric programme needs to be done carefully and for no longer than the prescribed time. It can take as little as 90 seconds to exercise the whole body.

The great advantage of isometrics is that you need no special equipment or facilities and the programme can be completed quickly, at any time.

Isotonics

In isotonic exercises, movements are performed against the body's own weight or some outside force: weight-lifting is a prime example. Muscles are strengthened and developed but women do not need to fear, for only if such exercises are practised frequently to a very high level will the muscle development be marked. Research has shown that muscle bulk depends on the male hormone testosterone, which is present only in a small quantity in women, not on weight-lifting.

As with isometrics, isotonics do not exercise the heart or lungs, so some additional form of exercise needs to be taken, such as swimming or jogging, to provide a rounded programme. Under instruction in a gymnasium you will progress slowly and safely without strain. It is important not to rush isotonics but to build up slowly, taking rests to allow the body to recover between sessions. You can take up isotonics at any time, but the younger you are the more beneficial they are likely to be.

You need the facilities of a gym and specialized equipment such as weights and an inclined board, which are found in most sports centres and health clubs.

Jogging

300 calories per half hour

Jogging is excellent for heart, lungs and circulation. The more you jog, the more calories you burn up and the stronger your muscles become. Almost anyone of any age can jog safely; even if your health is poor, provided your doctor approves, you can jog. No tuition is needed because the human body is designed for running and the action of jogging comes naturally. It becomes easier with practice and as you lose self-consciousness and learn to relax. Keeping the fingers slightly curled helps to promote relaxation, as does a good landing; you should land on the heels and pivot off from the toes.

You do not have to achieve any particular speed, nor is it necessary to jog every day. Build up gradually to 15 minutes three times a week, more if you can manage it and as you become more proficient.

Shorts and T-shirt are fine for good weather; trousers and sweater or tracksuit are ideal for cool days. Shoes should be proper jogging shoes with thick pliable soles, good padding round the ankles and instep support. They vary considerably in price but what matters is how they feel while you are jogging.

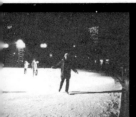 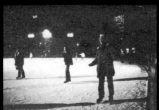 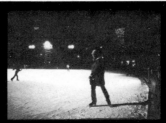 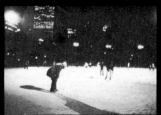

Jogging can be done anywhere, at any time of year, but grass is easier on the feet than pavements.

Judo

A form of exercise that uses all the muscles in the body, judo improves mobility and muscle strength and benefits the heart and lungs. The Japanese sport of judo was developed from Jiu-jitsu, a Chinese system of unarmed combat. Knowledge of judo does not mean that you can beat off an attacker, as it is not in itself a form of self-defence (for this see **Karate**) – translated, judo means 'the gentle way'. However, many courses, especially those for women, also include instruction in self-defence.

Although strength does count, the aim of judo is to overbalance your opponent and throw by skill. Judo is safe if practised properly and only on others who have a knowledge of judo. The first principle taught is the correct way to fall without hurting yourself.

The only equipment needed is a thick canvas jacket and thinner trousers, both white, tied with a belt, the colour of which denotes your level of achievement. Judo is practised on special rubber mats and is generally taught at clubs and adult education classes.

Karate

Karate is a form of unarmed combat with the same beneficial effect on overall muscle strength, mobility and the heart and lungs as judo. It consists of kicking, punching and striking techniques with the blocking required to defend against them. If you are interested in self-defence – karate is a martial art – take up karate. However, in karate as a sport, all the potentially damaging movements are controlled and body contact is light and limited.

Karate sounds difficult, but is not, and women are often better at it than men. Many of the exercises involved are stretching, keep-fit type, which appeal to women, and the movements are graceful. It is not necessary to be particularly strong, as strength is built up as you learn speed and agility. You do need to be fit, however, and it is hard work for anyone over 30 who is unused to sport.

As with judo, contestants progress through grades, or 'dans', denoting prowess and indicated by the colour of the sash worn on the waist.

Other martial arts: Aikado; Jiu-jitsu; Kendo; Kung Fu; Tae Kwondo; Tang Soo Do.

Lacrosse

★250 calories per half hour

Good for muscle strength and flexibility in the arms and legs and energetic exercise for the heart and lungs, lacrosse is one of the fastest outdoor team games.

You need to be fit and strong, although you can build up both these qualities through the game.

The men's game is more dangerous than the women's and for this reason men often wear protective masks; played properly the women's game is neither dangerous nor hard to learn.

The game is played by two opposing teams of twelve a side or increasingly seven a side (this version also varies in other respects). Each team tries to score goals into the opponents' net at either end of a pitch 92 m (300 ft) long. Each player holds a 'crosse', a stick with a triangular net at the top, and the solid rubber ball is caught in this net and thrown to another player. In a good game the ball hardly touches the ground.

Equipment, which can be hired from clubs and groups, consists of a stick and ball, socks and canvas boots with indented rubber soles, skirt or shorts.

Traditional lacrosse is played outside throughout the winter but the seven-a-side game can be played indoors with a softer ball.

Netball

★250 calories per half hour

Good for mobility and heart and lungs, netball strengthens the leg muscles and, because it involves jumping and stretching the arms, improves posture.

It is played on a hard-surfaced court between two teams of seven. Players may pass the ball by throwing it, but may not run holding it. The object is to score goals by aiming the leather or rubber ball through a ring at the opponents' end of the court. Players are restricted to certain areas of the court.

Dress is shirt and shorts or short skirt and rubber-soled shoes.

The season is officially through the winter, though play often goes on all year. Play can be indoors but is more usually outside.

Variations: basketball; team handball; speedball.

Parachuting

Of those daring enough to parachute, 85% do it only once, so the physical benefits of parachuting are hardly of paramount importance. However, even on that one

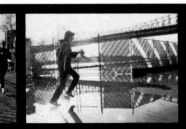
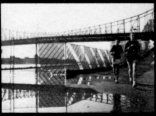
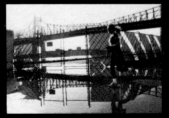
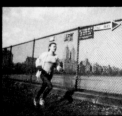

unforgettable occasion, the novice will find it involves more physical exercise than might be thought necessary: there is a lot of walking there and back. It is unsuitable for anyone with any serious health problem and it is preferable to be fit and not overweight.

Parachuting must be embarked upon under specialist instruction and it is best to join a club. Because of the lengthy instruction given before a jump – a minimum of six hours – it is very safe. At least six descents must then be made before you are allowed to go freefall and 65 descents to obtain the equivalent of a licence, the highest qualification.

All the equipment and clothing is provided by the club where you have instruction. This includes parachute, helmet, heavy boots and overall. Even experienced parachutists are discouraged from owning equipment as clubs prefer to trust their own equipment, which is submitted to regular safety checks.

Riding
175 calories per half hour

The physical benefits of riding, if it is simply hacking or trekking, are minimal. Jumping can be very energetic, as can long fast riding. Aching thighs will tell you which muscles are getting the exercise.

Riding is as dangerous as driving a car and possibly more so as you are exerting control over an animal rather than a machine; even the most apparently docile horse can behave unpredictably. To ride well and have good control you should start as a child, as this gives you time to acquire a 'natural seat'. However, if you just want to amble along country lanes you can take up riding later, although you cannot expect to reach a high level of horsemanship. Keeping a horse is expensive. A stable will provide you with a horse and all its tackle and a hard, protective hat. You do not need breeches – comfortable trousers or jeans will do. Wellingtons can get stuck in the stirrups, so if you do not have leather boots, wear gym shoes.

Variations: show jumping; three-day eventing.

Roller-skating
175 calories per half hour

Good for general mobility and for strengthening the legs, roller-skating is fun and easy to learn. It is best to start young when you have a good sense of balance.

You can hire roller-skates at a rink or buy your own, preferably at a rink where you can get advice as to fit.

There are different types for dancing and racing. No special clothing is needed, provided it does not impede movement; protective knee and elbow pads can be worn. For roller disco dancing, body-stockings, leotards or tight jumpsuits are the usual wear.

It is possible to roller-skate anywhere where it will not cause inconvenience or danger to pedestrians. While there are several purpose-built roller-skating rinks, public parks often have special areas and tracks for roller-skaters with smooth concrete or asphalt surfaces. Many rinks have clubs and offer coaching. You can specialize in figure or pair-skating.

Rowing
420 calories per half hour

Rowing is good all-round exercise for the muscles and the heart and lungs. Although it strengthens and develops muscles, below competition level it is unlikely to produce any unfeminine bulges, only the benefits of increased fitness, stamina and strength. Medical research has shown that muscle bulk is dependent on the male hormone testosterone, present only in a small quantity in women. You do, however, need to be strong to participate in rowing, the best preparation being participation in some other sport to ensure fitness.

The best way to take up rowing is to join a club, where you will have all the facilities of a clubhouse, training and, of course, a boat. You simply provide your own shorts, vest, tracksuit and rubber-soled shoes.

Rowing is usually a summer sport but for enthusiasts it involves regular land training throughout the winter.

Running (see also **Athletics**)
450 calories per half hour

Excellent all-round exercise for the heart and lungs, muscle strength and endurance, running is only for the fit and healthy. It is unsuitable for anyone over the age of 40 unless they prepare for it with another sport or regular jogging. In any case you should build up slowly to your goal, whatever time and distance you set yourself, and begin by using a mixture of jogging, running and walking to avoid strain on the muscles and heart.

When you have been practising on your own for some time and feel in need of a challenge, consider joining a local club for the fun of running in a group and trying out new terrain.

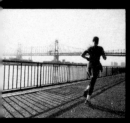 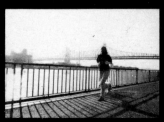 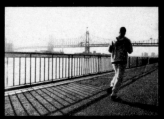 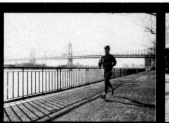

Shoes for cross-country running vary with the surface. For an all-grass course you need short spikes; for a hard surface, rubber studs. You should wear light woollen socks and heel pads. Shorts and a T-shirt are suitable for warm weather; a loose pullover may be needed in colder weather.

Sailing
200 calories per half hour

Exhilarating and reasonably energetic – depending on your ambition and the amount of wind – sailing calls for a degree of fitness and strength. It develops the muscles of arms and thighs in particular. The ability to swim is essential.

Sailing is not dangerous, but it is important to know some theory before beginning, simply to understand the instructions given in the 'language' of sailing. You can pick this up from a book or by taking a course; clubs often run beginners' courses. Practical experience is best acquired by crewing for seasoned sailors.

The most common choice of first boat is a dinghy. These come in all sizes, made of wood, fibreglass and plastic, and there are inflatable rubber ones; many can be powered by an outboard motor as well as being rowed or sailed. Most sailing clubs hire out a selection. For summer sailing you need shorts and a wool sweater over a T-shirt, with socks and canvas shoes with thick rubber soles. In winter you will need trousers and an anorak. It is always wise to overdress and essential to wear a lifejacket, which can usually be hired at a club.

Skiing
300 calories per half hour

Skiing is one of the best sports for all-round fitness, but you must be fit and have a sense of balance before starting. It involves the whole body in twisting, bending, pulling and pushing and is excellent for flexing knees and ankles. If you ski energetically, you will lose weight and work your heart and lungs hard.

Skiing is quickly learned and can be taken up at any age, although the younger the better. The risk of falling is lessened if you are fit and stop when you are beginning to tire. Older people sometimes prefer langlauf, the Nordic cross-country skiing, which requires different boots and skis. It is, however, just as energetic as downhill skiing. Lessons on a dry slope help to give the feel of skis and speed up the learning process before you go on to snow.

Boots and skis, made of fibreglass or plastic, can be hired at a ski resort. It is vital that the bindings that keep the boots on the skis are good and properly adjusted when you hire or buy. Boots should fit tightly, especially round the ankle. Waterproof nylon suits are the best skiwear, worn over a sweater. Ear-covering hat, strong gloves and goggles or sunglasses are essential, as is suncream. It is worth hiring all the major items of equipment the first time you ski in case you do not take to the sport.

Skipping
*400 calories per half hour

Skipping can form part of a bodybuilding programme to strengthen muscles or it can be used to shape the figure by tightening muscles and loose flesh, making the thighs and the calves firmer and more shapely and improving posture. Either way, skipping is a good warm-up activity, promotes stamina and coordination and is good exercise for the heart and lungs. Aching muscles and breathlessness are normal side-effects, but if you are over 35 and know you are unfit, go easy on a skipping routine and take rests when you need them.

When you skip, try to develop a good rhythm and keep the back straight, lifting the feet just enough to clear the rope and landing gently on the balls of the feet. Breathe through the nose and turn the rope as smoothly as you can, using a steady wrist action. Vary your skipping by jumping backwards and forwards, landing on alternate feet and passing the rope twice round as you jump. Aim to build up to 15 minutes a day.

A real skipping rope is an asset. Made of leather or heavy fibre, it has ball bearings in the head for smooth turning. Loose clothing and rubber-soled shoes are important. If you can, skip on a soft surface.

Squash
300 calories per half hour

The fastest game on two legs and the fastest-growing sport in Britain, squash used to be only for the boys. Today, more and more women are discovering the exhilaration and convenience of squash. Playing for half or three-quarters of an hour will help you lose weight, make you more supple, faster on your feet and improve your staying power.

The dangers of collapsing on court are few if you are fit and healthy and take it easy to begin with. The other

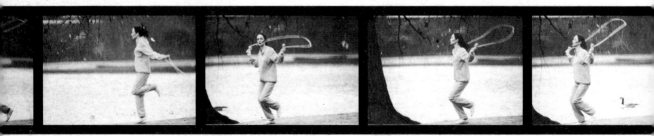

danger, that of being hit by the ball, is probably more of a threat: in the U.S.A. eye shields are increasingly worn to protect the eye-socket. Strained muscles and ligaments are common results of over-exertion and/or insufficient fitness.

Speed is more important than style, which makes squash relatively easy to master. The aim is to put the small rubber ball out of reach of your opponent, within the guidelines drawn on the walls of the four-walled court. The winner is the first to reach nine points and a match is the best of five games.

White shorts or skirt, shirt, socks and shoes are generally obligatory and there is a ban on black-soled shoes as these mark the expensive wood-strip floor. Rackets are smaller and lighter than for tennis. Wooden rackets should be stored in a press to maintain tension.

Being an indoor game, squash is played throughout the year, although it is uncomfortable in very hot weather. Public courts abound in sports centres, but most people enjoy the social facilities of a club even though membership and court fees can make squash an expensive game.

Variations: fives; court handball; paddleball.

Surfing

*250 calories per half hour

Anyone with average build, a sense of balance and coordination, plus determination, can succeed at surfing. As well as the exhilaration, the benefits are that it strengthens the arm muscles and back considerably. It also involves some swimming as you paddle out to catch a wave – this is hard work in strong surf so for such conditions you need to be a strong swimmer. Provided you are not over-ambitious to begin with and practise only in fairly shallow water rather than the 3 m (10 ft) breakers favoured by the experts, surfing is not necessarily dangerous; it does, however, require perseverance to master the technique properly. Even when you have acquired some expertise, always be prepared to give in to the prevailing conditions.

The aim is to ride the waves, either by lying prone on the surfboard, kneeling or, ultimately, standing. Knowledge of how the waves behave is vital, so surfing is best learned from an experienced instructor. Surfing is an all-year-round sport. As the best waves come in winter, a wetsuit is essential. You can hire this and a surfboard when you attend a beginners' course.

Boards are made of polyurethane foam with a top layer of fibreglass. You will also need a leash, a safety device binding your ankle to the board so that you do not injure other surfers when the board escapes.

Swimming

175 calories per half hour

Excellent for the heart and lungs, general mobility and strength, regular energetic swimming builds up endurance. The crawl is the most energetic stroke, followed by the backstroke; the breaststroke is the least demanding. Gentle swimming is good for convalescents and for trimming the figure after pregnancy. As no great strength is needed due to the buoyancy of water, swimming is also good exercise for the elderly and physically handicapped.

The only dangers to be avoided are cold dips, which can raise blood pressure, and too much exertion, which can be a strain on a weak heart. Other than these, there is far greater danger in not being able to swim. Most pools offer beginners' classes.

Variations: diving; scuba diving; synchronized swimming; water polo.

Table tennis

180 calories per half hour

Exert yourself at table tennis and you use your whole body, as demonstrated by the muscular appearance of the champions. On a lesser level the game exercises the heart and lungs, gets you on your toes and improves coordination. Provided you have an eye for a ball, it is easy to pick up and fun for all ages.

As with tennis, the aim is to hit the ball across the net in such a way that the opponent or opponents cannot return it, the difference being that the game is played on a table 2.7 m (9 ft) by 1.5 m (5 ft). A game is played to 21 points and a match is the best of three or five games.

You can play table tennis in any loose, light clothing and rubber-soled shoes. You need a racket or bat made of wood with a surface of raised rubber dots. The small ball is plastic or celluloid.

Most sports and social clubs have a table tennis table; collapsible tables can be bought for home use.

T'ai Chi

T'ai Chi is an ancient Chinese form of meditation expressed through slow, graceful and dance-like

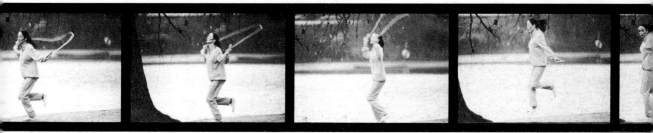

movement. It involves and benefits the mind and body. Improved concentration, self-awareness, co-ordination and balance, inner peace and relaxation, better breathing and circulation are just some of the benefits.

It can be learned only from a trained instructor. Every movement is precise and calls for inner strength: to the Westerner it is either completely alien or a revelation. There are up to 128 complete movements, 37 basic postures.

T'ai Chi is taught at health clubs and dance centres. No two teachers teach exactly the same technique. Any loose comfortable clothing is ideal. The whole idea of T'ai Chi is that you can do it any time, anywhere.

Tennis
220 calories per half hour

A gentle game of mixed doubles tennis is fun, a hard game of singles burns up calories, exercises the heart and lungs, increases suppleness and helps tighten the stomach muscles in particular, and can still be fun.

Although tennis can be played and enjoyed at many different levels, some degree of skill is needed to produce the serve and strokes and coaching is helpful. The aim is not merely to get the ball over the net and within the white lines of the court but to play winning shots.

Standard tennis wear consists of white shorts, skirt or dress, shirt, socks and white rubber-soled shoes. When buying a racket you need expert advice in order to get the right weight and balance for your size. Always store a wood-framed racket in a press. Public courts are adequate for the occasional player but for the best facilities you must join a club.

Tennis is traditionally a summer game played outside on grass, although indoor courts make it possible to play throughout the whole year.

Tenpin bowling
135 calories per half hour

Tenpin bowling does not really exercise the muscles, it merely strengthens the bowling arm. It can be taken up at any age and does not require any particular level of fitness. The technique of propelling the ball with a smooth under-arm swing comes with experience rather than strength. The ball has finger holes for gripping, which most bowlers do with three fingers.

Tenpin bowling can be played by two or four people or by teams of up to five a side. Each player rolls a rubber composition or plastic ball, aiming at ten wooden pins set out in a triangle at the end of the wooden-surfaced lane. Points are scored according to the number of pins knocked over.

The only stipulation as far as clothing is concerned is that it should be loose enough to allow freedom of movement. Soft-soled bowling shoes should be worn to avoid damaging the surface of the approach to the lane. Equipment is hired out by the bowling alley, although some keen bowlers may prefer to have their own shoes.

You can go tenpin bowling all year round at indoor purpose-built alleys.

Volleyball
175 calories per half hour

Good for mobility and strength, beneficial to the heart and lungs, the stretching and jumping movements in volleyball are good for posture too. Until you have become reasonably experienced, the punching of the ball with the hand, head or any part of the body can be painful and bruising.

Two teams of six players each propel the leather or rubber ball over a raised net, the top of which is 2.4 m (7 ft 11 in) above the ground. They can use any part of the body above the waist to do this, but generally it is the clenched fist. The opposing team must not allow the ball to touch the ground on its side of the net. Points are lost if the ball fails to clear the net or goes out.

Dress is shorts or short skirt and shirt, rubber-soled shoes, or bare feet.

Play can be indoors or out and although the season is usually a summer one, it often goes on all year.

Walking
175 calories per half hour

When 4,000 doctors in 20 countries were asked in a survey what they considered the simplest way to improve health, the majority said 'walk'. Walking improves the circulation, stimulates the heart and lungs, loosens the joints and helps the walker lose

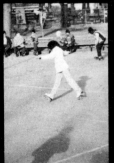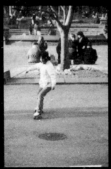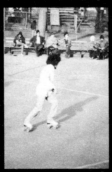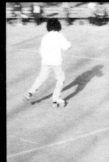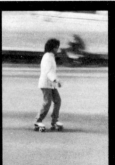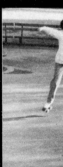

weight. None of these effects is dramatic – walking is not violent exertion, but it has the advantage of being something that can be done every day, and by almost anyone, regardless of age and state of health.

The more you walk and the fitter you are, the more you will enjoy it. If you are interested in doing more than weekend walking, the way to progress is to join a group or club, which will provide advice about equipment and clothing. Stout shoes are fine for weekend walkers, but a good pair of waterproof leather walking boots is essential for the serious walker. You will also need thick socks, and layers of clothing rather than one bulky sweater, so that they can be adjusted according to conditions. It is always advisable to take too much clothing and to be prepared for bad weather rather than be caught out with inadequate covering. Wool trousers or breeches are preferable to denim jeans, which become cold when wet. A waterproof cagoule or anorak is essential, as are hat and gloves. If you are going on a day's expedition a small rucksack is the best method of carrying food, map, compass, extra clothing, etc.

Water skiing
240 calories per half hour
Fun and exhilarating, water skiing is good for trunk, arm and leg muscles. You need a strong back, a good sense of balance and a good level of general fitness. You must be able to swim in case you fall off the tow rope. Many water skiers wear light lifejackets.

The beginner's best way to learn is to take a course, which is also probably the least expensive way to learn an otherwise costly sport, the main cost factor, apart from the skis, being an experienced driver and the fuel for the boat.

A club will lend you skis and provide a towing boat and tuition. Skis are made of wood or fibreglass and have 'pouches', which are release bindings to hold the foot. Their length varies from 1.5–1.8 m (5–6 ft) depending on your weight and height. You may be able to hire a wetsuit, essential for skiing in winter. In summer a one-piece swimsuit is safer (from a modesty point of view) than a bikini.

Most water skiing is done in summer, but land training in winter is important.

Windsurfing
★250 calories per half hour
This new and exciting sport combines many of the skills of skiing and hang-gliding, with the addition of high-speed sailing. It requires a good sense of balance, strength, fitness and the ability to swim. It develops agility, muscle strength over the whole body and is very energetic. It is recommended only for the young and athletic, preferably those with experience of dinghy sailing.

The windsurfer sails her board by standing on it and holding on to a guard rail running along both sides of the sail. It is generally done fairly close to the shore. Learning balance and how to use the wind is not easy – beginners spend a lot of time in the water. It is a good idea to take a short course of instruction from a special windsurfing school.

The board, usually available for hire from schools, is made of fibreglass or plastic and the sail has clear plastic windows. Except on hot days, a wet or dry suit is advisable. A lifejacket should always be worn.

Windsurfing does go on all year, on lakes and the sea, but it is wiser to do it in the summer unless you are very experienced.

Yoga
Hatha yoga is the branch of yoga concerned with physical and mental control and involves the practice not of exercises but of a series of postures called 'asanas'. Regular practice promotes a relaxed and supple body and an appropriate state of mind. Anyone can take up yoga, whatever their age or state of fitness. It is totally uncompetitive: you do just as much as you comfortably can. Many people find that it helps them to overcome specific problems such as smoking or drinking.

To practise yoga successfully and satisfyingly, it is best to have some tuition. This will inspire you and set you on the right path and will also help you to master the correct breathing technique, which is important. Yoga must be learned slowly, avoiding all strain.

For yoga postures to try out, see pages 163–165. No special equipment is needed, although a mat is helpful – just a quiet room with no interruptions and comfortable loose clothing and bare feet.

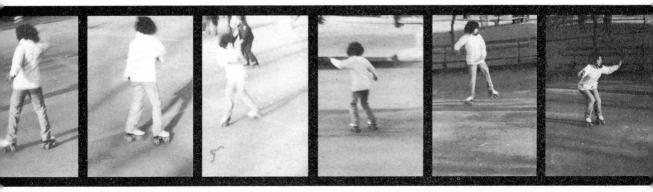

Yoga

Yoga is a vast philosophy with its roots deep in Indian mystical thought. There are many different paths or forms, perhaps the one most commonly practised in the West being Hatha yoga, with its emphasis on physical postures. Unfortunately, although the West has embraced this tradition with enthusiasm, it has at times vulgarized it. It is important to understand that yoga is not merely athletic contortions or self-hypnosis but a disciplined practice of precisely defined movements resulting in precise effects. It is no exaggeration to say that, when done correctly and regularly, yoga postures bring not only health but an inner radiance and beauty.

Postures

Of the eight limbs of yoga first described, in about 200 BC, by Patanjali, the collator and systematizer of yoga philosophy, the most widely practised are asanas, the physical postures, and pranayama, breathing exercises. Unlike sports and many other forms of exercise, asanas seem to be almost static positions, held for some seconds with normal breathing. Within this apparently static position, however, the body is still moving, extending dynamically as you concentrate on every limb and muscle of the body. By exercising every muscle, nerve and gland, yoga asanas promote a well-toned, strengthened and healthy body; the concentrated effort helps to discipline the mind and calm the nerves, so making yoga an invaluable antidote to the strains of modern life.

Although medical opinion is divided over some of the more extravagant claims for the benefits to be derived from correctly performed asanas, it is generally felt that yoga postures can have a prophylactic effect; that yoga promotes a good standing and sitting posture; and that specific asanas may alleviate such medical conditions as backache, depression and insomnia. Yoga can be practised by all – men, women, old and young, the stiff and the supple. If, however, you are pregnant or suffer from back disorders, dizziness, heart trouble or any other serious medical condition, consult your doctor before taking up yoga.

Pranayama, or breathing exercises, is as important as postures. The word 'prana' symbolizes breath and vitality, pranayama denotes the extension and control of the breath. Slow rhythmic deep breathing soothes the nerves and brings about a healthy mentality. The quiet and meditative state induced by pranayama should never be confused with self-hypnosis, chanting or mindless candle-gazing. Like meditation, pranayama can be dangerous unless practised within the context of serious study. These exercises are not generally suitable for complete beginners as it is important to master a good standing and sitting posture in order to breathe correctly.

Practising yoga

Although the postures can be learned from books, it is preferable to be guided through them by a good teacher. The course of standing, sitting and relaxation postures outlined here is intended as a starting point and as a reference and is based on the teachings of B.K.S. Iyengar, world authority on yoga and author of the influential *Light on Yoga*. Bear these points in mind when practising:

- breathe normally through the nose.
- do not expect to be able to do all the postures immediately – regular practice will bring noticeable improvements and it is better to attempt a posture intelligently, even if hampered by stiff joints and weak muscles, than merely to achieve a superficially graceful effect.
- hold a posture only for as long as is comfortable – aim for about 30 seconds initially in standing and sitting postures.
- wear loose clothing that enables you to stretch fully and comfortably and practise in bare feet to prevent slipping.
- always practise on an empty stomach – allow about four hours after a large meal.

A busy mother can practise yoga asanas at home, in a small space with the children sleeping or playing or even with them joining in. Equally, the working woman, especially if coping with the hectic pace of city life, recuperates and derives energy from the relaxation and non-competitiveness of yoga.

Beauty is an elusive quality depending upon cultural standards and yet a strong body with good posture and a clean and healthy appearance seem to be universally admired. Yoga develops all these attributes and furthermore promotes a more balanced personality.

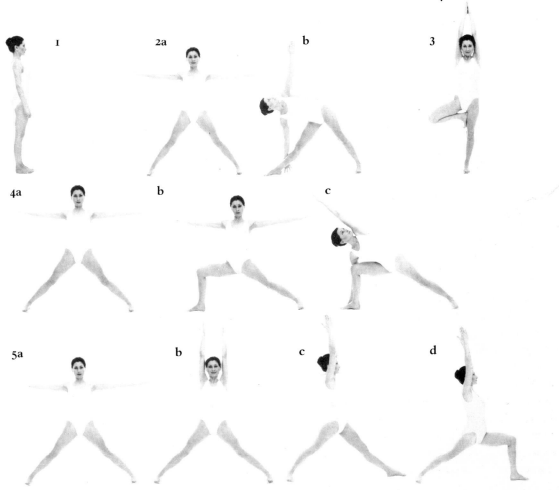

1 Tadasana

The basic standing pose. Stand with heels and big toes touching. Spread all the toes to give firm support. Tighten knees, contract buttocks and lift up from pubis so abdomen flattens. Stretch spine, including back of neck. Keep chest open and drop shoulders.

2 Trikonasana

Removes stiffness in legs and hips, relieves back and neck pains. From Tadasana jump feet 1 m (3–3½ft) apart and stretch arms out (a). Turn left foot slightly in and right foot out at 90°, lining up right heel with left instep. Exhaling, hinge sideways from hip, keeping back of head and hips in a line, arms and spine fully stretched and knees tight (b). Hold posture, breathing evenly; come up and repeat on other side.

3 Vrksasana

Tones muscles and improves sense of balance. Stand in Tadasana. Bend right knee and place heel at root of left thigh, toes extending down. Balance on left leg, turning right knee out but keeping hips facing forwards, to give a good opening at the hip. Stretch arms over head without bending elbows and stretch up out of hips. Repeat on other side.

4 Utthita Parsvakonasana

Develops chest, reduces fat round waist and hips, relieves sciatic and arthritic pain; aids elimination and digestion. From Tadasana, jump feet 1.3 m (4–4½ ft) apart, toes stretched and in line. Stretch arms at shoulder level, palms down (a). Turn left foot slightly in and right foot out at 90° as in Trikonasana. Bend right knee to make right angle, keeping thigh parallel to floor (b). Stretch trunk on to right thigh. Extend left arm over head and look up (c). Keep head, chest and hips in line; stretch from left heel to fingertips.

Breathe normally and repeat on other side.

5 Virabhadrasana I

Reduces fat on waist and hips, relieves stiffness in shoulders and neck. Strenuous, so do not attempt until strong in 1 to 4. From Tadasana jump feet 1.3 m (4–4½ ft) apart, arms outstretched (a). Stretch arms up (b). Turn right foot in, left out as in Trikonasana and turn trunk fully to left (c). Bend left knee to form right angle (d). Do not push lumbar spine forwards but bring waist back to ensure a good stretch from base of spine to crown of head. Keep chest open. Repeat on other side.

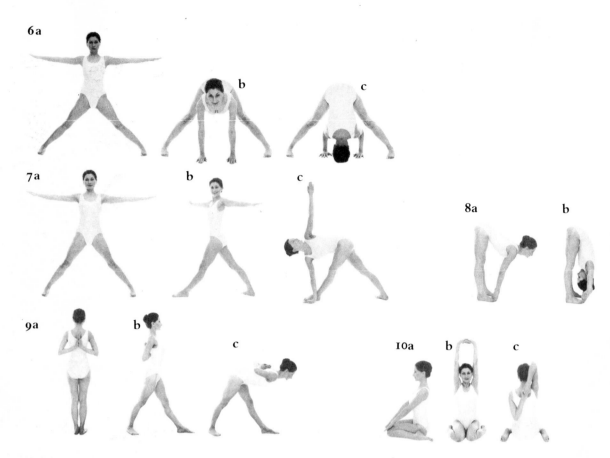

6 Prasarita Padottanasana

Develops hamstrings and abductor muscles, aids digestion. Spread legs 1.5 m (4½ ft) apart (a), hands on waist. With knees tight, bend forwards from hips, stretching spine from pelvis and keeping back concave. Place palms on floor between feet (b). Exhaling, bend elbows back and bring head down between hands (c). Keep weight on legs not head.

7 Parivrtta Trikonasana

Relieves lower back pain, develops chest and strengthens hip muscles. From Tadasana jump feet 1 m (3–3½ ft) apart and stretch arms out (a). Turn right foot slightly in, left foot out at 90°, keeping kneecaps pulled up. Exhaling, rotate trunk to left, especially right side of pelvis (b). Place right hand on floor against outer side of left foot and stretch left arm up (c); keep arms and spine fully stretched. Beginners can put right hand on a brick or rest fingertips on floor. Repeat on other side.

8 Padangusthasana

Tones abdominal organs, activates digestion and liver. Stand in Tadasana with feet about 30 cm (12 in) apart. Exhaling, bend forwards from pelvis, keeping back concave, and catch big toes between thumbs and first two fingers (a). If you are stiff and cannot make your back concave, place hands on shins and stay in (a); also stay in this position if you have spinal injuries. Otherwise, exhale and bring head down as far as possible, keeping knees tight (b).

9 Parsvottanasana

Removes stiffness in wrists and shoulders, tones abdominal organs, improves breathing. Stand in Tadasana with palms joined together on back. Draw shoulders and elbows back (a). Spread legs 1 m (3–3½ ft) apart, turn right foot out at 90°, left foot slightly in and turn trunk to right (b). Exhaling, extend trunk forwards from hips without bending knees (c). As you become more flexible, place head on shin. Repeat on other side.

10 Virasana

Cures rheumatic pains in knees, corrects flat feet by strengthening arches, relieves rheumatic pains and stiffness in shoulders. Kneel on floor, knees together and feet apart with toes pointing back and touching floor; lower buttocks on to floor or sit on a cushion if stiff (a). Interlock fingers and stretch arms over head, palms up and elbows straight (b). Repeat with opposite interlock of hands. Rest hands briefly on knees. Extend right arm up, bend elbow and bring fingers down between shoulder blades. Bend left arm up back to hold right fingers (c). Keep head and neck erect. Repeat, starting with left arm.

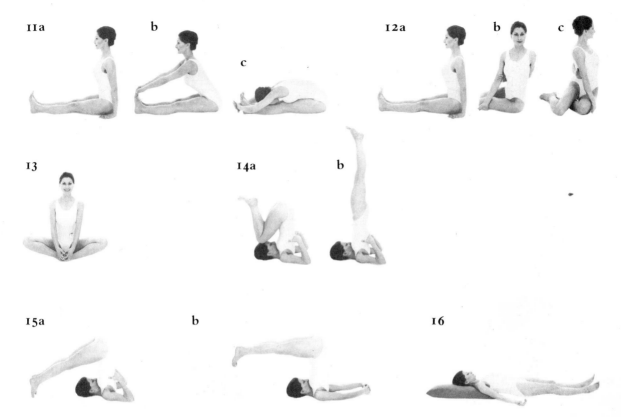

11 Paschimottanasana

Tones kidneys and abdominal organs, energizes spine, beneficial for heart. Sit on floor, legs stretched straight in front, hands on floor by hips. Stretch spine and back of neck upwards (a); do not tense shoulders. Extend spine forwards, keeping back concave, and grasp toes (b); hold a belt round your feet and do not bend forwards if your back makes a hump. Stretching from the pelvis, bend forwards flat on thighs (c).

12 Bharadvajasana I

Works on lower back, makes stiff backs more supple. Sit on floor as in 11 (a). Bend knees to right and bring both feet to right hip. Keeping both buttocks on floor, turn to left, bringing chest in line with outside of left thigh (b, c). Rest right hand on outside of left knee and bring left hand across back to touch right elbow.

13 Baddna Konasana

Particularly recommended for urinary disorders, relieves sciatic pain, regulates menstruation, helps ovaries function properly. Sit on floor, bend knees and bring feet together against pubis. Hold feet, widen thighs and lower knees as far as possible.

14 Salamba Sarvangasana I

Beneficial for the whole system, mentally soothing, restores energy after illness; the chin lock regulates blood flow, promoting a healthy thyroid gland. Do not attempt when menstruating. Lie flat on back with a folded blanket under head, shoulders and elbows if desired. Exhaling, bend knees and, supporting upper back with hands, bring trunk up perpendicularly until chest touches chin (a). Straighten legs and lift spine from shoulder blades (b). Aim to hold for 5 minutes once the posture is comfortable.

15 Halasana

Benefits as 14; do not attempt when menstruating. From Sarvangasana take legs over head so toes touch floor (a). Rest your feet on a box or chair if you are a beginner or have a stiff back (b). Try not to collapse spine but increase height of trunk from chin to pubis.

16 Savasana

Quietens the brain and leaves both mind and body refreshed and relaxed. Lie flat on back, with a cushion under head and shoulders if desired. Drop shoulders down and rest arms a little away from trunk, palms facing up. Close eyes and let breathing become fine and deep. Concentrate on the exhalation and let go every part of the body and face, so that you gradually relax completely. Stay in the posture for 10–15 minutes.

Exercise Machines and Equipment

Any well-equipped modern health club or gymnasium will have a range of exercise machines. They fall into two groups: the passive exercisers and the active exercisers.

The passive exercisers include vibrator belts and machines that stimulate the muscles electronically. These provide an easy way of taking exercise, letting the machine do all the work, but their benefits are limited. Although it is possible to trim the areas treated and firm up flabby muscles, there is no evidence that weight loss results, or that general fitness is improved. Such machines can, however, have a very relaxing, soothing effect and electrical stimulation of the muscles has proved effective in cases of insomnia. Active exercisers, on the other hand, can make a valuable contribution to fitness if used regularly, vigorously and with due awareness of the particular benefits of individual apparatus. Far from being an easy method of taking exercise, they are physically exhausting, but are a quicker and often more convenient way of keeping fit than playing any form of sport.

Various types of exercise equipment can be bought for home use: they range from full-sized apparatus, such as cycling and rowing machines, to simple aids like chest expanders, dumb-bells or weights, which can be strapped to the wrist or ankle. A flat, padded exercise bench can be used with a variety of weighted attachments to exercise arms and legs. Weight-training is good exercise and will not build bulging muscles in women because this development is dependent on the male hormone testosterone. Weights are versatile; the size of weight and the way they are distributed can be varied to suit different ages, builds, degrees of fitness and desired effects. Use small weights and many repetitions of each exercise for weight loss, medium weights and a moderate number of repetitions to tone the body and heavy weights with few repetitions to strengthen and build up muscles.

It is important to establish which parts of the body the chosen pieces exercise: the equipment is expensive and it may not give a complete workout. It may be convenient and a good incentive to have, say, a cycling machine in the bathroom, but unless you make a point of doing a variety of exercises on it, you will not use all your muscles. It might be wiser to spend the money on a subscription to a health or sports club where there should be a large and varied array of machines. The variety will make it more likely that you will stick at it – you should reckon to exercise three times a week for about half an hour.

A good club will make a fitness assessment of each new member and tailor a programme to suit individual needs. Trained staff encourage perseverance and demonstrate how to exercise in the best way, so that there is less danger of strained muscles. The social benefits of a club are an added incentive.

Whether you use an exercise machine at home or in a gymnasium, do not expect miracles: the machine is only as good as the effort you are prepared to put into it.

Abdominal sit-up board (1) flattens and firms abdominal muscles. Lie face upwards on the inclined, padded board and practise sit-ups with feet wedged under the bar or in the strap at the raised end; the incline can be increased as you become stronger. Alternatively, grip bar or strap with hands above head and raise and lower legs from the waist.

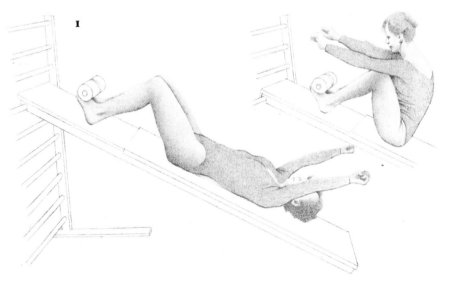

I

2

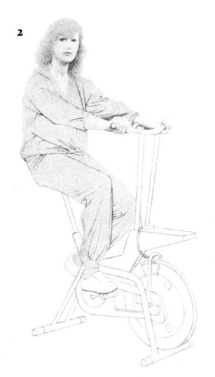

Twist machine (3) trims and tones waist. Stand on disc and push against fixed metal T-bar to right and left to swivel from side to side. Move from waist upwards only – keep legs and hips stationary.

3

Hack squat or pre-ski trainer (4) firms thigh muscles. Squat with lower back against the padded board and raise the weighted bar, attached to the frame, as you stand up. Lower the bar as you squat and repeat, raising and lowering the bar rapidly.

4

Cycling machine (2), good for general warm-up and an excellent machine for improving the efficiency of heart and lungs; also improves the strength and endurance of leg, hip and back muscles and shapes up thighs. A stationary cycle, it usually has one wheel, but it may be just a frame, pedals and handlebars. Resistance is provided by a braking force on the wheel or pedals and can be increased as you get fitter. More sophisticated models have meters to measure pulse rate and the 'speed' and 'distance' achieved.

5

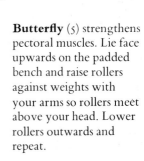

Butterfly (5) strengthens pectoral muscles. Lie face upwards on the padded bench and raise rollers against weights with your arms so rollers meet above your head. Lower rollers outwards and repeat.

Relaxation

Relaxation of tense muscles has become a recognized way of dealing with stress. It has been found that people who can relax at will have more energy to pursue their chosen activities and are less irritable or aggressive. The ability to relax in this way may also help to reduce dependence on cigarettes or alcohol.

Muscles work when we give the order from our upper brain to perform some activity such as 'walk' or 'dance' and so they are called voluntary muscles. The conscious brain does not order the muscle work. This has already been learned and stored in the brain. But voluntary muscles also sometimes work as a result of a stimulus from outside. If an object comes towards us, we automatically close our eyes or blink. This is a reflex action. Body health is maintained by many such actions. For instance, we unconsciously shiver when the temperature suddenly falls in order to keep ourselves warm by the muscular activity.

If a situation arises whereby we feel threatened and insecure, the body becomes dominated by a complicated response known as the fight or flight reflex, so that we may be able to defend ourselves or run away. This is a very primitive reaction, which animals share. Stress, however, is not caused by one sudden event but is a prolonged state in which tension gradually builds up so that the responses of the fight or flight reflex are inexorably perpetuated.

Build-up of stress
Tension can be caused by manifold factors, either singly or in combination: emotional upset, family worries, failing health, problems arising from work – an uncongenial atmosphere, promotion to a strange environment, or a demanding job coupled with heavy family responsibilities – can all trigger off a state of stress.

A certain amount of stress acts as a good stimulus but it is impossible to say what is the optimum for any one person. This may vary from day to day and any unexpected burden, such as illness in the family, may suddenly prove too much; the tendency is then to strive still further and so the stress becomes worse. If the pressure goes beyond a healthy stimulus and is continued, the build-up of stress can have serious results, such as insomnia and ulcers, and it may even be a contributory factor in heart disease.

This is because adrenalin pours out into the blood stream, the heart speeds up, blood pressure rises and sugar is released into the blood from the body stores. Extra blood is directed to the muscle groups, which work in a pattern for fighting or running. In consequence, less blood is available for the digestive organs and for the brain, which normally receives 15 per cent of the blood pumped out of the heart at each beat. Because of the strong static muscular activity, the temperature tends to rise and so the body sweats to control this. Carbon dioxide and lactic acid in the blood increase as they are given off by the working muscles, and this affects the breathing, which becomes first deeper and then faster.

All this rearrangement of bodily functioning is very tiring and unproductive since we neither fight nor run – indeed we are not even aware that this reflex has taken control of us. Moreover, it has been proved by Dr Herbert Benson of Harvard Medical School that increased lactate in the blood heightens anxiety, thus perpetuating the state of stress and creating a vicious circle.

Just as an emotional stimulus causes this physical response, so it has been found that physical relaxation of the tense muscles can cause an emotional feeling of ease. As the relaxation spreads and the fight or flight reflex subsides, the physiological symptoms of stress, such as the increased heart rate, return to normal. This is the reason for the search for safe relaxation techniques; a selection of the most commonly practised ones is given below and on the following pages.

Comfort
A simple method to try out either on yourself or on someone else. Make the person comfortable with cushions and warm covers on a warm bed, in a room with lowered lighting and music if desired. Then, in a soporific voice, repeat the word 'relax' frequently. By experiencing ease in this way, people who have never given themselves time to enjoy bodily comfort may find that rest and relaxation are both pleasurable and an important and necessary part of their everyday life. This technique is not suitable for acute stress.

Visualization

As in Comfort, with which this technique can be combined, the person is made comfortable. Then, in a soothing voice, they are asked to visualize calming pictures – perhaps a still lake, a flight of birds against a moonlit sky or kittens playing. Interspersed with these instructions are general recommendations for calmness and enjoyment of ease. This can be very beneficial both at the time and in everyday life.

Massage

This can be done in conjunction with Comfort and Visualization. Stroking combined with general massage, continued for about an hour, can give great relief, but does lead to dependency on the masseur or masseuse. Self-massage of the face, particularly the forehead, helps to relieve facial tension and insomnia and encourages feelings of ease (see pages 176–177).

Distraction

This can be anything from painting and amateur dramatics to gardening, knitting or going to the cinema. Engrossment in such activities can bring temporary relief and may even help to promote a more positive and balanced viewpoint afterwards.

Playing with 'worry beads' can also help to soothe the mind and stop tension building up. Made of substances such as stone, ivory and glass strung on a suitable cord, they are much used in Greece and Eastern countries.

Tranquillizers

These can certainly be useful for some pathological conditions for a defined period of time. They can, however, lead to addiction. They should always be prescribed and carefully supervised by a physician, who will try to lessen the dose when possible.

Breathing

This involves becoming aware of breathing and trying to use the diaphragm and lower ribs while slowing the rhythm. When tense, the tendency is to breathe only with the upper chest or to hold the breath. This is often helpful at times of known stress, such as when driving, attending interviews and making public appearances.

Hypnosis

There are various methods of hypnosis. Typically, the hypnotist induces a trance by repeated suggestions in a low voice; the subject then responds only to his instructions and may continue to respond to suggestions – to remain relaxed, for example – after awakening. Hypnosis should be administered by a reliable practitioner; for it to work, the subject must be responsive (see also page 236). Self-hypnosis consists of inducing peaceful alpha brain waves at will by repeating such phrases as 'I am relaxed'.

Meditation

An ancient way of quietening the mind, which takes on many different forms. It can involve special positions of the body, such as yoga asanas, specialized forms of breathing or the repetition of selected sounds or mantras, as in transcendental meditation. It can take the form of the 'relaxation response', as described by Dr Herbert Benson in his book of that name, or it may merge into prayer as in Christian or Buddhist groups. Devotees of meditation insist on daily practice and stillness, to promote a tranquillity that flows over into daily life, so making them less vulnerable to stress.

Exercise

Sustained exercise may result in a feeling of well-being, which, although different from true physiological relaxation, may be confused with relaxation; it may be associated with tiredness or simply be the contrast of relief from work. It is, however, valuable to experience this feeling, especially if it encourages learning other ways of obtaining voluntary control of relaxation that may be used in daily life.

Progressive relaxation

Sometimes called 'tense and let go', this method was developed by Dr Edmund Jacobson in the United States in the early 1930s. It consists of recognizing when muscles are tense or relaxed and learning to produce either state at will. This takes some time to learn, all the main areas being gradually trained over several months, with close supervision by an instructor. Dr. Jacobson recommends between 12 and 30 hours training for the arm muscles alone.

Physiological Relaxation

This technique for relaxation, which is also known as the Mitchell method, was developed from 1957 onwards and is now practised in 25 countries including the United States, Canada, Australia and Denmark. It is so called because it applies modern physiological knowledge of how voluntary muscles work.

Recent research has shown that the conscious brain cannot feel the muscles working, and you can prove this for yourself by taking a step. You will find that, whereas you can feel the joints working and the skin pressure on the sole of your foot, you cannot register the movement of individual muscles.

The key to physiological relaxation is to learn to recognize the positions of stress in every part of the body. This is easy to do, since special nerve paths constantly convey the sensation of the position of the joints and of the pressure on the skin directly to the upper conscious brain.

Self-orders

Another physiological fact is then applied. When the brain gives an order for any activity, one set of muscles is ordered to perform the work and the opposite set of muscles is ordered by the central nervous system to relax. To activate the opposite muscles from those working to maintain the stress position, the Mitchell method employs a series of self-orders for the various parts of the body and face. All the orders are in lay language so that they can easily be memorized and have been carefully chosen to obtain the exact result required, whether you are leaning forwards at a desk, sitting back in a chair or lying on your side in bed. They are all specific and positive as the conscious brain obeys only precise instructions; words such as 'relax' are not used as they are not sufficiently precise. It is important therefore to use exactly the same words as those in the key instructions below.

To start with, try out the method either sitting in a high-backed chair with arms or lying on the floor on your back with a pillow under your head and your hands on your tummy. There are three stages to each order: first, make a small movement; then stop; finally, feel the resulting position and pressure in your joints and skin. Do not attempt to feel muscles. Follow the sequence given below; the key instructions are in italic.

Typical external signs of stress include raised shoulders, bent elbows, clenched hands, head and body somewhat bent forwards and a tensed face, with clamped jaw or even grinding teeth. The stressed person either keeps compulsively on the move, or if sitting, crosses her legs, curling one foot around the other leg or flapping it up and down. The greater the stress, the more complete is this picture.

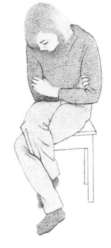

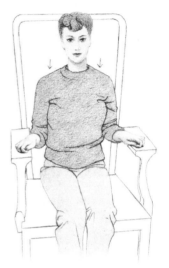

Shoulders
Pull shoulders towards feet Immediately the muscles below the shoulders start working and those holding them up have to let go. *Stop* The muscles stop pulling down and all the muscles round the shoulders are relaxed. Register the new position of the lowered shoulders.

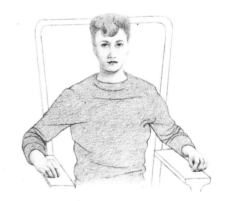

Elbows
Out and open Push your elbows out from your body to the sides and open the angle between the forearm and upper arm somewhat. Keep them touching the floor if lying down or the arms of the chair if sitting up. *Stop* Feel the position of the elbows 'out and open' and register the pressure of your skin touching the support.

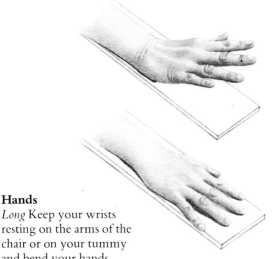

Hands

Long Keep your wrists resting on the arms of the chair or on your tummy and bend your hands back at the wrists, opening the fingers and thumbs up in the air so they are as long as possible. This instantly undoes the clenching in tense hands. *Stop and supported* The stretched out fingers and thumbs fall on to the support (your tummy if you are lying down or the chair arms if sitting up). Register the motionless fingers and thumbs touching the support and the new positions of all the joints. This is pleasant and easy to do, as the fingers and thumbs have proportionately the widest area of all parts of the body for registering feelings in the whole conscious brain. Take as long as you need to teach yourself how enjoyable the relaxed positions are, for it is this registration in the brain that is the essential training. Never hurry it – it may be a totally new feeling.

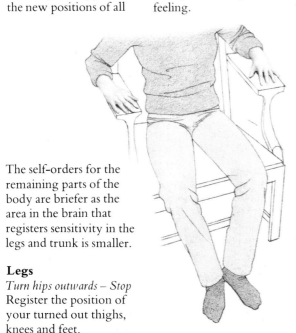

The self-orders for the remaining parts of the body are briefer as the area in the brain that registers sensitivity in the legs and trunk is smaller.

Legs

Turn hips outwards – Stop Register the position of your turned out thighs, knees and feet.

Knees

Move knees very gently until they are comfortable – *Stop* Feel the comfort you have induced.

Feet

Push feet away from face – *Stop* Feel the weight of your feet dangling down from your ankles.

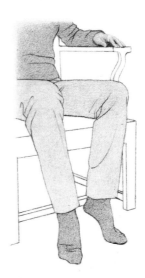

Body and head

Push body and then head into support – Stop Feel the weight of your body and head and the pressure of your skin on the support.

Breathing

There is no need to do deep breathing as the tensed muscles are now relaxing instead of working and so do not need much oxygen; nor do they need to get rid of excess carbon dioxide. It is important, though, to make sure your diaphragm is working, if only very gently: take a gentle breath in and expand just above the waist in front, while lifting the lower ribs out to the sides and up towards the armpits. Breathe out easily and feel the ribs fall down again. Repeat only once.

Face

Spend as much time as possible releasing the tension on your face into ease because, here again, there is a large area of the brain that registers feeling in the jaw joint and the skin of the face, especially the mouth.

Draw jaw down With the lips just touching and no tightness round the mouth, separate your teeth slightly. *Stop* Feel the mouth soft with the jaw open. *Place tongue in middle of mouth – Stop* Feel the tongue lying loosely inside the mouth.

Close eyes Make sure that you do not screw them up but just lower the top lid. *Stop* Enjoy the darkness.

Smooth forehead upwards Try to feel your hair being pushed up, over and down the back of your head.

You should now be completely relaxed. Stay still and either go slowly over all the self-orders again, stopping and feeling as you go, or occupy your mind to stop worries and problems creeping in by slowly recollecting some pleasant happening in the past.

You can repeat the whole sequence as often as you like, either fully, to have a proper rest or to go to sleep, or in parts, while you are working or whenever you feel any part of your body become tense.

Massage

Although massage can be performed by various means, including a vibrator or other specially contoured appliances, there is no apparatus so wonderfully made as the human hand for sensitivity of touch, receptivity of sensation, temperature control and adaptable shape; it is therefore the ideal manipulator and the following suggestions are based on the use of the hands to perform massage on someone else or on oneself.

Massage can be used to affect:

• the skin: to encourage sensitivity and increase circulation.

• the fat just below the skin: to encourage increased blood supply. Massage does not reduce fat deposits unless accompanied by a reducing diet and increased exercise.

• the small blood vessels (capillaries) and tissue fluid in which all the body cells are bathed: to hasten circulation towards the heart.

• the muscles attached to bones: to stretch tightened areas and increase circulation. It does not affect muscle tone; this is improved only by regular exercise.

• the points where bones are attached to each other: to increase circulation. Great care must be taken to handle all joints gently.

• some organs such as the stomach and possibly the intestines: to disperse air pockets.

No massage should cause any pain or even, in general, discomfort. It should be enjoyable and engender a feeling of well-being.

Manipulations

There are two main groups of techniques:

A Effleurage; kneading; picking up; skin rolling.
B Stroking; vibrations.

All these manipulations can be performed separately, but if you want to give a general massage to any part, such as the back, use those in section **A**, in the order given and finishing with more effleurage. Stroking and vibrations can be added anywhere in the sequence or be done on their own. They are primarily to give ease and pleasure.

There is also a series of movements grouped under the heading Tapôtement. These are all forms of clapping, pounding and so forth and can cause injury if not performed by an expert and for a specific medical purpose. They have therefore been omitted except for light patting of the face.

Never give massage to the back or abdomen after a heavy meal. It is perfectly safe, however, to treat the face, neck or limbs at any time. No massage should ever be given to anyone with a raised temperature or suffering from any pathological condition except by a fully trained physiotherapist at the request of a physician.

Preparation

The nails should not protrude beyond the fleshy part of the fingertips: no one enjoys being prodded by spikes. The hands should be warm and clean, neither sweaty nor greasy. If you find it easier, sprinkle a very little talcum powder on the hands, and then shake it off. But any powder, cream or lotion tends to make your touch less delicate and sensitive, as it forms a barrier, however slight, between your hands and the surface they are touching.

It is better not to wear any jewellery as it may jangle, and to wear a sleeveless dress or shirt, for even a rolled-up sleeve edge can trail on to the part being massaged and be ticklish and annoying. You should be relaxed and able to concentrate on what you are doing and on your partner, who should be concentrating on what he or she is feeling. It is not a time for chat. The skin is the most sensitive organ of the body; appreciate its sensations.

Your partner should be loosely clad and should lie on the floor or on a bed. Have lightweight warm covers handy to slip on or off as required, and some extra pillows. The room should be warm and the part being massaged must always be supported and relaxed. For example, it is impossible to give a satisfactory massage to the back of the neck if your partner is sitting on an upright chair with head held up. The muscles of the neck will be working continuously to support the head, which weighs about 5 kg (10–12 lb).

Sit on a chair beside the bed – not on it – or kneel on the floor beside the other person, so that you transfer your weight on to the chair or floor. Otherwise, unwittingly, you may transfer your weight through your arms on to your partner, thus making heavy clumsy movements. If you work through your hands and arms only, they will remain perceptive to what they are doing, which is of the utmost importance.

Effleurage

(right) Helps to drain blood from the smallest blood vessels (capillaries), which immediately fill up again with fresh blood. Tissue fluid is also dispersed and quickly replenished from the blood. All strokes are made in the direction of the heart, pushing blood towards it. One or both hands can be used.

Place the hands gently on the skin so the thumbs and fingertips fit the depressions between the muscles, while the palm encloses them gently. Exerting pressure, push the hands along, towards the armpits if massaging the arms or back, towards the back if massaging the tummy and towards the groin if working on the legs. The pressure should be continuous and as deep as is comfortable. Lift the hands and begin again from below, or stroke gently back to the starting position and repeat. Gradually work over the whole area.

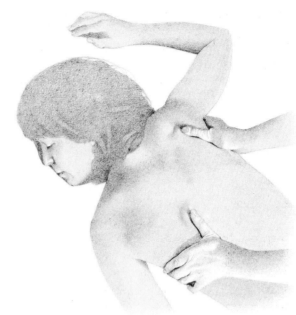

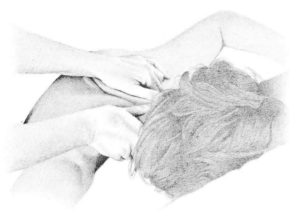

Finger kneading

(below) To massage your neck, rest the elbows on a firm surface, support the head with one hand and lightly knead the side and back of the neck with the fingertips of the other. Change hands for the other side.

Kneading

(left) Affects muscle and fibrous tissue. It can be performed in any direction, with one or both hands. On smaller, delicate surfaces such as the face or hand, knead only with the fingers.

After some stroking or effleurage, let the hands lie on the muscles and alternately press and relinquish pressure from the palms on the parts beneath, gradually wriggling the hands fairly vigorously along the mass of muscle. Let the fingers trail, exerting pressure.

To knead your lower back (below), place the hands palms down on the back with the fingers meeting at waist level, thumbs pointing forwards. Knead comfortably up and down and from side to side; then knead the sides of the waist. This can be done over clothing.

Picking up and Skin rolling

Affect fat and fibrous tissue, helping the circulation and also stretching the tissues. They will not reduce fat unless accompanied by suitable diet and exercise. If working on an arm or leg, support it with one hand and work with the other; otherwise, use one or both hands.

Picking up

(right) With the wrist raised and the hand relaxed, dangling down, seize the flesh between the thumb and forefinger and lift it away at right angles from the bone. Drop it and repeat, moving your hand along, grasping handfuls as you do so. Do not hurt by undue dragging or merely skim over the skin. When you have covered the whole area, begin again, giving some effleurage in between.

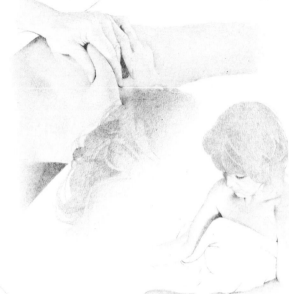

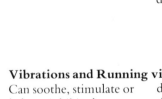

Skin rolling

(left) First grasp the flesh as in Picking up. Roll the thumbs flat on the skin, exerting gentle but firm pressure below, so pushing a roll of the underlying fat towards the forefingers. Repeat all over the area in any direction.

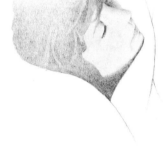

Stroking

(below) Affects skin sensitivity only. Often an instinctive demonstration of affection, it can be soothing or stimulating, depending on the depth, rate and length of the strokes; it can establish a rapport between two people.

Place the palm of the hand gently on the skin and immediately move it, in any direction, followed or even overlapped by the other hand, to give the feeling of a series of hands. Both hands should slide easily on to the area being massaged, closely follow its contours and just as delicately leave it, to alight elsewhere. Vary the depth, rate and direction of the strokes.

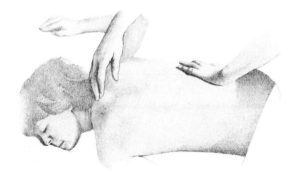

Vibrations and Running vibrations

Can soothe, stimulate or help an inhibited partner enjoy skin sensations. The latter may, however, be irritating, so use this technique only if your partner enjoys it. It can also be quite difficult to do well; do not try too hard or keep it going for too long; stay relaxed; do not hold your breath. Use one or both hands.

Position the hand comfortably, palm down, on any part of the skin with fingers and thumbs very slightly outspread; bend the wrist, elbow and shoulder to preserve sensitivity. Send a shiver down the arm through the hand to quiver on your partner's skin. For running vibrations, let the hand trail gently over your partner's skin as you do this. Lift the hand and repeat elsewhere.

Foot massage

This is a highly delectable experience, which everyone seems to enjoy. Although it is possible to give oneself a fairly simple foot massage, (see page 93), the more thorough method outlined below cannot be adapted for self-massage.

It is important to ensure that the feet have just been bathed as they easily become sweaty because of the concentration of sweat glands. If necessary, sponge them quickly with warm water and soap and pat them dry with a warm thick towel before you begin.

Sit opposite your partner who should be leaning back in a comfortable chair. Have a towel on your lap and support one foot on this.

1 Place the palm of one hand on the sole of the foot as though you were going to shake hands. Place the other hand gently on the top of the foot and stroke both hands calmly up towards the heel, swivelling the top hand downwards and backwards when you get to the ankle. Repeat the stroking a few times, making sure that only the fingertips begin the stroke and then gradually hugging the foot closely with both palms.

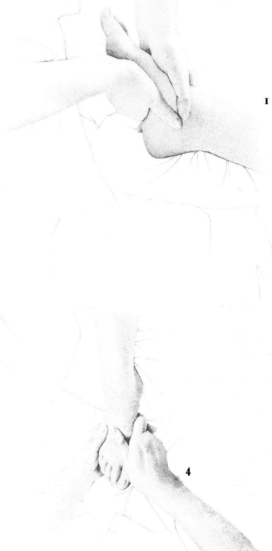

I

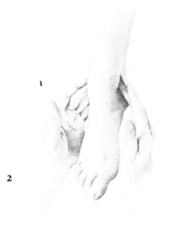

2

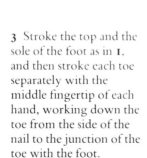

3

2 Place the tips of your three middle fingers just in front of and below each ankle bone and finger knead (see page 173) deeply and thoroughly all round the indentation between these bones and the heel. This is where swelling tends to gather in tired feet and the pressure should be applied carefully upwards. Repeat several times, gradually making your fingertips fit deeply but comfortably into the channel on either side of the ankle joint.

3 Stroke the top and the sole of the foot as in **1**, and then stroke each toe separately with the middle fingertip of each hand, working down the toe from the side of the nail to the junction of the toe with the foot.

Repeat any or all of **1** to **3** and finish, if you wish, with some effleurage and kneading of the lower leg (see page 173). Repeat the whole routine with the other foot and leg.

4

4 Place your hands so that the palms are across the sole of the foot and the two thumbs across the roots of the toes. Following the contours of the foot carefully, knead towards the ankle with your thumbs; do this fairly lightly, as the top of the foot is rather bony. Repeat as wished.

Facial Massage

This is both extremely pleasurable and a good way to help circulation of the blood. It can be done in any of these positions:

1 Sit at a dressing table or in front of a mirror standing on a firm surface. Plant the elbows on the surface to take the weight of the arms off the hands and so ensure a delicate touch.
2 Lie on a bed propped up on pillows, with your head and elbows resting against them.
3 Sit in an armchair with a tall back. Rest your head against the back and your elbows on the arms. For the last two positions, hold a hand mirror in one hand and work with the other.

Massage lines

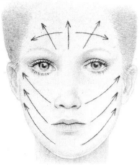

To start with, it is important to look carefully into the mirror all the time, to be sure that you follow the right lines. Never stretch the delicate skin round the eyes, especially round the sockets below as this is where bags so easily form. When you have learned the technique and have felt your way about your face discriminately, you may discard the mirror and perform all the massage by the sensation of the fingertips and face. Do not be in a hurry to do this: you will learn a great deal by looking at what you are doing and registering the feelings in your skin as you work.

For greater accuracy use only one hand, whichever you know to be the more expert. The same hand can be used for both sides of the face, or you can gradually train the less agile hand to massage its own side or the opposite one. The following methods are given for one hand at a time. Moisturize your skin as you massage by dipping your three middle fingers in smooth skin cream or moisturizing lotion. Follow the directions indicated in the diagram above for all manipulations and massage techniques.

Effleurage

This helps to drain the local fluid under the skin.

Place the fingertips on the centre of the chin and, exerting pressure inwards and upwards, push them towards the ear, creating a little bulge of flesh in front of the moving fingers. Raise the hand and begin again. Repeat two or three times until the skin feels pleasantly moistened with the cream. Work alternately along the jaw and just above it.

Repeat the movement, following the lines on the diagram: work from the corner of the mouth to the ear and then from the nostril to the ear. Always work up and out, never down. Never massage the eye socket in this way as the area is delicate, with little supporting fat and muscle.

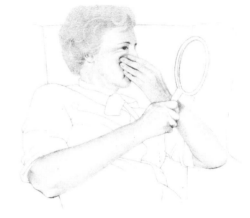

Finger kneading

Place the tips of the three middle fingers on the centre of the chin and make small circular movements, pressing and releasing pressure alternately as you very gradually move towards the ear. As you do this, do not move on the skin but rather make the fingers adhere to it, so that all the pressure goes through to the muscles below, which run in all directions.

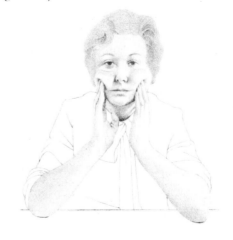

Patting

With the tips of the three middle fingers, hit the skin smartly and quickly, flapping the hand up and down from the wrist; keep the fingers relaxed and the elbow supported. Move the hand along very slowly so that numerous little pats rain down on the skin. Do not drag the skin, simply hit it at right angles with tiny blows and remember it should be pleasurable and not punishing. Keep the hand moving.

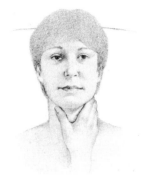

Neck massage

Correctly done, this has an enchanting soporific effect, which can alleviate insomnia. Sit up or lie down with your head supported on pillows to ensure the neck muscles are relaxed. Use both hands, one immediately after the other, so the right hand massages the left side and vice versa.

Smooth cream on both palms. Place the fingers of one hand along the mid line of your neck, exactly under the middle of your chin. Sweep them upwards under the jawline to the opposite ear, leaving the thumb touching the other side of your Adam's apple. Curve downwards to the root of the neck, smoothing the fingers back lightly to the mid line. Repeat to cover that side, then massage the other side with the other hand, developing a rhythmic movement between the hands. Finish with patting all over as for the face.

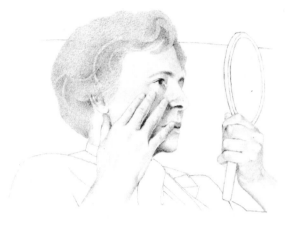

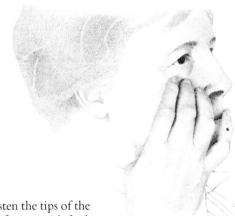

Eyes

1 Moisten the tips of the middle fingers with fresh skin cream if necessary before beginning the massage. Place the middle fingertip on the socket of the eye beside the nose and very lightly trace the edge of the socket out, up and round, passing just under the eyebrow and finishing against the nose just above the inside corner of the eye.

2 Within this circle pat alternately with the first and middle fingertips very lightly all over (above). Keep the wrist still and work only from the fingers, as if drumming them on a table. To practise this, curve the fingers, lift them and let them fall, moving quickly and gently from the knuckles only. You can also massage the forehead in this way, using three fingers.

Facial exercises

Now that you have massaged the skin of your face, hastened the blood and fluid circulation and treated the muscles, it is a good idea to use these muscles fully, to try to make them firmer. The following exercises will help achieve this; repeat them all as often as is comfortable (for further exercises see page 146 and for an alternative view on facial exercises see page 243):

1 Screw your eyes up tightly, then open them as widely as possible and repeat. Stop immediately the muscles begin to fail in their work and rest with closed eyes.

2 Twitch one corner of your nose upwards, then drop and repeat on the other side.

3 Lift the corner of your mouth upwards and outwards, drop it and repeat on the other side.

4 Slightly open your mouth and waggle your chin gently from side to side. Do this carefully to avoid injuring your jaw.

5 Looking in the mirror, brace your chin back strongly so that all the skin and the fine sheet of muscle just below stand out tense and strong. Let the jaw go loose. This helps to keep the throat and jawline neat.

Now you should have a beautifully poised head on a strong neck and a face you are proud to show.

Sleep

Said Winston Churchill, a man needs six hours' sleep, a boy needs seven and only women and fools need more. Marisa Berenson, although she might not care to be bracketed with fools, would be the first to agree with that. She reckons on nine hours' sleep a night to keep up the appearance that has earned her the reputation of one of the world's most beautiful women.

Most newborn babies sleep for perhaps 15 hours out of the 24 and require less sleep as they grow older. By the time a child is ten, he or she may need no more sleep than an adult. At the other end of the age range, there are septuagenarians who catnap through the night and yet are still sprightly the next day. For the majority of people, the need to sleep decreases with age.

Research has shown that the physiology of sleep is complicated. The brain has two centres that are involved in the process – one makes us go to sleep, the other keeps us asleep. The first is triggered off by a variety of factors, for example, darkness, habit, what others around us are doing, physical or mental tiredness. It is thought that the second is set off mainly by chemical reactions occurring in the body and brain cells.

It is useful to think of sleep as resembling the recharging of a battery and it seems that, for most people, between 16 and 17 hours of wakefulness are sufficient to run down the battery.

Dreaming

Sleep plays an important part in the way the body recovers from a day's activity. However, scientists believe that it is through dreaming that the brain prepares itself for the next day.

If you think of the brain as a computer constantly absorbing, sifting, channelling, analyzing and synthesizing information, then it is obvious that if the channels become clogged with information, a fuse will blow. One attractive theory about dreams describes them as the mechanism by which the brain discharges redundant information, or, in other words, clears the circuits. According to another recent theory it is during dreaming that our brain cells manufacture the essential chemicals needed for intellectual functioning. Thus, if we are deprived of dreams, these chemicals are not synthesized. This theory is supported by experiments that have shown that if people are woken up every time they start to dream (this is checked on an electroencephalograph, which shows how the pattern of brain waves alters at the point when dreaming begins), they quickly become exhausted. Moreover, this exhaustion occurs even if they have the requisite number of hours' sleep.

The only conclusion to be drawn from this is that we do not just need to sleep, we need to dream. Indeed some scientists even say that we sleep only in order to dream.

While we are asleep other things are happening in the various parts of the body. The heart rate slows down and there is a drop in body temperature of $0.5\,°C$ ($1\,°F$). In other words, we are in a state of partial hibernation. Breathing also becomes very slow, which means that the body is relatively deprived of oxygen. The result is a concentration of carbon dioxide in the blood, making the body slightly more acid than it is during waking hours. The small amount of urine produced in the night is therefore very acid so that the body's pH (the balance of acid and alkali) is maintained at a level of around 7.4. Digestion proceeds as normal but the body produces less of an important hormone called cortisol, which at the higher daytime levels is responsible for activity and alertness.

Insomnia

It is extremely rare for anyone to lie awake the entire night. Although you may imagine you have not slept at all, it is probable that in fact you did drop off for a few fitful hours. But insomnia, however it hits you, is unpleasant and if it goes on for more than two or three days can be debilitating. The most prominent effect is extreme muscular fatigue, while conceptual thinking, which is necessary for making decisions, may become impaired.

Insomnia has many causes and many patterns. The person who cannot get off to sleep is usually tense, insecure or anxious about something. The most common emotion that stops people sleeping is resentment – if you feel you have been unfairly treated, you may lie for hours plotting retribution. There is also the sleeplessness that hits you when you have been dozing nicely, wake up and just cannot get back to sleep – the first snooze has blunted your need for sleep and you have to lie awake long enough to build up a debt of tiredness. There is yet another kind where you wake very early in the morning and wait for the dawn chorus; this type of early wakening is associated with depression and is one of the classic symptoms that doctors look for in a depressed patient.

A special form of insomnia can occur in pregnancy. Paradoxically, one of the first signs of pregnancy is fatigue and the need to catnap at any time of day. At the same time, nocturnal insomnia may strike and is probably associated with hormonal changes that occur within a week or two of fertilization. The body metabolism picks up speed as a result of pregnancy and is no longer responsive to the braking system that normally occurs late at night. After all, the baby does not stop developing just because it is dark and the body involuntarily maintains its maternal responsibilities, hence insomnia.

There are a number of drugs that affect the sleep centres in the brain. Drugs that make you sleep (hypnotics) act either on the centre that sends you off or on the one that keeps you asleep, or on both. The older hypnotics prevent dreaming, which accounts for the hangover commonly experienced after taking barbiturates. The most widely used barbiturate is a short-acting one (between four and six hours), but in overdose it is rapidly fatal. Most of the newer hypnotics, which are related to minor tranquillizers, enable you to be alert if you wake up, but stimulate the second centre sufficiently for you to go back to sleep. They also allow you to dream more naturally.

Many people think, wrongly, that alcohol is a good sleep inducer. It may send you off to sleep for a short time, but as the alcohol is absorbed into the blood it acts as a stimulant that can wake you up, with your mind active and racing, so that you cannot get back to sleep again.

Below are a few things you can do yourself to improve your chances of having a good, and comfortable, night's rest.
- Make sure your bedroom is as well-ventilated as is comfortable for you and neither too warm nor too cold.
- Invest in the best mattress you can afford. If you tend to have trouble sleeping you will never get a good night's rest on a sagging or lumpy mattress.

- Try to do something relaxing before you go to bed. Yoga is excellent, as is a short walk. If that is too strenuous, sit and scan the newspapers in a leisurely fashion. Many people find that a book or a quiet half hour of television is the ideal soporific, but do not choose anything too exciting, or it will set your mind turning again.
- Make sure that all dripping taps are turned off and that squeaking doors are closed.
- Do not wear a constricting nightie or pyjamas.
- Take a warm drink at bedtime (a milky one, rather than coffee or tea, which contain stimulants). This has nothing whatever to do with 'night starvation', which is a fiction invented by advertisers. However, some food on the stomach diverts blood from the brain and makes you feel drowsy.
- Have a warm bath. It works in a similar way to a warm drink, the blood being diverted from the brain to the skin.
- Give yourself a facial or neck massage (see pages 176–177).

Have your own personal relaxation routine ready. Lie in bed and do the following:
- Check every part of your body systematically and make a conscious effort to relax any muscles that feel tense. Tense muscles can prevent sleep (see also pages 170–171).
- Slow down your breathing by taking one long breath in and then out again where you would normally have taken two.
- Try to empty your mind of all thoughts – count sheep if you like. A good trick is to think about black velvet.

Should all these things fail and you find yourself lying awake next to a snoring partner, do not lie there and let your resentment bottle up. You may as well use the night to do something productive, so get up, go downstairs, make yourself a cup of tea and do some job that you were not able to fit into the daytime.

If insomnia is a chronic problem you should consult your doctor. Everyone needs sleep and everyone should have sleep. Sleeping pills taken over a short period to re-establish your routine are a necessity for some, but you should stop taking them once old sleeping patterns are established. Sleeping pills should never be relied upon as a long-term measure.

A Facial Statement

Appearance counts: there is no doubt that, for most women, how we look is important both to us and to other people. The ideal is to be both healthy and beautiful and one easy way to enhance and show off to best advantage a healthy body and face is through the use of cosmetics.

The function of make-up is manifold. It can be used to camouflage flaws – the practical side of cosmetics that should not be underestimated; to make a statement about our personality; to transform the image we present to the outside world; to boost the morale. It can act as a disguise, a mask to hide behind. It also provides an opportunity to indulge in fantasy, to create a look that nature alone cannot achieve. The use of cosmetics has a long history. Kohl, for rimming eyes, has been found in excavated Egyptian tombs as far back as 3000 BC. Roman matrons used coloured powders kept in narrow-necked bottles and long-handled bronze spoons for extracting and mixing their own cosmetics. Making-up has long been associated with loose women: a book of etiquette written at the turn of the century declares sternly that 'the Eastern habit of brightening the hue of the lips is generally recognized as confined to the stage and to a certain class of wholly artificial creatures, with whom no good woman or pure young girl wishes to be confounded.' Happily, attitudes have changed in recent years and all women, wicked or otherwise, can enjoy using cosmetics with impunity.

The cosmetic industry is big business and advertising and packaging tend to raise unrealistic expectations. It is sensible to be aware of this but, as buying make-up should be a boost for morale, a prettily packaged product can be part of the enjoyment. There is no need to buy an extensive range of products, but it is important to learn how to apply them correctly: an expert make-up artist can work successfully with a limited range of products and colours. Moreover, an astute buyer can find successful products at very little cost by shopping around for the shades and effects she likes in the cheaper ranges, which often use similar formulae to the more expensive ones. Some women find they are allergic to many make-up lines, for it is impossible to manufacture make-up that is safe for everyone because allergic reactions are so individual and unpredictable. However, if your skin is prone to reaction, choose from the ranges of hypo-allergenic cosmetics designed to exclude ingredients that cause allergies.

Make-up

Equipment and Accessories

A successful make-up needs three ingredients: products that suit the colouring and personality of the wearer, a confident, well-practised hand and the right equipment. This does not mean an array of expensive items hardly used, but practical tools that will give the finished face a professional look.

The most important aid for a successful make-up is good lighting. The best lighting is daylight, but not direct sunlight, in front of the work-table. Artificial light should be evenly distributed; soft lighting, while flattering to the face, is unsuitable for applying cosmetics and fluorescent light, unless designed to simulate daylight, has a tendency to distort colours. Strong light from one side, which throws hard shadows, should also be avoided.

A make-up table should be well lit, functional, clean and tidy, with everything that is needed close to hand. A free-standing mirror and a hand-held one, to be brought in close for more detailed work, are both useful; remember to check the finished work from both sides. Unfortunately, a bathroom, which often has good mirrors and lighting, is not the best place to keep cosmetics, as they react badly to the steamy atmosphere and sudden temperature changes.

Keeping make-up tidy encourages creativity – having all the products easily to hand can be an inspiration to try out different ideas and to mix products and colours. There are special boxes with pull-out trays for holding cosmetics, which, although useful, can be expensive. Look instead at the practical boxes made for fishermen's equipment, which are ideal for storing make-up and can be painted a bright colour to soften their utilitarian look. A cutlery tray divides the products into compartments for easy reference.

Brushes

Fingers are important for getting to know the face and the textures and spreading qualities of make-up, but they are not always the best tool for applying make-up. Brushes are necessary for precision in fine work or for a very light touch, required for applying powder for instance. You will need several sizes for different tasks: the selection illustrated here shows the ones that are used most often. Many cosmetic departments sell brushes for make-up, but as they should be functional, not decorative, probably the best place to buy them is from an art shop, as all the sizes you need will be there. Some sizes are used for more than one task, so it is sensible to have two or three of each. For example, a very fine tip can be used to outline the mouth, apply liquid eyeliner or disguise wrinkles; a medium tip can be used for both powder eyeshadow and contour colour. Not all the brushes have to be expensive: a baby's toothbrush is excellent for shaping eyebrows and for separating eyelashes after applying mascara. When choosing any size of brush, look for one with soft bristles – sable are the best – and for brushes that do not shed hairs.

Other useful equipment

Among other essential items on the work-table are tissues, preferably large, for blotting, removing make-up and keeping hands, brushes and the work-surface clean. Cotton wool should always be at hand; balls are convenient, but are too small for applying face powder, so a roll is probably better and certainly cheaper. Cotton wool buds, or swabs, make good applicators and, like sponge-tipped applicators, are particularly suitable for powder eyeshadows. Sponges, either natural or synthetic, are useful for make-up that must be diluted for application and can also be used for applying foundation. Synthetic or cotton puffs can be used instead of brushes or cotton wool for applying powder. Swansdown puffs are a luxury for putting on loose powder and give a light touch, which helps avoid clogging and unevenness of finish. Include hairbands and grips in your list of equipment, for it is difficult to apply make-up evenly with loose hair hanging round the face and the hair will become greasy if it comes into contact with the products. Tweezers, scissors, eyelash curlers and a pencil sharpener or safety razor blade may also be useful.

Finally, no artist would be complete without a palette. The best palette for make-up is the hand. Try out powder shadows and creams on the back of the hand, turning it about to check the intensity of the colour and to see how the make-up reflects the light.

Keep all brushes absolutely clean by frequent washing in water and mild detergent or by dipping them into an alcohol solution after use. Stand them upright in a pot to dry.

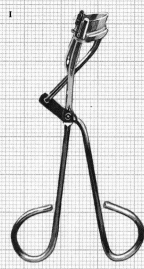

Eyelash curlers (1) make eyelashes look fuller and longer and eyes look bigger.

Tweezers (2) come in two sorts. Use those with slanted tips, above, to pluck stray hairs and eyebrows. Use square-tipped ones to apply false lashes.

Eyebrow brush (3) for training brows and for brushing surplus powder from them; can be used instead of a mascara wand to separate made-up eyelashes.

Eyeliner brush (4) for liquid eyeliner, disguising wrinkles and acne pits and also for outlining lips. Short, feathery strokes give greatest accuracy.

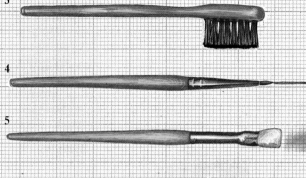

Lip brush (7), the most accurate tool for applying lip colour.

Contour colour brushes (8, 9), the easiest way to apply powder blushers, shaders and highlighters; they help to keep colours subtle and to blend away hard edges. Use the large brush for cheeks, the smaller one for more intricate work.

Sponge-tipped applicator (5), often supplied with powder eyeshadows; gentle for the eye area. You need several for different colours of eyeshadow.

Eyeshadow brush (6), an alternative to the sponge applicator, useful for applying and blending any texture of shadow. You need a few for different shadows.

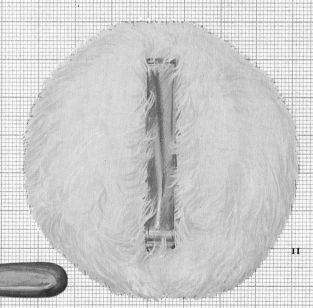

Powder brush (10), an alternative to a powder puff. Brush upwards to buff the skin for a natural sheen; finish with a few downward strokes to smooth the natural down on the face.

Powder puff (11), available in various forms – synthetic, down and cotton – ranging in size and quality from the small puffs that come with compressed powder compacts to the large swansdown variety illustrated above.

... the basis of a successful ... like cleansing and mois- ... ential part of the make-up ... e an ideal surface to receive ... also helps to even out the ... ect the imperfections of tone or bloto... which the skin of the face, because of its vulnerability to the elements, is so prone. It acts, too, as a barrier between the skin and atmospheric pollution. A spotty skin is often better with a foundation to protect it from dirt.

It is important to remember that foundation should always rest on the skin's surface and never be absorbed or rubbed into it. That is why moisturizer should always be applied before the foundation, as its emulsion stops any moisture in the foundation being absorbed into the skin, so leaving the colour pigment behind in unattractive patches; foundation also flows more smoothly on to moisturized skin. If put on properly, found-ation should last throughout the day without needing to be retouched.

Ingredients

Whatever the type of foundation, the basic ingredients include colour pigment, derived from iron oxide and titanium oxide, and, to enable foundation to run smoothly and evenly over the skin, a natural wax such as bees' wax. They also include an emulsifier and a form of cellulose, which thickens the mixture and gives it adhering qualities. Hypo-allergenic foundations contain only allergy-tested ingredients. Perfume, the main cause of allergic reactions, is cut out and the preservatives essential to stop foundation going bad are kept to a minimum. Lanolin, also a suspect ingredient, is omitted from many hypo-allergenic products.

The first thing to establish when buying foundation is skin type, for although moisturizer temporarily corrects a skin's inherent dryness or oiliness, the skin gradually reverts to type during the day (see pages 22–23). So women with an oily skin should not choose a foundation with extra moisturizing properties, and those with a very dry skin should choose an oil-based rather than a water-based brand. Liquid foundation, which usually comes in bottles, gives a light coverage and is especially suitable for fine skins or young skins that tend to form fine lines. Most foundations have a creamy base and are packaged in tubes. These are the easiest to apply and suit a wide range of skin types: some include moist-urizer, others give a powdery finish. Be wary of medicated foundation, which may cause allergies. Hypo-allergenic foundations are excellent for sensitive skin. Solid foundations, which come in stick or cake form, give a dense cover and can help to camouflage badly blemished or scarred skins (see pages 205–207). Finally, for even-toned, tanned skins there are bronzing gels or tinted moisturizers. An ideal cosmetic kit should contain more than one type of foundation: a natural cover for daily use, a denser base for night time to counteract the harshness of artificial light and a bronzing gel for a tanned skin. The simplest way to apply foundation is with the fingers; a small sponge, squeezed almost dry, may also be used.

Choice of colour

Foundation should match the natural colouring of the face as exactly as possible. A more dramatic change of colour can be achieved by the addition of highlighters, blushers and shaders over the neutral base of foundation. However, it is possible to complement the skin colour with foundation. For example, a florid complexion can be toned down with a beige shade and a sallow one enlivened with a slightly pink hue. To find the correct colour, try it on the skin, preferably on the side of the hand, along the thumb, as this area shows a typical range of skin tones. Always put a little moisturizer on first because the way the foundation takes to the skin is an essential part of its success. Check the effect under natural and artificial light.

Coloured women often have difficulty finding the right colour for their skin tone, which can range from pale bisque to black with an almost blue sheen. Other products can be used to adapt the colour. Brown-shaded cream eyeshadows can add depth of colour to a pale foundation. A dark blusher or tawny lipstick can intensify and warm the tone. Alternatively, a little dark blue eye-shadow may bring a foundation nearer the skin colour. Experiment by mixing the different colours together in the palm of the hand, where the warmth will aid blending.

Applying foundation

You will need: a clean face, with hair pinned or tied well back; foundation and tissues; a small sponge (optional). The face must be freshly moisturized. Oily skins are usually better left for a few minutes after the moisturizer has been applied; but with drier skins, the foundation can be put on immediately. Shake the foundation container and squeeze or pour out about a teaspoonful of foundation into the palm of the hand you are not going to use.

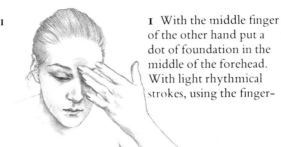

I

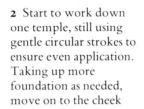

2 Start to work down one temple, still using gentle circular strokes to ensure even application. Taking up more foundation as needed, move on to the cheek

I With the middle finger of the other hand put a dot of foundation in the middle of the forehead. With light rhythmical strokes, using the finger-

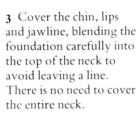

and then the eye area, covering the lid up to the eyebrow and the skin under the eye. Then work towards the jaw, remembering to go right to the ear.

tips, blend the foundation with gentle, circular movements on to the entire forehead area right up to the hairline.

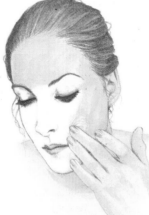

2

3

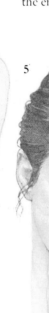

3 Cover the chin, lips and jawline, blending the foundation carefully into the top of the neck to avoid leaving a line. There is no need to cover the entire neck.

4

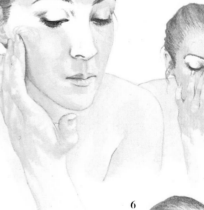

5

4 Work up the other side of the face, from the cheek to the area round the eye, and on to the temple, blending the foundation into that on the forehead.

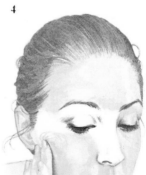

6

5 Put a streak of foundation down the length of the nose and blend down both sides. Move closer to the mirror and check the whole face for streaks, bare patches or uneven colour, correcting any imperfections with small dots of foundation well blended into the rest.

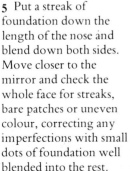

6 Remove any surplus foundation on the neck, and give yourself a massage at the same time, by using the backs of the fingers in light upward strokes under the chin and round the jaw. Check the face once more, then wipe off the foundation in your hand with a tissue.

Powder

Although foundation is the basis of a good make-up, providing a neutral surface to work on, it has to be fluid for application and so must be fixed with powder. It is tempting to miss out the powdering because foundation has a pleasing sheen without any additions but powder lends a bloom that is more natural than foundation alone. When it is badly put on, it can look clogged and floury, but manufacturers now mill their powder so finely that it is possible to retain a sheen on the skin's surface while cutting out shine, so powder is particularly useful for countering the shine on oily skin. The only instance when powder is not needed is when a bronzing gel is worn.

Products

Powder comes in two forms: loose and compressed. Loose powder gives a subtle, even finish and any surplus is easily removed. Solid, compressed powders are convenient to carry and are useful for touching up problem areas such as a shiny nose. However, they need careful application because the effect can become uneven. It is also important to clean the puff regularly to ensure an even transfer of powder on to the face.

The range of powder colours is more limited than that for foundation and the most popular brands are the lightly tinted translucent varieties, which give texture and finish but add no colour. If you use a non-translucent powder, choose a colour a few shades lighter than your foundation; remember that powder looks darker in the compact than on the skin.

Ingredients

All powders are based on talc; other ingredients include chalk compounds for absorbency, perfume and colour. However, hypo-allergenic ranges include powders in which perfume, the main irritant for allergy-prone skins, is omitted or kept to a minimum. Baby talcum powder can be used quite effectively: its initial whiteness on the face, which can be off-putting, disappears when all the surplus powder is removed. Translucent powders have a finer texture than most baby talcum powder; oxide colours are mixed into the finely milled talc to create a tinting effect.

Compact powders are usually mixed with a small amount of oil or wax and then compressed. These solid powders give denser coverage than loose powders and must be more carefully used. A good way to apply them is to fold the puff to form a ridge. Press this lightly on to the powder and with a gentle twisting movement press the powder on to the face. Whether loose or compressed, powder should never be rubbed or smeared on to the skin as this disturbs the foundation and results in a patchy finish.

Applying powder
You will need: hair tied or pinned back; loose powder, preferably translucent; tissues; a large piece of cotton wool or a large soft brush or a powder puff.

1

2

1 Scatter a generous amount of powder on to a tissue and press the cotton wool, brush or puff over it gently. With a rapid twisting movement of the wrist, cover the face with powder, including the crevices of the nose and lips and all round the eye area. The powder should rest on the surface of the foundation, so that the face looks floury. Do not try to rub it in.

2 Ensure that the powder is distributed evenly over the face. With a fresh piece of cotton wool, a brush shaken clean or the reverse side of the puff, remove the surplus powder with rapid upward strokes. This restores a natural texture to the skin and buffs it to give a subtle sheen. Knock any loose powder off the applicator and finish with a few downward strokes to settle the down on the face. Blend the edge around the jawline. Clear the brows of any powder with an eyebrow brush.

Contour Colour

Blushers, shaders and highlighters are often bracketed together under the name contour colour. They perform two functions: they bring life to the face with colour and shine and they shape it by emphasizing the underlying bone structure. A simple principle to remember is that colours paler than the skin tone bring features forwards, while darker colours make them recede. Try to be flexible with the products you buy: the colour of your skin is more important than the label on the product. For instance, something labelled shader or contourer might be a good highlighter for a black skin, whereas a pink-tinted highlighter might be an excellent cheek colour for a pale complexion. There are no firm rules about colour but texture sets limitations. Any make-up with shine or frosting catches the eye, while matte colours look shadowy.

Unlike lip and eye make-up, contour colour should never be noticeable, but must be blended with a light touch until there are no harsh lines. There are two techniques for applying colour. The first is to apply a broad sweep of colour rapidly and lightly, using fingertips or a brush and then to blend away any edges without shifting the colour. The second, useful for smaller areas, is to take up a little colour on the fourth finger or on a small brush and finger-print or stipple the colour on to the skin until it merges with the rest of the make-up. With the exception of transparent gel blusher, which looks good applied directly to tanned skin, contour colour should be worn over foundation set with powder, to aid blending.

Ingredients

Contour colour comes as gels, liquids, creams, sticks, pencils, or as loose or cake powder, in standard or hypo-allergenic ranges. Gels and liquids give colour to the skin without dense coverage and look particularly good on a tanned skin, while creams, sticks and pencils give more coverage. Creams and gels consist of colour mixed with a greasy agent such as beeswax or cocoa butter. Liquids are based on a formula similar to foundation. Sticks and pencils have a stiff wax base with added mineral oil and oxide colours. Powders are easiest to apply, as colour can be built up gradually. Their formula is similar to face powder but with a higher colour content; highlighters sometimes contain a small proportion of powdered metals to catch the light.

The colour can look strong in the container but only a little is needed to give a natural look. An excess of colour can be gently wiped away with a tissue; powder colour can also be removed with a clean, dry brush.

Exploring your face

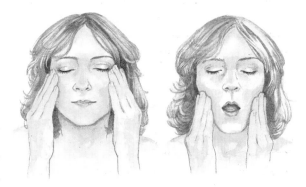

Even the lightest film of contour colour must be precisely located to achieve the right effect, so it is important to know the strengths and weaknesses of your face. Fingertips, which have great sensitivity, help in this facial anatomy lesson. Place them on the forehead and run them lightly down towards the eyes. The forehead often bulges to the front or side – are these bulges enhancing to the face or could they be made less prominent? Is the forehead broad or narrow in comparison to the rest of the face? When the fingers reach the browbone, slide them round to the temples at the side of the eyes. Discover where the hairline starts. Now place the fingertips directly under the lower lashes and run them lightly downwards, feeling the swell of the cheekbone.

Open the mouth slightly and continue down the face. Directly under the cheekbone there is a hollow – you may have to press a little to find it. The structure of the face round the chin is important. Does the jawbone jut or recede? There are often unattractive hollows beneath the corners of the mouth, which perhaps you have not noticed before. Do not be surprised if the face is slightly different on each side as few faces are entirely symmetrical.

Finally, shine a strong light directly on top of the head to exaggerate the slopes and valleys of the bone structure. Pull the hair away from the face and look in a well-lit mirror. Is the basic shape of the face good? Without giving the shape a label such as square or round, decide whether its proportions are pleasing. There is no such thing as a correct face shape: every face is unique and this frank assessment is necessary to decide how to capitalize on what you have. With this intimate knowledge of your face it will be much easier to use contour colour.

Blushers

Of the three contour colours, blushers are possibly the most useful; even a face that has no need of contouring can benefit from the warmth that blusher lends to the skin. Blusher is another name for rouge, which has been used for centuries to give warmth and vitality to the face, although modern products come in a much wider range.

Although they are designed to colour rather than shape, blushers can help to give proportion to the face, particularly by defining the cheek area. They can even out a patchy skin tone – useful if the skin is tanned and a gel blusher is applied directly to the skin. A blusher is particularly important for bringing life and colour to a drab skin. It can also bring out the delicate quality of a very pale skin, which can look bluish. Sallow skins are greatly improved by colour, especially Oriental skins where the use of a peachy tone can enhance the ivory colour. Even black skins can look drab and grey and can benefit from blushers in shades of plum and dark red, which complement their natural lustre: you may find the best tone in a lip colour.

It is important to place blusher properly, particularly on the cheeks. If the colour is too near the nose, it can draw the whole face inwards, making it look older. Although more intense colour should be worn in the evening because of artificial lighting, the placement is still important, as electric light tends to drain colour and leave merely the tone. If cheek colour is placed near the nose, it can make the area look sunken rather than rounded. So always work away from the nose and blend towards the hairline; at night, a blusher with shine helps to counteract a shadowing effect.

Applying blusher
You will need: blusher; a brush if using powder blusher.

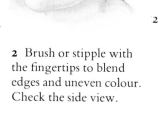

2 Brush or stipple with the fingertips to blend edges and uneven colour. Check the side view.

Blusher on the forehead
Apply a light touch of blusher in a small circle in the centre of the forehead. Blend away the edges.

Blusher on the cheeks
1 Apply a band of colour along the most prominent part of each cheekbone, starting below the outer corner of the eye and working out towards the hairline.

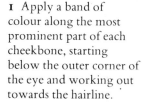

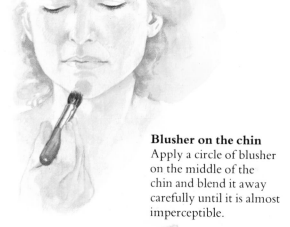

Blusher on the chin
Apply a circle of blusher on the middle of the chin and blend it away carefully until it is almost imperceptible.

For a healthy glow
Apply a little matte powder blusher round the hairline from the right ear to the left. Brush it in towards the face and blend carefully.

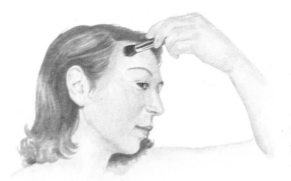

Shaders

Expertly applied, shaders can create hollows, emphasize bone structure and improve the appearance of features such as a wide nose or forehead. It must be stressed that shading should be subtle and that the effect should be an impression rather than a statement. Crude handling of contour colour can be counter-productive, emphasizing weak points rather than improving them. The more delicate shading techniques, such as fining down a wide nose, require some practice: it should be impossible to tell that a shader has been used.

For daytime wear, beginners should use a shade of blusher darker than the skin tone rather than deeper browns, since warm colours look more natural than neutral-coloured shaders, especially on full cheeks, which do not generally have shadows. Naturally high cheekbones can be shown off by a streak of neutral shader drawn with a finger or brush under the bone and blended towards the hairline; but on a round face use the softer technique of applying a matte blusher in a fat triangle.

Use dark, neutral shades for evening, or for more dramatic remodelling if you have a skilled touch. These products are dark and can look drab and uninteresting on the palette – but remember you are making shadows. If your skin is very dark, you may have to use highlights to do the work of shaders – highlighting the centre of a wide forehead instead of shading the temples, or highlighting cheekbones to define the structure of a round face instead of shading cheeks.

Applying shader
You will need: shader, preferably in powder form; a brush, the width depending on the area to be covered – fine for the nose, broader for the cheeks.

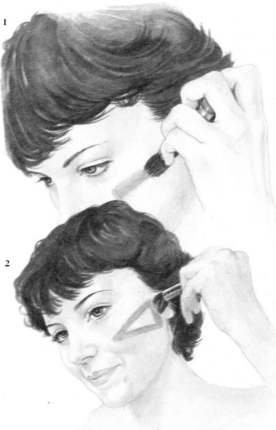

1

2

A basic technique for shading cheeks
1 Using a warm tawny shade, draw a fat line under each cheekbone towards the top of the ear, starting below the centre of the eye.

2 Draw a second line towards the bottom of the ear, starting from the same point as the first line. Complete the triangle with a third line drawn upwards beside the ear. Fill in the centre of the triangle using the same blusher and blend away all edges.

To enhance the jawline
Brush a line of shader just under the jawbone all along its length.

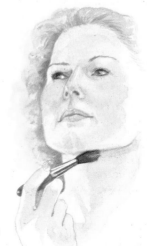

To narrow the bridge of the nose

Draw a line down the side of the nose from the eyebrow, stopping on a level with the corner of the eye. Blend.

To fine down a wide nose

(below) Draw a line down the side from the inner corner of the eye to the bottom of the nose. Blend well.

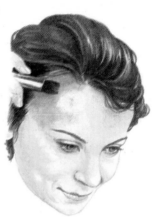

To narrow the nostrils

(above) With a fine brush, apply shader in a crescent-moon shape round the crease at the side of each nostril. The band of shader should be widest and darkest at the widest part of the nostril; fade out the edges.

To give a wide forehead better proportions

(below) Apply shader in a warm tone to the temples, from where the forehead slopes back to the hairline. Blend well.

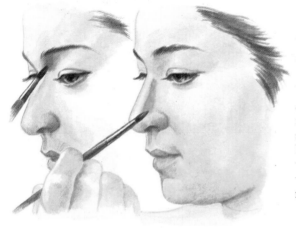

Highlighters

Highlighting is the positive part of contour colour. Use its light-catching qualities to draw attention to a feature that you are proud of, such as eyes, cheekbones or chin; try a line down a perfect straight nose or a dab in the middle of a classic forehead. Highlighter has a practical use too: any ageing wrinkle or groove on the face, such as the line from the nose down to the mouth or the hollows at each side of the chin, can be filled out by lightening the shadows. Dead white products are hard to use, so instead try those with pink or cream tones, which blend more easily with the natural skin tone. Bronzes, golds and darker pinks with added sparkle can also be used and look especially good on darker skins. Natural colouring dictates the choice of colours – the darker the skin, the wider the range of products that will highlight it. On the other hand, a very pale skin might need a pure white product. Remember that added shine intensifies the effect and that a light touch of highlight is most effective.

Highlighter is particularly important for complementing eye make-up. The cheek and browbone form a natural frame for the eyes and a touch of light on the top of the cheekbone as well as just under the brow helps to make a strong eye make-up blend in with the rest of the face.

Applying highlighter

You will need: highlighter; a brush or sponge-tipped applicator (optional).

Highlighting the chin

(below) For a well-modelled chin or to bring forwards a receding one, apply highlighter on the front of the chin and blend.

To highlight the browbone

(below) Draw a fine line just above the eyebrow along the length of the brow and blend well.

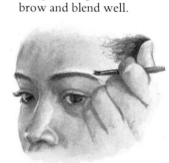

To emphasize cheekbones

(below) Apply a line of highlighter from the outer corner of each eye above the cheekbones to the hairline; blend.

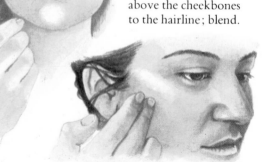

Using contour colours together

It is no accident that these three make-up techniques are so closely associated. They can be used separately but they complement each other so well that they work best in conjunction with each other. Although the main function of blusher is to add colour, it also helps to link highlighter and shader, softening the contrast between them and completing the total effect by adding warmth and glow. Blusher will tinge a highlighter with its colour and warm a cold shader to give a much more natural effect. For example, after shading full cheeks with a dark shade of matte blusher, a lighter blusher suitable for creating a natural glow can be used on the cheekbone to soften the effect and draw attention to the bone structure.

Shader and highlighter are essentially complementary and, since they must always be used as subtly as possible, the way in which they complement each other is important. If, for instance, shader is being used to narrow a wide jaw, a touch of highlighter on the chin will divert attention from the sides of the face. Just as highlighter brings out the good points, a subtle touch of shader can draw attention to good bone structure by darkening the natural shadows. Above all, when using contour colour, do not be afraid to experiment or to exaggerate unusual features that express your personality.

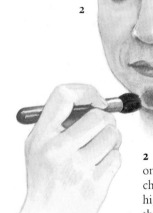

To soften a pointed chin

1 Feel the slight indentation at each side of the chin under the outer corners of the mouth and smudge a little highlighter, about the size of a thumbprint, into the hollows.

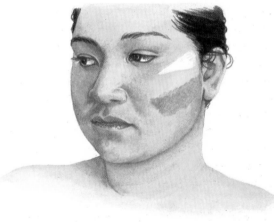

2 Brush a circle of shader on to the front of the chin. Blend both the highlighter and shader thoroughly.

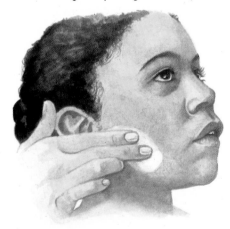

To soften a pointed face

Apply a dark matte blusher to the outer half of the cheekbones, taking it out towards the ear. Blend well. Use a subtle, matte highlighter on the outer part of the jaw, blending it up to the middle of the cheek and back towards the ear.

To slim a full face

A round face needs both shader and highlighter to change the shape. Well-defined, interesting eye make-up also helps to divert attention from full cheeks. Shade the cheeks at their fullest, between the cheek- and jawbones, taking a wide line of shader from below the centre of the eye out towards the ear. Apply a diagonal line of highlighter above the cheekbone from the outer corner of the eye to the hairline; broaden the highlighted area as you work outwards. Blend away any edges to ensure a natural look.

Eyes

Eyes respond well to make-up: they are often the most interesting feature and the lightest touch of mascara can transform the entire face, throwing the eyes into new emphasis and giving them sparkle and brightness. Shaded lids draw attention to the colour and shape of the eye, and highlights and shadows can suggest a better bone structure. Bad points can be played down and good ones brought into fresh emphasis; with a little practice it is even possible to change the eye shape quite dramatically, though it is often more effective to exploit the natural shape, for most have potential. Study this shape and understand it. Rather than making the eye conform to fashion, try enhancing its intrinsic value. Ideas can be gleaned from magazines or by studying other people's eye make-up. Such is the versatility of eye make-up that it is possible to pay court to a new look while stamping it with your personal touch.

The most comprehensive range of cosmetic products available is for the eyes. The entire colour spectrum is represented in rows of glittering shades. Whereas make-up for lips and cheeks is limited to certain colours and shapes, there are no firm rules for eyes. They can be dark and sultry, pale and ingenuous, dramatic, subtle, matte or shiny – it is entirely a matter of personal choice and individual skill. However, this freedom means that there are hazards, for it is tempting to choose sparkling, unusual colours that catch the attention rather than those that suit the eyes, skin tone and bone structure.

Textures

The form of the products is, however, the most important consideration, as the range of colours is available in every type. Find a texture that suits your eye and lifestyle, and you are likely to find it in the colour you want. Powder eyeshadows are often sold in blocks with sponge-tipped applicators; looser powders often come with a dipstick. Shadows also come as creams, gels, liquids, solid water-colours or pencils: the list is endless. Most mascara is sold in tubes with wand applicators. Some brands have added fibres to make the lashes look longer and thicker, others are water-resistant.

For a beginner, the problem is making the colour stay in the right place and not drip, cake or crease. Powder colour is the easiest to apply and often stays on longest. Water-colour shadows, which can be worked into a thick cream or diluted with water into a thin wash and then applied with a brush, also last well but are quite difficult to apply. Eye pencils are easy to work with and versatile. Use them to outline the eye or, for a more subtle effect, smudge and blend them over the entire eyelid with the finger; look for the softest. Liquid eyeliner is also easy to blend, but to line the inner rim of the bottom lid, kohl or an eye pencil is essential.

Ingredients

The manufacturers of eye products are bound by strict rules about ingredients. Under the United States Food, Drug and Cosmetics Act, the use of coal tar colours in preparations to be applied in the area of the eyes is forbidden, even when those colours have been certified for use in cosmetics. Various blacks, such as carbon and oil black, are allowed in the E.E.C., provided they are pure colours containing no chemical additives. This applies also to pure vegetable dyes. Mineral and earth colours are allowed but again are subject to strict rules regarding their purity, as are finely powdered metals, which are often used in shadows. Eye products are carefully screened for any possible long-term harmful effects, so although the more adventurous might like to experiment with artists' crayons (see page 204), it is safest to use proper eye products, or hypo-allergenic ones if you have a history of allergy.

Cream shadows consist of colour suspended in a waxy base, such as cocoa butter, beeswax or petroleum jelly, with added preservative. Liquid shadows and eyeliner are coloured by oxides suspended in an emulsion. Kohl is also coloured by oxides in a base of talcum powder. Powder shadows are much the same as cake rouges or compressed powder but with a stronger colour; highlighters often include finely powdered metals and iridescent material to give a glittering effect. Eye pencils and eyebrow pencils are based on a similar formula to lipstick but with a higher proportion of beeswax or another high-melting constituent to make a firmer texture. The colour range of mascara is limited by the type of pigments suitable for use; in the U.S.A., the addition of organic dyes is prohibited. A water-proof mascara is made by adding a resin in which the colour is suspended. Cream or liquid mascara is made with the addition of small quantities of greasy agents such as cocoa butter and beeswax. Cake mascara is based on a soap-like ingredient plus oils, waxes and colour. False lashes are made either of human hair or nylon, depending on the quality required.

Cosmetic cleansers and lotions are formulated to dissolve and remove these ingredients and are more effective in doing so than soap (see page 199 for how to remove eye make-up). Use an oil-based cleanser for removing waterproof mascara.

Colours

Choice of colours is so personal that it is hard to lay down rules. For instance, some people like to emphasize very blue eyes with a vivid matching shadow, while others feel that a bright shadow detracts from the natural colour and that neutral shades are better. Try out different effects and you may find that surprising colour combinations do most for your eyes. It is important to put on eye make-up accurately. Nothing looks worse than an unflattering colour haphazardly applied.

Skin tone must also be taken into account when choosing colours. Very fair skins can be over-whelmed by too positive an eye make-up and are better suited to the delicate watered-silk colours. The darker the skin and hair colour, the more dramatic the eye make-up can be: intense glowing shades can be used without being overpowering. A pale shadow appears darker over a dark skin, though frosted colours reflect the natural sheen of a black or brown skin to great effect. However, frosted colours can be difficult to wear, especially on crepey lids.

An ideal starter's kit consists of a neutral shade in a matte colour, a highlighter for the browbone, kohl or a pencil for definition, mascara and a light-catching colour shadow. Choose mascara in a shade that complements your hair colour: avoid black and dark brown if you are blonde, aiming instead for mid-browns, blues and greys. When practising different effects and colours, try making up one eye only to see how it contrasts with the other.

The application of eye make-up can be tricky, for the area to be worked on is small and has many creases and has a tendency to develop fine wrinkles. Pulling it encourages crow's-feet; care must also be taken to avoid getting make-up into the eyes. Furthermore, the make-up for both eyes should match, which can be particularly difficult for anyone with short, or near, sight. Practice will enable you to experiment with confidence and to find the effects that suit your features and personality best.

Glasses and contact lenses

For those who wear glasses it is worth bearing these points in mind. Lenses for long, or far, sight make the eyes look larger; those for short, or near, sight smaller. In both cases use several coats of mascara to give the eye definition and keep make-up as natural as possible. Unusual colour combinations and geometric lines do not look right behind glass. Where the eye is magnified, a wash of matte colour on the lid looks effective. If the eye is already prominent, use neutral shadow and a kohl liner on the inside rim of the bottom lid. A clear bright eye pencil in silvery blue or green looks particularly good on an older woman with grey hair (see pages 208–209).

If you wear contact lenses, avoid greasy products as they tend to run and can cloud the lens. Soft, loose powders can be as irritating as a handful of dust thrown into the eye, especially those with metallic glitter added. Solid powder shadows over a non-greasy foundation or water-colour shadows are best. Pencil liner can be difficult to apply, particularly on the upper lid, because the pencil can press painfully against the lens; it is better to use a liquid liner and blend the edges to soften the effect.

Hay fever sufferers face particular difficulties: try a light application of waterproof mascara and the ranges of water-resistant shadows.

Eye make-up can be what you make of it. A natural-looking eye can take as much time and effort as a dramatic one. On the next few pages, some techniques for basic and more advanced eye make-ups are shown. However, these are intended simply as guidelines; experiment with a wide variety of textures and colours to discover your personal preferences and try not to be bound by habit or fashion.

Eyebrows

Surprisingly effective in framing the eye, the eyebrows can alter the entire face if their shape is improved, but the whole face must be taken into consideration before deciding on the ideal shape. Fine features on a small face look better with a subtle brow, whereas stronger features are balanced by a thicker one. Although it is tempting to pluck bushy brows quite drastically, fine adjustments are usually most successful. Always work with the natural arch of the brow.

Eyebrow pencils can be used to thicken or darken brows; choose a colour that matches your natural brows or one only a little darker. If you have sparse brows, avoid being heavy-handed, as the effect will be harsh and unnatural. Try to get into the habit of brushing your eyebrows and tweezing any stray hairs every day.

1 To find the ideal span of the eyebrow, place an eyebrow pencil beside the widest part of the nostril and hold it vertically by the side of the nose. The inner boundary of the brow should fall where the pencil crosses it.

2 To find the ideal outer edge of the eyebrow, swing the pencil over to make a line from the nostril to the outer corner of the eye. There should be no stray hairs beyond the point where the pencil crosses the eyebrow.

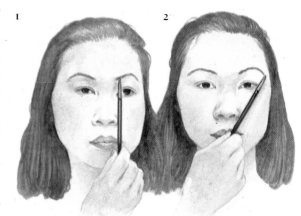

3 To trim and shape the eyebrows, pluck each hair with a swift, sharp movement using slant-tipped tweezers and holding the skin taut above the brow with the other hand. Always pluck from underneath the natural arch of the brow and in the direction of the hair's growth.

4 Brush the eyebrows upwards and outwards with a small stiff brush.

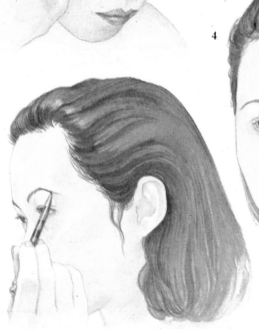

5 An eyebrow pencil gives definition to the brow. Imitating natural hairs, pencil in short, feathery strokes. To create an illusion of fullness, draw a wide line along the brow in beige before pencilling in the fine strokes.

Basic eye make-up

You will need: a neutral base covering the eye area; eyeshadow in two shades, one slightly darker than the other – powder shadows are easiest to use; powder highlighter; an eyeliner pencil; a mascara wand; applicators according to personal preference and the texture of shadow and highlighter (see pages 182–183).

1 Cover the upper lid and then the socket with the lighter shadow, working out from the nose. Do not extend the shadow above the socket. Take a narrow band of colour round the outer corner of the eye and under the lower lashes, fading it out half way along the lid. Blend gently with a fingertip.

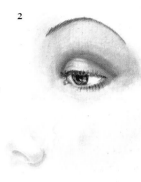

2 Define the eye socket with a contour shadow a few shades darker than the first. Extend the shadow slightly above the crease and down on to the top of the lid. Blend with the fingers.

3 Highlight browbone under the brow, following the natural curve; blend carefully with a fingertip.

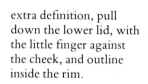

4 Steady the hand on the cheek. With the eyes open, outline the bottom lid close to the lashes. Lower the lids and pencil an outline along the top lid close to the lashes. Blend both lines. For extra definition, pull down the lower lid, with the little finger against the cheek, and outline inside the rim.

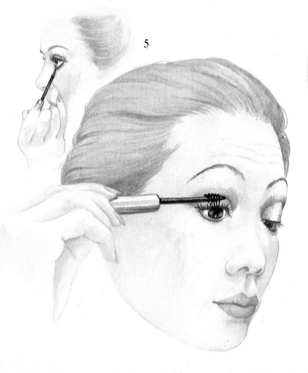

5 Apply mascara in several thin coats to prevent lashes sticking together. Use the wand until almost dry, then separate the lashes with it. Coat the inside of the top lashes, holding the wand horizontally. It is easier to coat the bottom lashes with the wand held horizontally, but try to hold it vertically instead, resting the hand on the cheek, so that each lash is coated individually.

Eyelashes

Most eyes are improved when framed by dark, curly lashes. Mascara is a compulsory item in a make-up kit: even a light coat draws attention to the eyes by separating and darkening lashes. A simple way to emphasize lashes is to curl them. False lashes, which come in a variety of designs, supplement short or sparse lashes, enhancing natural lashes subtly or creating a dramatic effect. For a natural look choose lashes only a few shades darker than your own.

False lashes

You will need: false lashes – full sets (1, 2) or individual lashes (3, 4); lash adhesive; square-tipped tweezers; an eyeliner pencil.

1 Practise positioning the lashes before putting on adhesive and trim to fit if necessary. Then, with the tweezers, grip the lashes firmly by the centre hairs and apply a thin line of glue to the inside rim. Lower them

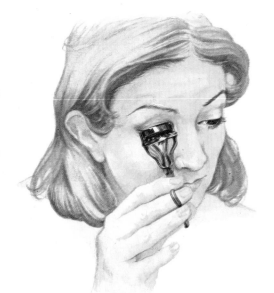

into position as near to the natural lashes as possible. Work from the middle of the eye out.

Individual lashes

These look natural as they can be applied only where needed and can be left on until they fall off like real lashes.

3 Apply the lightest possible dot of adhesive to the knotted end of each lash.

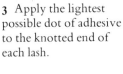

Eyelash curlers

(left) Prepare the lashes with a thin coat of mascara for protection. With the eyes slightly open, holding the curlers like scissors, place the opened curlers close to the eyelid, so that all the upper lashes peep through the gap. Close the curlers and squeeze gently for two seconds. Open them and see if the lashes have curled. Thick lashes might need another squeeze. Repeat with the other eye. Try not to be heavy-handed, as eyelashes can break off easily.

2 Use an eyeliner pencil to disguise the line formed by the lashes on the lid. Mingle natural lashes with the artificial ones by applying mascara to the tips of both.

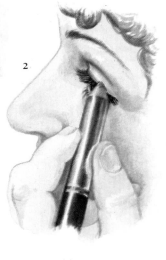

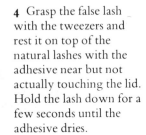

4 Grasp the false lash with the tweezers and rest it on top of the natural lashes with the adhesive near but not actually touching the lid. Hold the lash down for a few seconds until the adhesive dries.

Eye shapes

Eyes come in remarkably diverse shapes and sizes. Unless they are blessed with black lashes and strong colour, they can be insignificant – this is where mascara and eyeshadow can transform. Although it is often more successful to emphasize the intrinsic shape, it is possible to change it with clever use of shade and colour. A young face also needs care, as heavy make-up can look unbalanced. Experiment with the following suggestions even if the eyes described do not exactly correspond to your own.

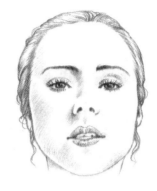

Make-up for a young girl

(left) Keep make-up light. Brush the eyebrows upwards each morning to train into a good shape. Apply a light film of pastel shadow over the entire lid up to the brow. Use a thin coat of brown or navy mascara.

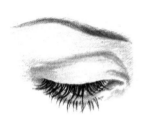

To enhance small or deep-set eyes

(left) Ensure the eyebrows are tidy and not too heavy. Use pale shadow on the lid, either powder or pencil. Wear several coats of mascara or false eyelashes.

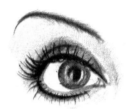

To make eyes less protruding

(right) Use a matte eyeshadow in a muted shade over the entire lid up to the browbone; avoid frosting, as it emphasizes the prominent shape, and very dark shadow, as it can make the lids look heavy and sleepy. Apply a matte highlight over the darker shadow on the browbone. Use eyeliner or kohl on both lids and blend away the hard edge on the top lid. Finish with a generous coat of mascara.

To make eyes look rounder

(above) This make-up suits most eyes. Apply dark shadow to the lid in an egg-shaped curve extending slightly above the socket on to the centre of the browbone; highlight the browbone. Use dark kohl or eyeliner all round the eye; blend. Apply plenty of mascara.

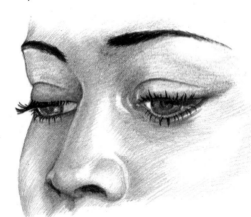

To emphasize a slant

1 Apply two diagonal bands of dark shadow from the inner and outer corners of the eye up to the eyebrow.

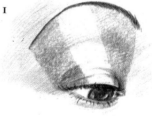

1

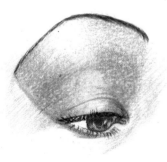

2

2 Using a paler shadow, fill in the central band up to the brow and blend carefully. Apply eyeliner to the bottom lid only, working out from the centre and taking it up to meet the outer corner of the brow. Soften the edge of the liner at the centre of the eye and blend it up into the shadow. Use only a touch of mascara.

To enhance heavy-lidded eyes

1 Brush the eyebrows upwards and define the shape with an eyebrow pencil. Apply mascara and curl the lashes with curlers. Use eyeliner on the upper lid and contour shadow in the socket.

2 Blend the liner up over the lid and blend the contour colour on to the browbone and down on to the lid to meet the contour shadow. Apply highlighter close to the brows. Pencil a faint brown line on the inside of the bottom lid.

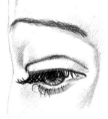
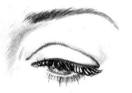
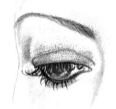
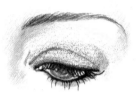

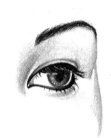
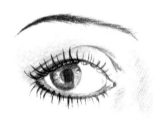
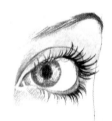

For wide-apart eyes

(left) Cover the lid and socket with a mid-toned shadow, blending up slightly above the socket. Take the shadow right up to the inner corner of the lid, but not beyond the outer corner of the eye. Apply a light touch of darker shadow near the nose up to the eyebrow. Use eyeliner or kohl along both lids.

For close-set eyes

(right) Thin the inner half of the brows. Cover the lid with shadow, going beyond the outer corner; apply paler shadow to the inner corner above the socket and on the lid. Highlight the browbone. Use eyeliner on both lids, from the centre out. Mascara the outer lashes.

Advanced make-up

Here is a make-up that makes the eyes the most important feature and looks effective worn with a simple hairstyle, a plain dress and the minimum of accessories. The time and patience required are rewarded by the final result.

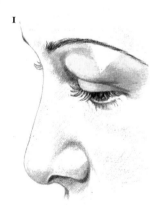

1 Ensure the eyebrows are tidy and well shaped. Apply a neutral-coloured foundation over the entire eye area to prevent the shadow from creasing or fading. Blend well. Mark a triangle of highlight on the most prominent part of the browbone above the centre of the eye. Do not blend as this is the focal point for the make-up.

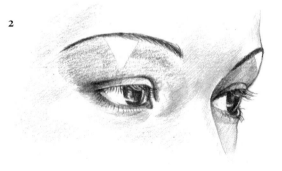

2 Cover the lid sparingly with a dark brown, grey or blue powder shadow; take the shadow up to the brow without covering the highlight and round in a narrow band beneath the lower lid, tapering it towards the inner corner of the eye and blending away any hard edges.

3

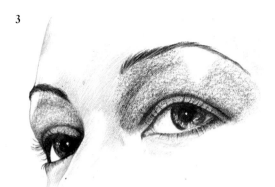

3 Cover the dark shadow with a thin coat of bright powder shadow, not necessarily in the same colour range, to give a shot-silk effect.

4

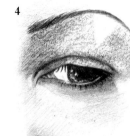

4 Pencil a fine line of bright metallic colour round the inside corner of the eye. Do not blend, but leave the eyeliner shiny and defined.

5

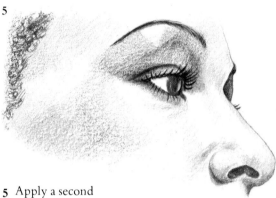

5 Apply a second highlighter along the browbone and take it down on to the cheekbone, blending it into the blusher; cover the first triangle of highlight. The range from plum to palest pink can be very effective. Apply a generous coat of mascara.

6

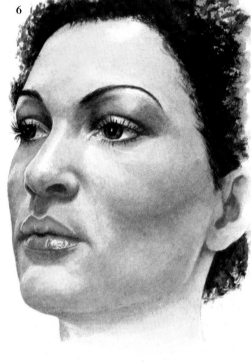

6 The finished look: intense glowing colour that is not crude or overdone. Shine is effective at night and intensifies colour. The secret is a light touch and frequent practice.

I

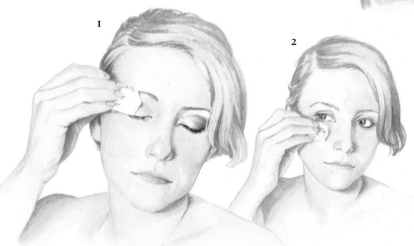

2

Cleansing
Remove eye make-up carefully: never drag at the skin. Soak a pad of cotton wool with eye make-up remover or cleansing cream and draw it outwards across the upper lid, with the eye shut (1). Open the eye and, with the clean side of the pad, cleanse the lower lid in the same way (2). Repeat until clean; remove surplus cream with a tissue.

Lips

Lip colour complements other make-up on the face, draws attention to an attractive mouth and, more practically, keeps the skin moist. It can give a boost to a dull complexion, which is particularly important for the older woman; it can also hide pigment variations on the lips, a problem for some black women. Moreover, lipstick is fun, a great lifter of the morale and the cheapest way to update your looks.

Products and ingredients

Lipsticks are arriving in ever-increasing varieties on the market. The solid stick is still the most popular form but there are also pencils, roll-on colour, lip pens, pots and gels. Almost without exception these products are intended to create a moist, shiny look; because they are based on mineral oil, they have less staying power than traditional lipsticks, which were intended to stain the skin but tended to cause allergies and to dry out the lips. The creamy texture of lipstick is achieved by blending oils, glycerides and waxes, a solvent for the dyes, perfume and flavour – lipstick is the only make-up that must be acceptable to the palate of the wearer as well as pleasing to the eye and nose. For the highly sensitive, there are allergy-tested products. Glosses have a high grease content and are only slightly tinted for a transparent finish.

The acid in some skins reacts with lipstick so that it turns bluish. If this happens, prepare the lips with a solid foundation rather than a liquid or cream and avoid colours with blue tones such as sharp pinks and burgundy shades.

Colour

The range of shades is seemingly limitless, with one to suit every type of face and personality. Several different shades are useful in a make-up box: remember that brighter colours are needed in artificial light. Skin colour should be considered. The darker the skin, the more vivid the lipstick can be, whereas a pale skin can be overpowered by too bright a shade. Yellow teeth can be made to look whiter by using bright lipsticks in wine or pink shades; avoid tawny colours. Although you may find that you prefer one range of tones, it is important to be flexible, as sticking to a colour that is no longer fashionable

can look dating. Even a subtle change of colour makes a great difference. Bear in mind clothes and other make-up when choosing a shade.

Application

A good lip make-up can be achieved only by applying colour with a fine brush, for a stick is too wide to create a precise shape. Using a lip pencil to define the outline of the lips is also an excellent technique to master, as the harder formula keeps the soft lip colour confined to the lips – particularly important for women with wrinkles running from the lips. Many women like to apply colour, blot and re-apply. This helps to keep the make-up on a little longer or to remove too much colour or shine but it does tend to blur a precise outline. To remove lip colour, blot with a tissue and then use cleansing cream or lotion. Apply a lip salve afterwards to prevent the lips becoming dry.

Lip shapes

Mouths give a strong clue to character and more often than not their shape is right for the face. However, small adjustments can be made. A wide mouth can be made to look smaller if the pencil outline stops just short of the corners and the lip colour is faded out to the sides, with gloss applied in the middle of the mouth only. Conversely, a small mouth appears wider with a pencil outline extended just beyond the natural corners and filled in with colour. Thin lips can be made to look fuller by drawing a pale pencil outline just beyond the natural line of the lips, filled in with a bright shade of lipstick and plenty of gloss. Full lips can be outlined with a darker pencil just inside the natural edge of the lip; very pale and very bright colours should be avoided and the lip colour can be blotted to cut down on the shine. If one lip is fuller than the other, this can be balanced with a lip pencil: both lips should be outlined to give a more subtle effect, and a darker colour should be used on the full lip than the thin one. Mouths that turn down can be made more cheerful by drawing the outline on the upper lip slightly above the edges at the sides and not taking the colour right down into the corners. Such adjustments require a certain amount of skill and patience but, if carefully done, they can be very effective.

Applying lipstick

You will need: lip colour; lip gloss (optional); a lip brush with a square end, preferably sable or a sable mix; a lip pencil and sharpener. Prepare the mouth with a neutral lip base if you are not wearing foundation and powder. To ensure a steady hand, place the elbow on a hard surface and rest the little finger against the chin.

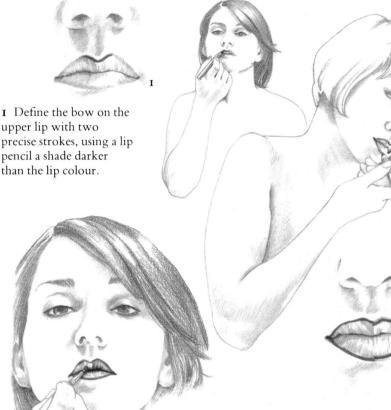

1 Define the bow on the upper lip with two precise strokes, using a lip pencil a shade darker than the lip colour.

2 Continue the outline of the upper lip towards each corner, keeping the mouth closed but relaxed. Use short, feathery strokes, which allow precise control. Repeat with the lower lip, working outwards to the corners. The outline defines the lips (left of detail). To slim full lips, draw just within the edge (right side).

3 Work some lip colour on to the brush and fill in the outline from the centre to the corners of the mouth. Work gradually towards the outline with short, controlled strokes, leaving the pencil line uncovered, or covering it for a softer effect.

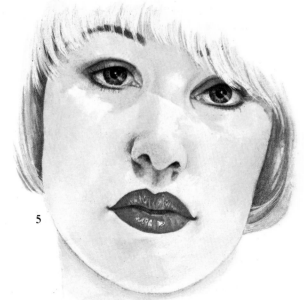

4 Open the mouth and carefully brush the lip colour into the corners, so that there are no unfinished edges.

5 For a shinier look apply lip gloss, but to the centre of the lips only, as it spreads easily. Lip colour complements eye colour and completes the make-up.

Party Tricks

Party time is the time to look special – to indulge in a little fantasy, to look not just good but sensational. The clothes we wear help to create the illusions, but what is worn on the face is important too. With skill and practice, every rule about make-up can be broken at night. Whereas during the day you probably want to look naturally beautiful, which restricts the choice of colours, at night artifice can be beautiful – electric light and candlelight make the use of shine, unusual colour and unusual placing far more effective. The kind of occasion and the lighting determine the make-up. For instance, a weird fantasy make-up would look out of place at an outdoor barbecue and a subtle, back-to-nature look would be lost in the flashing lights of a disco. As your colour sense develops, more exciting possibilities will become apparent.

If the plan is to be adventurous, it is important to practise beforehand; do not embark on a wild make-up five minutes before the party starts. Check the finished look in the appropriate light, if possible. Remember the practical limitations of make-up, too, and make sure the creation will not run, smudge, change colour or irritate the skin. There should be no need to keep retouching.

Two evening make-ups on the same face show that it is possible to achieve totally different looks. Both use a combination of shine, unusual colours in unusual places and exaggeration. Use the ideas for inspiration, without feeling obliged to follow each step exactly.

The dark look
The focus of this make-up is the curve of contour colour on the temples and cheeks, which adds colour and enhances the shape of the face. Use aubergines on cheeks, shades of violet on eyes. Blend away all edges.

1 If you do not have a real tan or dark skin, apply fake tan with a sponge. Use no foundation but cover whole face, including lips and eyes, with translucent powder.

2 Dark aubergine under cheekbone and on to temple.

3 Dark aubergine at hairline, if hair is swept back.

4 Mid-aubergine on cheekbone and temple.

5 Aubergine highlight under outer corner of eye up to eyebrow.

6 Aubergine highlight on outer half of browbone.

7 Light violet on inner half of lid, up to nose and brow.

8 Mid-violet covering area between highlight and light violet.

9 Dark violet to line both lids, extending a little beyond outer corner. Take colour along outer quarter of socket line and blend downwards to form a triangle.

10 Brush dark violet into eyebrow.

11 Black mascara, or blue if you are blonde.

12 Plenty of lip gloss over dark aubergine lip colour.

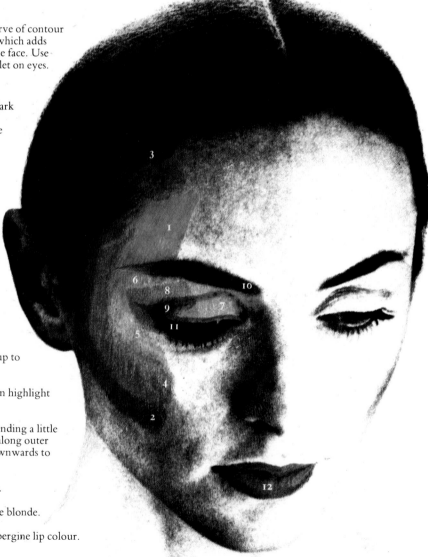

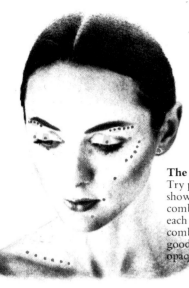

Colour combinations

Experiment with unusual combinations such as apricots for cheeks and aquamarines for eyes, or clear reds and pinks for cheeks and blues for eyes.

The glitter look

Try positioning glitter as shown, following one of the combinations indicated – each colour represents a combination. Glitter looks good with gold or silver opaque highlight.

The pale look

Contour colour is applied to emphasize the cheekbones, counteracting the flatness created by the white powder. Use brick reds on cheeks and greens on eyes. All edges must be thoroughly blended.

1 Cover a light-toned foundation with talcum powder. If skin is very pale, omit foundation and use translucent powder. Remember to cover lips and eyes.

2 Dark brick red under cheekbone and on to temple.

3 Dark brick red at hairline, if hair is off the face.

4 Mid-brick red on cheekbone out to ear.

5 Pale pink highlight above and along top of cheekbone.

6 Pale pink highlight on inner two thirds of lid and under eyebrow, taken round to meet cheek highlight.

7 Mid-green over uncovered outer corner of eye and in hollow at side of nose.

8 Dark green to line lower lid and socket, taken slightly beyond outer corner of eye and blended on to edge of lid.

9 Brush dark green into eyebrow.

10 Opaque gold highlight on centre of lid and under arch of brow.

11 Opaque gold highlight on Cupid's bow.

12 Generous coat of black or dark green mascara.

13 Warm red lip colour; no gloss.

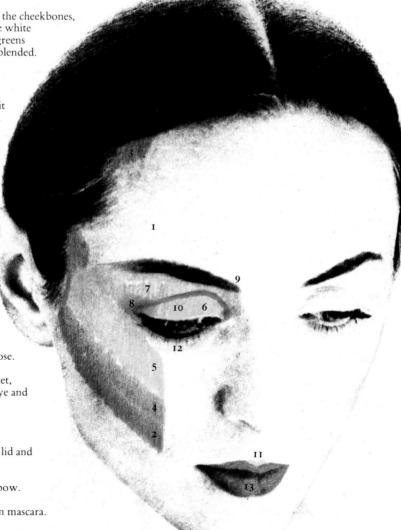

Shine and glitter

This is the quickest and easiest way to transform an everyday make-up into an evening one.

Supplement shiny lipstick with extra gloss for a shimmery look. Use roll-on lip gloss: warm it a little beforehand, then roll some on to the palm of the hand and apply it with a brush so as not to smudge the lip colour already applied. Use the same gloss on the cheeks, on the browbone, to outline the bow of the lips or in the centre of the eyelid.

Powder eyeshadows and blushers can be bought with added glitter. Apply them over matte colours for a subtle effect or on their own for more shine. For maximum shine try not to rub the glitter too much into the skin, although any hard edges must be blended away.

Every make-up box should include a gold or silver powder: gold looks good on everyone; silver is especially effective on pale skins. Use these on the eyes and also on the bottom lip, to define a pretty Cupid's bow, on the temples and on the shoulders and arms if you are proud of them. Gold powder on the earlobes sets off earrings and glittery streaks in the hair look particularly good on a swept-back style.

Pearlized products give a high shine and smooth, dense coverage. Try a multi-coloured iridescent highlighter, which throws out different colours at different angles.

Glitter comes in many other forms such as sequins or little gold stars. Try tiny pearls, trimmings from old dresses, rows of rhinestones, Christmas card glitter, even the fluorescent stars and moons sold to children to liven up their nursery walls. Fix them in place with a dab of eyelash adhesive.

Unusual colour combinations

Whereas during the day foundation should complement the natural skin tone, at night it is possible to experiment. Create an expensive-looking tan with a foam fake tan, applied with a damp sponge over the entire face and any part of the body that is exposed, and set with a dusting of translucent powder. Remember that it will rub off, so avoid wearing it next to white or black fabric. For a really white look, use a pale foundation set with talcum powder. This is more

difficult to achieve on the body than the face but works well if the skin on the body is pale and has not been exposed to the sun.

Choose unusual colours by using a starting point, such as the colour of a dress, hair, eyes or even an unusual skin tone. Try not to be tied by eye colour, though, for blue-eyed women often look wonderful in bronze and gold, brown-eyed ones in purple and amethyst. Water-soluble conte crayons have a wide colour range but it may be necessary to warm them slightly so they do not pull the skin; if there is a history of allergy, stick to proprietary brands.

Beginners should try three shades of the same basic colour, as unusual colours need to be related. Eyebrows and lashes look most effective if included in the colour scheme and brushed faintly with the darkest shade. A complementary colour can offset the rest of the make-up. For instance, aquamarine can look marvellous with a range of colours in apricot and terracotta, or try a range of blues with clear reds and pinks.

Exaggeration

Make-up should be strengthened for the evening, if only to maintain the same effect as during the day, for artificial light permits the use of more intense colour, deeper contrasts of light and shadow and more precise outlines.

The shape of the eye can be exaggerated with free use of pencils and shadow; two extra coats of mascara can be surprisingly effective, or try false eyelashes.

Changing the shape of the lips is most successful at night. Experiment with exaggerating a Cupid's bow or a sensual lower lip. Use a densely-covering foundation to blur the natural outline and apply colour with a lip brush for greater precision. If the mouth is your best feature, play it up with bright colour and extra shine. Use a darker colour than usual to emphasize cheek hollows.

Exaggerate shine by using a glittery high-lighter, applied like powder over the entire face. Or try a matte look on a velvety complexion, with powder pressed generously into the skin and not buffed, smoky powder shadows round the eyes, sooty kohl, mascara to define lashes and blotted lipstick.

The Art of Camouflage

Although make-up should be used primarily to make the most of good points, it can also camouflage weak ones. While eyes and lips can be enhanced with clever use of colour, some skin defects can be completely erased with a careful cover-up technique. Research into ways of improving the appearance, by means of cosmetics, of victims of serious burns and scarring has benefited everybody who has a problem that they wish to disguise, for the techniques perfected as a result of this research can be used by anyone with a mark or blemish on the skin. The film industry has also contributed to this field. Film stars' demand for densely-covering skin bases with great staying power and in a wide range of shades has led to the creation of products that are ideally suited to disguise less than perfect skins.

It is easy to become depressed about a blemish, especially on the face, and to exaggerate its importance and conspicuousness. Surgery is a possible solution for more serious problems (see pages 220–224) but the first step should always be to try cosmetic disguise, for make-up can be just as effective and is, of course, cheaper and safer.

Products

Not all the products that are useful for this aspect of make-up will be advertised as such: most are to be found in ordinary make-up ranges. The principle is to buy products that give a dense cover. These cosmetics can look surprisingly natural – remember that many seriously disfigured people are men who do not want to look as if they are wearing make-up at all. On a woman, only the area that needs a disguise will be covered, the edges blended into an ordinary make-up.

The most useful tool in the art of covering-up is a solid make-up base. Usually sold in sticks like greasepaint, it is based on lanolin, wax or oil and is therefore resistant to water – it is important for the reassurance of the wearer that any make-up used to cover should not wear off quickly. These bases are sold in a variety of shades, so choose the colour nearest to the natural skin tone. For pigmentation disorders where the skin appears piebald, select a mid-tone.

Other effective camouflage products include the small sticks of concentrated pale colour, which many cosmetic houses sell and which are designed to disguise dark shadows under the eyes and to iron out wrinkle shadows. These are handy to carry about for instant touch-ups. Solid powder compacts can also be used to touch up small areas. Similar sticks come in a range of flesh tones designed to disguise unsightly pimples and can also be used to camouflage small birthmarks, moles, brown age spots or the odd broken vein. There is, incidentally, no totally safe and effective bleaching cream for treating age spots. Some creams contain allergy-provoking ingredients and may irritate the skin and discolour it further.

Covering make-up, even if worn every day, cannot exacerbate spots, blackheads or acne. To remove it before going to bed, use a cleansing lotion or cream, which is more effective than soap and water. For how to cleanse see page 23.

Powder-based, waterproof make-up that is applied with a wet sponge gives a natural finish on areas such as the arms and legs where foundation is not normally used. Powder is necessary to fix the make-up, baby talcum powder being cheaper to use over a large area than face powder. Powder blushers help to give added brightness: no skin is the same tone all over and some very covering make-ups can look rather flat. Blusher lifts and varies skin tone, creating a more natural look. Natural or synthetic sponges, preferably small and easy to hold, tissues, cotton wool buds, or swabs, and large and small brushes are useful too.

Application

The way in which these products are applied is important for their success. Anyone with a serious disfigurement should seek professional advice from a cosmetic house in order to gain more confidence and expertise in applying make-up. Keep the cover-up simple. The make-up should be applied and then forgotten, except for the occasional quick touch-up with a powder compact or a covering stick. Whereas getting caught in the rain will not damage the make-up, being constantly fingered or rubbed against material will. So keep clothing away from the make-up; you may also find it helpful to avoid wearing stark, plain colours close to the blemished areas. Remember also to make the most of your good points as well as covering up the bad.

A basic cover-up

This technique is used to disguise discolouration over a large area, such as varicose veins, brown liver, or age, spots, large birthmarks, burns, scars, broken veins, or even freckles. Do not moisturize just before applying densely-covering make-up, as the base adheres best to a dry surface. When covering a large area, allow some time for the make-up to settle before going out. You will need: solid foundation base; cake make-up; powder, preferably applied with a puff; tissues; a sponge and a bowl of water.

1 Take up a generous amount of solid foundation base with the fingertips and cover the entire blemished area with a light film.

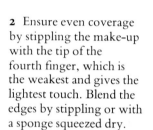

2 Ensure even coverage by stippling the make-up with the tip of the fourth finger, which is the weakest and gives the lightest touch. Blend the edges by stippling or with a sponge squeezed dry.

3 Dust with powder to set before application of cake make-up. Buff lightly with a puff to remove any surplus.

4 An application of cake make-up restores even skin tone and texture. Wet the sponge thoroughly, so that the make-up flows evenly on to the skin; work the dripping sponge into the solid cake and apply quickly with long, even strokes over the area covered with base.

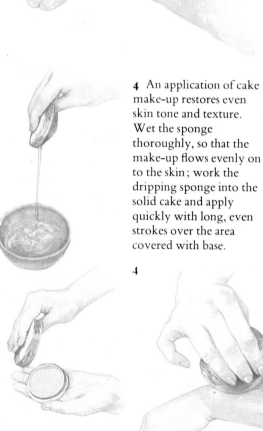

5 Carefully blot the damp make-up with a tissue until completely dry and dust with powder to set, as in **3**.

A cover-up for the face

Use to cover birthmarks, flat scars, chloasma, burns, vitiligo, freckles. This is the same as the basic cover-up technique to disguise skin discolouration on the body, except that foundation is used instead of cake make-up. Cover the blemish with a light film of solid base, as in **2** of the basic cover-up. Set with powder and then apply foundation to the entire face.

Wrinkles

Use this technique for fine wrinkles such as frown lines. For heavier lines, use a stick of solid base in a pale tone, applying the stick directly to the skin. Apply foundation beforehand.

1 Take up a little colour from a pale stick of solid base with an eyeliner pencil and paint a fine line exactly in the crease formed by the wrinkle.

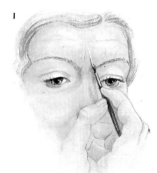

2 Working from top to bottom, gently roll the brush inside the wrinkle to blend the colour.

3 Set with powder, folding the puff for accuracy.

Broken veins and red complexions

Apply a thin film of green-tinted moisturizer over the area to be toned down and cover with a beige foundation over the whole face.

Acne pits, chicken pox scars, etc.

(below) These are hard to disguise effectively, but with practice can be softened after making up the face with foundation and powder.

1 Accurately paint a dot of pale-toned solid base into the indentation using an eyeliner brush. This should lighten the tiny shadow formed.

Abnormal pigmentation

The basic cover-up technique for a large area can also be used to camouflage pigmentation disorders where patches of light and dark skin create a piebald effect. Darken the light skin and lighten the dark skin with a mid-toned solid base. Apply cake make-up to tone with the natural skin colour.

Raised marks

The principles of contour colour come into play here. Any raised mark on the face catches the light. After applying foundation and powder, use a solid foundation in a slightly darker shade and dot it on the raised area with a fingertip or paint it on with a fine brush. Blend into the rest of the foundation and then powder.

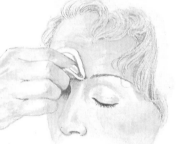

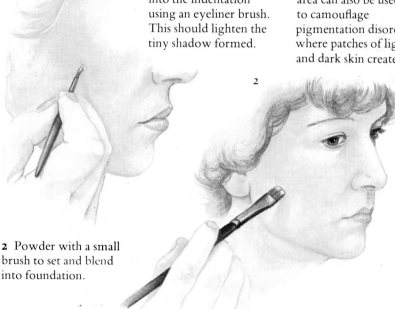

2 Powder with a small brush to set and blend into foundation.

The Older Face

Skin tone and texture

Foundation helps to correct any unevenness in texture and colour that may develop: beige or peach tones are more flattering than pink tones. Use plenty of moisturizer beforehand. Apply foundation carefully in two stages, the first for general coverage and the second to correct uneven skin colour, using further dots of make-up blended into the rest. Set with translucent powder.

Some skins fade with age. Do not try to correct this with an over-hectic foundation but brighten the skin colour with a blusher applied afterwards. Avoid complicated contour colour and highlighting effects, as these can look unnatural on a wrinkled skin; concentrate on enhancing colour and replacing a healthy glow.

Broken veins, age spots, pigment variations and any discolouration of the skin can in fact be camouflaged (see pages 206–207).

A sagging jawline can be subtly shaded to firm the lines of the chin but this needs a skilful touch (see page 189).

Wrinkles and hollows

Not all wrinkles can be disguised, but deep frown lines can be made less severe (see page 207). Hollows, especially round the chin and mouth, can be ageing. Using the fingertips, stipple a solid base in a light tone into the hollow to lift the shadow, before applying foundation and powder. Dark circles can be treated in the same way.

Hair colour

This has a great influence on the shades of make-up you choose and when hair fades it is not easy to adapt to a new colour range. Use soft, clear colours with no gimmicks or bizarre colour combinations, taking particular care to adjust to paler tones when dark or auburn hair turns grey or white.

Lips

Lipstick lends colour to an older face. The natural lip line tends to become less defined as you grow older, so redefine it with a lip pencil. A pencil also helps to prevent the soft lipstick running into wrinkles beyond the lips; a base of foundation and powder helps to disguise fine wrinkles on the lips. If wrinkles are especially noticeable, stop the lip colour short of the pencil line and use lip gloss sparingly. Colour should be carefully chosen: pale shades can look washed out, dark ones can be ageing. Bright coral and sharp pink can look surprisingly good.

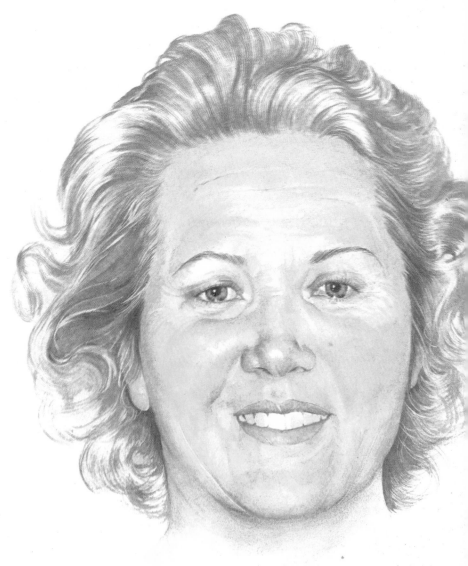

There is such emphasis placed on staying young and healthy that it is natural to find the process of growing old dispiriting. The gradual loss of the skin's elasticity as the collagen disintegrates (see page 12) can be particularly upsetting for the woman who cares about her looks. But there are also positive rewards in growing older: age brings an intriguing blend of serenity and experience to the face, which can be more beautiful than any youthful bloom.

Perhaps the most important gain is increased confidence in oneself and a knowledge built on years of experience of exactly what colours and styles suit the face. There is, however, a trap here too, because this knowledge can lead to an inflexible approach to a beauty routine. As the face changes its shape, texture and colour with age, its requirements and indeed the beauty products available change. Make-up is by its nature ephemeral and the older woman must experiment with new colours and techniques just as a young girl experiments with her first make-up box.

The object should not be to look young, but to look your best. Good looks can no longer be taken for granted: thorough and regular moisturizing is essential to keep the skin soft and glowing (see pages 21–22, 24), and it is never too late to start.

It is important to consider the textures of beauty products because of the inevitable wrinkles and bags. Always look for moisturized make-up: many foundations, lipsticks and even eye products will boost the moisturizer that must be worn under the make-up. It is possible to disguise with clever use of light and shade (see pages 187–191, 207) but it is more important to develop a skilled technique for using standard products. A lesson on the application of make-up is well worth while, for a sure touch helps when there are problems such as new spectacles or unsteady hands to contend with. Cosmetic houses and beauty counters in department stores are generally willing to offer advice; a professional lesson may give inspiration and a fresh approach.

Eyebrows

These tend to become rather sparse. It is important to keep them well shaped by plucking stray hairs but they are unlikely to need thinning. Supplement them, if necessary, with an eyebrow pencil, in a soft and natural colour. Avoid blacks and dark browns unless your skin is very dark. On a pale skin, a gingery brown creates a subtle effect; you may find the right shade in a lip pencil.

Eyelashes

Lashes are important as a frame for the eye. Apply a soft natural-looking shade of mascara in thin coats and use a stiff brush to separate the lashes. Experiment with false eyelashes, trimming them to a natural length, and matching the colour with your own lashes. Best of all are individual lashes, strategically placed to substitute for missing real ones. If eyelashes become grey, they can be dyed professionally.

Eyes

This is the area that wrinkles most easily because it is so mobile, with little supporting fat and muscle. Prepare with foundation and powder over the entire lid to prevent eyeshadow creasing into wrinkles. Avoid cream shadows, which crease easily, and contours, frosted shadows and highlights, as these draw attention to wrinkles. Be wary also of bright colours. Use a thin wash of shadow, either powder or water-colour, and then powder again with a fine translucent powder to set the colour. An eye pencil is easy to use and a line of colour on the upper lid, blended to a soft edge, brings light and sparkle to the eye; a silvery green or aquamarine is a good choice if the hair is grey. This looks particularly effective behind spectacles.

Choosing colours

The range of tones should be subtle. Strident colour overpowers an older skin and draws attention to lines and bags. There may be quite definite changes in skin and hair colour and use of make-up should reflect this. For instance, grey hair can have a draining effect on the face but blusher can replace a natural glow. Sometimes skin can become ruddy: to correct this, use a green base worn underneath a beige foundation to cut out the florid tone. The eye area is the first to become wrinkled, so avoid heavy eye make-up as this only draws attention to the fact.

Above all, keep a positive approach to beauty and enjoy making-up. Your best points will not change; if your eyes have always been large and interesting, then carry on making them so. Do not stop being amused and curious about make-up, but use it as never before to bring attention to your best features.

Improving on Nature

No matter what our physical and psychological birthright, we can all enhance our natural potential. Although basic body shape, complexion and emotional make-up are fundamentally unchangeable, there is always a way to make the best of them. An effort to optimize good points and minimize bad ones can greatly improve the raw materials we began with. Although some hard work is the sine qua non of self-improvement, there are plenty of sources of help open to those who take the trouble to look for them. No one should feel reluctant to consult an expert or inadequate for doing so. Most people love to give advice and we can spare ourselves a lot of wasted time and effort by consulting people who are in a position to make sound suggestions.

Professional

The quality of help is important here: the best kind comes from the best people. Second-rate expertise is simply not worth heeding, so make sure that those you ask for help are qualified to give it. Find out what their formal qualifications are and whether these are recognized by any reputable institutions. If in doubt, telephone a professional association or a well-known institution and make inquiries. Help, advice and support are available at many different levels. At one end of the scale is the scientific help orthodox medicine offers, at the other end are some beauty salon practices that come little higher than witchcraft. As long as the witchcraft does no harm, makes no extravagant claims and raises no false hopes, then you have nothing to lose – except money – by giving it a try. However, there is no need to chase up blind alleys when there are guaranteed ways of making the most of ourselves. Turn the page to see how to begin.

Treatments

The Range of Possibilities

The first principle of self-improvement is to achieve and maintain good health. A good sound diet and sufficient exercise are the starting points (see Chapter 2 for guidance on these). Any doctor can lay down the outline of a sensible diet and exercise programme, but orthodox medicine is so overburdened with the problems of failing health that most doctors have little time to give advice on achieving or maintaining health. For detailed advice on these subjects it may be necessary to turn to 'alternative' medicine. This heading covers numerous practices – to get an idea of the scope of the field see pages 232–237.

If there is a reliable practitioner in a particular area, the local doctors are almost sure to know of him or her. Many doctors now work hand in hand with practitioners of alternative medicine, such as chiropractic and osteopathy, and are happy to refer patients to them. Next best to a recommendation from a doctor is one from a friend who has found the treatment helpful. Ignore any person who advertises medical services: advertising is unethical for a medical practitioner and quite unnecessary for a good one.

One of the best ways to get to grips with alternative medicine is to make a visit to a health farm (see pages 238–241). Choose a good place, one that takes diet, treatment and medicine seriously and steer clear of health spas that place the accent on beauty. Books are another good source of information, although it is as well to avoid authors who have an axe to grind. I can strongly recommend Linda Clarke's books for a balanced and knowledgeable review of the whole gamut of alternative medicine.

Something we can all do, even without help from the experts, is to reappraise our diet, exercise programme and lifestyle. Common sense is often enough to point out where alterations could be made for the better. Carrying these through is one of the very few certain ways to achieve the goal of looking and feeling better. Provided we stick to our good resolutions, the effects on health and appearance can be long-lasting – which is more than can be said for most beauty clinic treatments.

Good health comes from within, but this is no reason at all why we should not improve our outward appearance with skilful make-up (see Chapter 3). Ask yourself what features need emphasizing, which playing down and try to use some of the tricks of the make-up experts. This kind of camouflage is not difficult and is one of the fastest morale boosters in existence. Cleverly applied cosmetics can make almost everyone look better and feel better as a consequence. Much the same argument may be made for cosmetic surgery if some bodily flaw is a constant source of embarrassment or misery to the owner. It takes courage to decide on cosmetic surgery, and even more to raise the subject with a family doctor who may not have a great deal of sympathy with cosmetic operations. However, it is essential to have any cosmetic surgery carried out by competent hands and the family doctor is the best person to ask advice from initially. If he cannot personally recommend a cosmetic surgeon, he is sure to be able to pass you on to a plastic surgeon who will be in a good position to offer sound advice. Do not follow up a newspaper advertisement: if you do, you may or may not end up with an able surgeon but you will certainly have to pay a high fee to the clinic that referred you to him. For further information see pages 216–229.

Feeling good also depends on emotional stability and fulfilment. Where emotional problems are concerned, both orthodox and unorthodox medicine may be able to help. The sensible first move is to talk to the family doctor. If he has not time to help you himself, he should be able to put you in touch with a psychiatrist, psychologist or psychotherapist who may be able to help you sort things out (see pages 248–251 for what psychotherapy involves). Whatever happens, do not be satisfied with repeated courses of antidepressants or tranquillizers, which treat the symptoms rather than the root of the problem. These drugs do help some people, but it is worrying to contemplate having to take them indefinitely and their long-term use should always be supervised by a doctor.

If the doctor cannot suggest anyone to help over an emotional problem, ask for names and addresses of institutions and organizations that might be useful. Help may come from a quite unexpected source. Your particular lifeline may be yoga or meditation – try a library noticeboard or a Citizens' Advice Bureau for the names of good practitioners.

Skin Treatments

In the search to find a way to stay happy, healthy and beautiful, try to keep as open a mind as possible. Consider the full range of professional help that is available. Try not to reject any possibility simply because it is unfamiliar or because of prejudice. Read about it, explore it, talk to people who have experimented with it and even go and have a try for yourself. It may turn out to be just the help you were looking for.

One of the most encouraging things is to take stock of the sources of help open to everyone – it makes quite a list.

• Orthodox medicine – for discussion and treatment of diseases, preventive medicine, referral to other medical practitioners and specialists, and advice on diet and exercise.

• Unorthodox medicine – for discussion and advice on lifestyle, diet, treatment of illness, and naturopathic treatments such as massage, heat and hydrotherapy.

• Health farms or spas – for rest and treatment the naturopathic, homeopathic or osteopathic way, information about alternative medicine, and discussion of fringe medicine.

• Cosmetic surgery – for the improvement of an unflattering feature such as a large nose, a facelift for a more youthful look, recontouring of the body for aesthetic reasons.

• Beauty clinics and salons – beware: nothing done here can have more than a transient effect or in any way slow the process of ageing. The most they can do is make you feel pampered, which can be an excellent morale booster.

• Make-up – to camouflage flaws and accentuate good points.

• Relaxation, meditation, yoga – to relieve tension and strain and to overcome insomnia.

• Psychotherapy – to give insight to cope with the problems in life that unresolved can make you look older or even cause physical ill-health.

There is no one route to a more relaxed, fit and attractive you: we all have to find our own individual recipe. In the search for it, do not be afraid to mix alternative and mainstream practices. Be eclectic. Go right through the list of options piecemeal and take advantage of any that seem to apply to you. Only you can make the choice and ultimately only you can take really effective steps to improve on nature.

There are several surgical and chemical techniques that may be used to alter or repair the surface of the skin. Without exception these treatments should be administered only by medical specialists such as dermatologists or plastic surgeons. Badly used they can damage the skin permanently and have serious side-effects.

Chemical treatments

Chemical skin peeling may be undertaken for either medical or cosmetic reasons. In both cases it is essential to go to a medically qualified professional for treatment.

A peeling agent in general use medically is phenol, which when painted on the skin causes coagulation, inflammation, swelling and peeling. Because phenol can be absorbed rapidly through the skin and may harm the kidneys, it should be used cautiously and infrequently and never be applied over a wide area. Hence its use is mainly in treating the pitted scars of acne and superficial complaints such as small spots and cysts.

In the past dermatologists also used resorcinol as a peeling agent, particularly to deal with itchy skin or to remove scales, and it may still be used today to treat acne. Resorcinol acts by breaking the chemical bonds that hold the scales of keratin on the skin's surface together, so that they peel away. It must never be used on broken skin: it can cause very serious effects if absorbed into the bloodstream. The use of resorcinol sometimes causes severe irritation of the skin or an allergy. For all these reasons dermatologists tend to feel that the dangers of resorcinol outweigh its advantages and that it should not be used.

Skin peeling for cosmetic purposes is a rather different kind of procedure, since the area to be treated may be fairly extensive (if so, a stay in hospital may be necessary). Expertly carried out, the technique can make blemishes, fine lines and wrinkles less obvious, can lessen pitmarks and may occasionally be used to treat discoloured areas of skin and freckles. Although it temporarily softens the facial lines most of us begin to collect by our middle forties, skin peeling does not stop the ageing process and the first rejuvenating effect wears off within a year, if not sooner.

Many dermatologists use an acid peeling agent such as trichlorocetic acid. The initial effect of the chemical is to produce a second-degree burn in the skin, turning it a whitish-grey colour. A brown crust forms within three to five days and when this drops off the skin beneath looks pink, tighter and has fewer lines and wrinkles. It is essential to test the peeling agent on the patient's skin before it is applied widely.

Never allow any person without medical training to administer a chemical face peel. Quite apart from the risk that the end result will be a scarred face, bear in mind the fact that a cosmetologist is not necessarily expert enough to recognize serious skin conditions that need medical attention.

Cryotherapy (freezing)

Freezing kills the cells within the skin and this is an effective method of dealing with superficial skin lesions such as warts, senile warts, or 'age spots', which usually occur on the face and the back of the hands, and small numbers of superficial veins.

The earliest skin freezing agent dermatologists used was ethyl chloride. These days carbon dioxide snow (solid carbon dioxide) is generally used, especially for acne scars, although liquid air and liquid nitrogen are popular.

Particularly in large clinics, liquid nitrogen is frequently employed to treat warts and verrucae. A cotton wool swab saturated with liquid nitrogen is applied to the wart for five to 30 seconds (verrucae are usually more deeply embedded and generally need a 60-second treatment period). One after-effect of this treatment is the formation of tiny blisters a few hours later, where the nitrogen burnt the skin. Recalcitrant verrucae may need further treatment.

Curettage

A curette is simply a spoon with a sharp cutting edge that can be used to destroy or remove certain well circumscribed and embedded skin conditions. Small curettes are used to enucleate small cysts and the larger curettes can be used successfully to treat warts and verrucae.

In the right hands, the procedure is quite straightforward. When the sharp edge of the curette is applied to the buried lesion correctly, it should separate easily from the normal surrounding skin and shell out without any bleeding. A caustic agent such as phenol may be dabbed into the crater after the treatment of warts and verrucae, in order to prevent regrowth.

Dermabrasion

This technique may be used to remove or improve pitted acne scars on the face, to treat large flat birthmarks and may even produce good results for stretch marks and the fine lines around the mouth. Dermabrasion requires the skill and experience of a medically qualified person who has specialized in the technique.

Abrasive methods of removing pitted scars and some birthmarks were first introduced in the 1930s. Today they are chiefly used to treat skin conditions on the face, where the generous supply of hair follicles and sebaceous glands allows the skin to regenerate quickly and usually without scarring. Care has to be taken not to destroy the hair follicles and sebaceous glands or the skin does not recover.

Great advances in dermabrasion have been made in the past 25 years, due especially to the use of a high speed rotary drill and better cooling techniques. It is important to adhere rigidly to the correct procedure during the operation, to avoid damage to both the patient and the operator.

For dermabrasion, the patient is first sedated or tranquillized and then the area involved is chilled with cold packs and cleansed, first with soap and water and then with spirit. Plugs of ointment-impregnated gauze are inserted into the ears and nostrils, the hair is carefully protected with towels and the eyes are covered with ointment and a lead shield or with more thick gauze held by an assistant. After the area to be treated has been frozen with a stream of cold gas, the drill is used to abrade the skin to the required depth. The degree of freezing and drilling needed can be learned only from experience and there are refinements too in the angle at which the drill is held and the direction and extent of the abrasion. The length of the whole procedure is controlled to a certain degree by the rate at which the skin thaws and recovers its sensitivity.

After treatment the area usually bleeds for 15 to 30 minutes. Non-adhesive dressings are used, which can be removed 12 to 24 hours later. The crusts that form at this point separate in around seven to ten days and subsequently the wound heals quickly if it is left open and dry. The same area can be treated again after about four weeks.

Although the dermabraded skin seldom becomes infected, sunlight or cosmetics may cause mild irritation for a few weeks and most patients are recommended to avoid strong sunlight for several months. Even after this time it is still advisable to use a sunscreen before exposing the treated skin to sunlight.

There are a few complications that may arise after dermabrasion, even if expertly carried out. The commonest ones are persistent redness, brown patches of pigmentation and lumpy scars. Some dark-skinned people develop light, de-pigmented patches, but these are nearly always temporary.

Electrodesiccation and electrocoagulation

It is possible to use a high frequency electrical current to destroy tissue in two ways: either by producing a spark that solidifies it or by heating it until it coagulates. In the first case all the cells in contact with the current are shrivelled and in the second they simply go solid in rather the same way as egg white does when boiled. The same apparatus is used for both processes and the required effect comes from varying the current.

This form of treatment is occasionally used on small broken veins in the skin of the face and legs, but it can also treat warts that stand proud above the skin surface. It is particularly valuable in dealing with small, protruberant skin tags, since it allows large numbers of these to be treated in one session without anaesthesia. Small tags are coagulated by momentary application of the apparatus and larger ones can be cut through at the base with the desiccating current. All this work needs to be carried out by a skilled operator in a hospital – preferably in a full operating theatre, or operating room, where proper anti-sepsis is routine and anaesthesia is available when required.

Although this type of treatment is not usually accompanied by bleeding, the area treated may become charred as a result of dehydration. As the skin heals, crusts form, which slough off in the following two or three weeks. Scarring is usually very slight, particularly on the face.

Excision

Certain skin conditions can be treated only by complete surgical excision of a piece of full thickness skin (including epidermis, dermis and subcutaneous fat). Only a dermatologist or plastic surgeon · can decide when this technique is necessary. As a general rule it is unwise to interfere in any way with a pigmented skin condition. Always see a dermatologist or plastic surgeon if you are contemplating having a pigmented mole removed: it is very important that this kind of excision should be carried out by an expert. It is usually performed under a general anaesthetic and takes no longer than an hour. A dressing is worn afterwards and, in general, alternate stitches are taken out in five to seven days, the rest in seven to ten days. Most scars fade in six weeks.

Soft X-rays (Grenz rays)

This type of X-ray can penetrate only one millimetre of skin. When its use is supervised by a dermatologist, it is a safe and logical form of treatment for some superficial skin conditions. Although there has been a move away from the use of Grenz rays in the United Kingdom, the popularity of this method is growing elsewhere. In chronic eczema, acne and some birthmarks it can be a good adjunct to other therapies.

Tattoos

A person who has a tattoo may later come to want it removed for personal or aesthetic reasons, but removal may also be medically desirable – for example, if the tattoo causes an allergic reaction or becomes the centre of a localized skin condition.

The only way to eliminate all particles of pigment entirely may be to excise the whole tattoo and cover the area with skin grafted from another site on the body. This is likely to be feasible only if the area involved is small. With a large tattoo dermabrasion may succeed.

Tattooing itself is a technique that has some cosmetic application, in that it can be used to camouflage pigmented areas of skin or birth-marks. Instead of coloured inks being injected into the skin, a special flesh-coloured fluid is used.

Varicose veins

For details of treatment see page 92.

Cosmetic Surgery

Under this heading comes a collection of operations whose primary aim is aesthetic rather than strictly functional. Over the past ten years this type of plastic surgery has gained greatly in terms both of availability and of acceptability. There are sociological reasons for this development as well as scientific ones. On the one hand, advances in surgical techniques have made the operations themselves less hazardous and more effective. On the other, an increasingly competitive environment has made personal success seem more and more dependent on self-image, and, with some people, on the possibility of bolstering it. While reconstructive plastic surgery can be seen as an attempt to restore normality, cosmetic surgery is essentially an attempt to supersede it.

The market for cosmetic surgery

Although it is by no means uncommon for a man to have cosmetic surgery nowadays, it is still mainly the province of women and is used above all in the pursuit of youth. Our culture has more or less forgotten what it is like to grow old gracefully. People are living longer and feeling fitter in middle age than they used to, and many have an understandable desire to look as young as they feel. For these cosmetic surgery has a powerful appeal. Social changes may underline this: many women now marry men years younger than themselves and turn to cosmetic surgery as a way of narrowing, superficially at least, the gap in ages. The men who consider cosmetic surgery come in the main from professions where appearance is of paramount importance – the theatre, modelling and films – but businessmen too may feel that looking young is an essential part of their job, and decide on a cosmetic operation to protect their career.

Of course, the desire to look attractive may be quite independent of any desire for a youthful appearance. Many people consider cosmetic surgery as a way out of having to live with a particularly unattractive feature, such as an oversize nose or a receding chin. Although some people adjust well to living with a deformity, few can cope with a really ugly feature without some degree of emotional trauma, especially in a society that places a high value on physical attractiveness.

The trauma shows itself differently in different people, but the most common reactions are feelings of inferiority, self-consciousness, hypersensitivity, anxiety, frustration and a general feeling of depression. These feelings may spur a person on to seek cosmetic surgery.

Popular attitudes to cosmetic surgery have undergone a substantial change over the past 25 years. Face lifts or rhinoplasty used to be considered rather frivolous. A woman who had her eyelids 'done' or her chin reshaped might be thought foolish by her friends and crazy by her family. This is no longer so, and many doctors too have become more aware that cosmetic surgery can contribute to a patient's overall well-being. This is particularly so among psychiatrists and psychotherapists, many of whom state that arresting the physical effects of ageing can be psychologically beneficial and rewarding to the patient, to her family and to society.

There is inevitably a danger, however, that people who are insecure or unhappy for quite unrelated reasons may blame these feelings on some imaginary flaw in face or body. They may seek cosmetic surgery not merely to transform their faces but to transform their lives and they are almost always doomed to disappointment. To avoid this danger, it is best not to decide on cosmetic surgery during or immediately after a crisis such as divorce or bereavement. Cosmetic surgery is no route to take when you are feeling lonely, guilty or disorientated.

The pursuit of youth, the accent on physical appearance and indoctrination by the media on what constitutes beauty have made cosmetic surgery in the United States both widely accepted and inventive. There is hardly a woman in her forties who thinks of cosmetic surgery as beyond her reach. There is hardly a cosmetic surgeon who will not take up the challenge to give his patient the nose, breasts, waist and bottom that she desires. The trend in favour of regarding plastic surgery as an acceptable cosmetic adjunct is strong in South America and Latin American countries, increasing in Scandinavia, the United Kingdom and Japan and developing in France, Germany and Italy too. In many other parts of the world the accent is still on the reconstructive aspects of plastic surgery.

What it costs

The fees for cosmetic surgery depend on the complexity of the procedures required and on where the operation is performed (New York and California are the most expensive areas). A simple operation to pin back protruding ears might cost around £100 in London, removing drooping skin from the eyelids might cost around £300, but an operation to reshape the breasts might carry a fee of more than £1000. Body contouring would carry a higher price still.

Before making a decision

There are four points to think about when trying to decide whether or not cosmetic surgery is worth it for you.

• All surgery carries with it risks. There is a risk, albeit small, of dying under a general anaesthetic and a risk that the operation will give the patient's system such a shock that it never recovers. Since many of the patients undergoing cosmetic surgery are no longer young and are less robust than people in their twenties, it could be argued that the risks associated with having cosmetic surgery are higher than normal.

• The operation may not work out exactly as planned. The results may be less good than you expected or frankly disastrous. There may be complications that delay recovery. In the hands of an expert surgeon these risks may be slight but they must still be taken into account.

• The immediate aftermath of any operation can be unpleasant. The area operated on may be uncomfortable or even painful for days or weeks. There may be a period of complete immobility or of severely restricted activity. Someone who is really sure she wants the operation is highly motivated to cope with these temporary phenomena, but it is as well to prepare for them in advance.

• Many operations are certain to leave behind them scars. These may be hidden under the hair or inside the mouth, but in some cases the scar will be apparent. If this aspect of cosmetic surgery worries you, it might help to talk to someone who has already had the operation, to get an idea of the likely extent of the problem. The more expert the surgeon, the more likely he is to take pride in leaving only the faintest of scars.

How to look for a good cosmetic surgeon

A woman who has saved the money and plucked up the courage to visit a cosmetic surgeon is in his hands once she enters the consulting room, so it is essential to choose a good one. The best possible recommendation is from your own general practitioner – he should be able to give a professional, objective opinion. Less reliable, but still a good bet, is a recommendation from a friend who has had cosmetic surgery. It is especially valuable if you can see the results and know what she looked like before the surgery. It is definitely not a good idea to follow up an advertisement in a newspaper or magazine: first, because it goes against the ethical code of doctors to advertise their services; second, because a good surgeon has no need to advertise.

To stand the best chance of ending up in the hands of a good surgeon, avoid the following:

• a surgeon who is willing to perform exactly the operation you want and offers no professional opinion as to what you actually need. A surgeon who is worth his salt will aim to do the operation that brings about the best result for you and is almost certain to offer his own suggestions about what should be done (you are not obliged to take his advice, of course).

• a surgeon who is not realistic about the potential results of the operation. No cosmetic surgery guarantees 100 per cent success – and no good surgeon will guarantee anything. He will explain in some detail what the operation involves and the effect he is trying to achieve, with a realistic estimate of the chances of bringing about the desired effect.

• a surgeon who will not answer questions in detail, with illustrations, and show you examples of his work in the form of 'before and after' photographs.

• a surgeon who does not wish to take many and detailed photographs of the area of your body that requires surgery. He needs the photographs to study exactly how and what to do to make the correction.

• a surgeon you do not like immediately. The relationship of a patient with a cosmetic surgeon is an extremely personal one. If you find that there is no rapport between you, think twice before entrusting yourself into his care.

Cosmetic surgery

Name of operation / What it means	In/Out-patient / Length of stay	Preconditions	Anaesthetic / Length of op	Post-op appearance and discomfort
Blepharoplasty / Reshaping eyelids, removing bags under eyes	In-patient / 3 days if possible	None	General / 1 hour	Soreness, bruising round eyes
Rhinoplasty / Altering shape of nose	In-patient / 3 days	18 years +	Local or general / 1 hour	Soreness inside nose, swelling of nose, bruising under eyes
Otoplasty / Pinning back ears	In-patient (child) or out-patient / 48 hours	None	General; local optional / 1 hour	Nothing abnormal, little discomfort
Cheekbone augmentation / Making cheekbones more prominent	In-patient / 3 days	16 years +	Local or general / 1–2 hours	Swelling and bruising under eyes or inside of mouth sore
Double chin reduction / Removal of excess fat and loose skin under chin	In-patient / 3 days	40 years +	General / 1 hour	Chin and neck red and swollen
Chin reduction / Correction of protruding chin	In-patient / 3 days	None	General / 1–2 hours	Soreness, swelling, possibly bruising
Chin augmentation / Correction of receding chin	In-patient / 3 days minimum	None	General / 2 hours	Soreness inside mouth, swelling of chin
Face lift / Lifting skin of whole face	In-patient / 3 days	40 years +	General / 2 hours +	Face red and swollen
Total facial rejuvenation / Face lift, neck lift, eyelid repair, dermabrasion for mouth wrinkles	In-patient / 5 days minimum	45 years +	General / Up to 4 hours	Face red and swollen
Breast augmentation / Enlarging the breasts	In-patient; rarely out-patient / 3 days minimum	Full discussion with surgeon to decide size and shape	General; rarely local / 2 hours	Occasionally soreness, bruising, tingling round nipple
Breast reduction / Making breasts smaller	In-patient / 5 days minimum	No strong desire to breastfeed subsequently	General / Up to 3 hours	Soreness, bruising, tingling and numbness of nipple
Breast uplift / Raising breasts	In-patient; rarely out-patient. 3 days	None	General / 2 hours	Soreness, bruising
Breast reconstruction / Building new breast(s) after mastectomy	In-patient / 3 days + for each stage	Psychological preparation No indication that cancer has spread	General / May be in 2 stages	Soreness, bruising
Abdominoplasty / Removal of folds of fat from lower abdomen	In-patient / 7 days	Wait until you have completed your family	General / 2 hours	Drainage tubes in wound for 3–5 days
Buttocks, hips and thighs / Recontouring of shape by removing fat and skin	In-patient / 5 days if possible	As much fat as possible has been lost by dieting	General / 2–3 hours depending on operation	Can move and sit same day but some discomfort likely for 2 weeks
Upper arms / Removal of loose fat and skin	In-patient / 48 hours	None	General / 1 hour	Hardly any discomfort
Total body lift / Removal of sagging skin from abdomen, buttocks, thighs, arms, neck and face	In-patient / 5–7 days on each occasion	As much fat as possible has been lost by dieting	General / 1–2 hours each session	Depends on operations
Hair transplants / Transplanting skin from back of scalp to bald area	In-patient / 7 days	None	General or local / 1–2 hours each session	Swelling and crusting

Stitches removed	Post-op restrictions Care and dressing	Time to full recovery	Complications	Results
48 hours	None Antibiotic ointment	3 months	Barely detectable scars which blend with skin creases	Very good. If you wear dark glasses can be back at work in 3 days
None	Do not blow nose Light dressings only	6 months	Stuffiness of nose for 3 weeks. Possible numbness for 2 months	Excellent
5–7 days	None Antibiotic ointment Possibly bandages for up to a week	2 months	None	Excellent
5–7 days for incision beneath eyes	None	4–6 months	None	Excellent
Some at 5–7 days rest at 2 weeks	None Large dressing for 48 hours	Swelling gone in 2–3 weeks	Feeling of tightness normally gone in a few weeks	Excellent
5–7 days	Diet of soft food for 10 days Dressings for 3–5 days	4–6 months	Swelling for up to 1 month	Excellent
None	Diet of soft food for 10 days Bandage for 10 days	3 months	None	Excellent
Some at 5–7 days rest at 2 weeks	Can eat immediately, fully active in 3 days Large dressing for 2 days	Superficial swelling subsides in a month	Feeling of tightness, usually gone in few months	Generally very good. Only fully apparent in 3 months. Lasts 8 years
Some at 5–7 days rest at 2 weeks	Can be fully active in 3 days Bulky dressings for 48 hours	Swelling subsides in 3 weeks	Tightness round neck and numbness round ears, subsiding in few months	Good. May take up to 6 months to see best effect
1 week	No active sports or stretching for 1 month Light dressing and antibiotic ointment	2 months	Hardening of implants Any bruising and discomfort usually gone in a few weeks	Very good with most up-to-date methods
1 week	No active sports or stretching for 1 month Dressing for 3–5 days	2 months	Rarely reduction in sensitivity of nipple Visible scars	Very good
1 week	As breast reduction	2 months	Rarely reduction in sensitivity of nipple Visible scars	Very good
5–7 days	As breast reduction	3 months	Swelling, discolouration, infection possible Visible scars	Good
14 days	Keep body bent for 3–5 days. Mobility restricted for 4–6 weeks Daily dressing	3 months	Scarcely visible scars	Good
7–10 days if non-soluble	Ordinary activities in 14 days. Sport in 1 month Light gauze and antibiotic ointment	2 months	Significant scars	Very good with most up-to-date methods
5–7 days	No stretching for 2 weeks Light gauze and antibiotic ointment	2 months	Visible scars	Very good
Depends on operations	Depends on operations Depends on operations	3–4 months after last operation	Significant scars	Good
7 days if used	Careful shampooing and combing Bulky bandage for 7 days	1 year	None	Better for men than women. Repeat may be needed

The Face

It is impossible to describe what would constitute the perfect face. Ideas of perfection change over time (sometimes with startling rapidity) and vary from race to race and culture to culture. Fashion, fad and media propaganda all have a hand in building up a picture of an ideal face for one particular society at one particular time. As well as this generally accepted current ideal there is a much more personal concept of beauty that will vary from person to person, so that a face that seems beautiful to me may not look exceptionally attractive to someone else.

Another complication if we are trying to arrive at an ideal face is that beauty is more than the sum total of individual features. While some women with quite plain features look beautiful when taken as a whole, others with good features might never be called beautiful. The old saying that beauty comes from within has a great deal of truth in it. Indefinable qualities of the spirit, the character and the disposition can combine to make quite nondescript features beautiful.

The current ideal

Always bearing in mind the caveats above, it is generally agreed that certain proportions go to make a beautiful face. In Caucasian peoples, the preferred shape of face is oval, with the eyes no higher than two thirds of the way up the face. It helps if the eyes are set wide apart and if there is at least 1 cm ($\frac{1}{2}$ in) between the upper edge of the eye socket and the eyebrow. The cheekbones should be high – this not only sculptures the face but makes it photogenic. To conform to the Caucasian ideal, the nose may be almost any shape, but it must be fairly small – a tip-tilted nose, narrow at the very end, is probably the most sought-after shape. Proportions often cited as ideal in beauty magazines are an identical distance from the tip of the nose to the tip of the chin and from the tip of the nose to the outer corner of the eye. It is currently fashionable to have only a short space between the nose and the upper edge of the lip (as Brigitte Bardot has, for example), giving the mouth a rather pouting look. The general shape of the lips is unimportant so long as they are full and generous. The chin should neither jut out nor recede but should balance the nose in profile and the forehead in full face.

No cosmetic surgeon will attempt to make a face conform to these criteria. It is essential that each person's face retains its own individuality after surgery and a good surgeon strives to make changes that are almost imperceptible. He aims to create an overall effect without pinpointing any single feature and he takes care to preserve the character of the face.

Removing the signs of age

Cosmetic surgeons say that typical face lift patients are not vain, rich women with nothing better to do with their money, but energetic, active people who are less interested in hiding their age than in looking as youthful as they feel. These patients feel that an obviously ageing face erodes self-confidence and may even cause panic. A typical question such a patient asks herself is 'Why should I go on looking like this when every other part of me feels young?'

Many women in their forties or fifties are not ready to resign themselves to being thought of as ageing. They feel that growing old would be easier to bear if they could avoid looking old in the process. Furthermore, they often feel it is unjust that they should begin to show signs of deterioration when they are just beginning to reach intellectual and emotional maturity. Consequently, when fine lines, wrinkles and sags appear on their faces, they decide to fight back.

A woman having a face lift does not want friends and relatives to gasp with surprise at their first sight of her afterwards. She would prefer a natural look, an almost indefinable improvement in her appearance. For this reason a totally smooth skin is not the desired outcome. If the skin is over-stretched, a false oriental look around the eyes may rob the face of much of its expressive qualities, including taking the spontaneity from the smile and producing an impression of continual tension. The best advertisement for a good cosmetic surgeon is a patient who looks naturally young for her age, not one whose smooth skin seems artificial.

Improving the features

In some instances the decision to have cosmetic surgery has nothing to do with ageing. Sometimes an obvious facial peculiarity, such as a long or bulbous nose, can have profound psychological effects that begin as early as adolescence. A teenager may find that no matter how she arranges her hair or puts on make-up, the flaw is still apparent. This situation may make a good student feel inadequate and too restless to continue education, or lead the school-leaver to try a succession of jobs.

At some point, matters reach a crisis: the patient may resort to psychotherapy, for example, because of her problems with self-confidence, indecisiveness and inability to enjoy sex. She may find it impossible to relax with people because of her consciousness that she is not looking attractive. Very often there is not so

much an intense desire to have the offending feature improved as a continual feeling of depression caused by the knowledge that she is not looking good. It is not unreasonable to expect many of these feelings to diminish sharply, if not to disappear, once the deformity has been corrected by cosmetic surgery.

The same feelings, of course, may arise from a flaw so trivial that scarcely anyone else is aware of it. Even in these cases, surgery can bring about a dramatic psychological improvement – although it is always possible that the patient's own feeling that her appearance has been altered for the better may vanish when no change in other people's reactions to her is apparent. The inner quality that

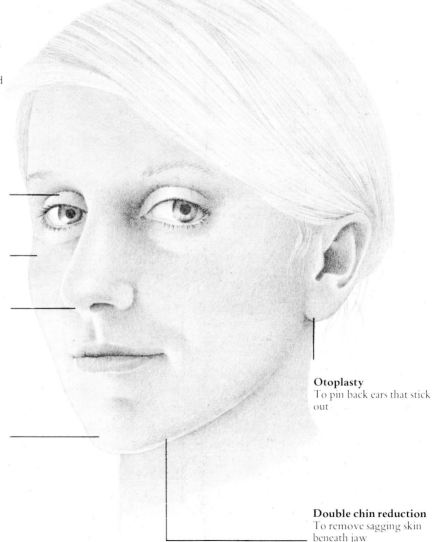

Face lift
To remove wrinkles and sagging skin over whole face

Total facial rejuvenation
Includes face and neck lift, blepharoplasty and dermabrasion of lines round mouth

Blepharoplasty
To improve drooping or puffy eyelids, remove bags beneath eyes or reshape eyebrows

Cheekbone augmentation
To make cheekbones more prominent

Rhinoplasty
To alter size or shape of nose

Chin reduction or augmentation
To alter size or shape of chin

Otoplasty
To pin back ears that stick out

Double chin reduction
To remove sagging skin beneath jaw

makes some people attractive is something no surgeon can give, and it is not necessarily linked with having beautiful features.

What to expect

It is important that a person who is going to have cosmetic surgery is highly motivated. If not, the chances are that she will not be happy about the outcome, no matter how successful the operation.

Before a person gets to see a cosmetic surgeon, she may have to overcome opposition from family, friends and possibly the family doctor too (some general practitioners give cosmetic surgery a very low priority and may be pessimistic about the chances of success). It is also necessary to prepare for the immediate after-effects of surgery, which can be quite a shock to the system. Many patients have lived for years with a physical flaw to which they have become emotionally adjusted. After the operation, the mind has to recover, as well as the body. Mild depression is a fairly common post-operative reaction – understandably, since the effects of the surgery are at that point completely buried beneath dressings. Even when the dressings are taken off, the face may look far from reassuring: it will be swollen, the skin bruised and there may be stitches. It may take some faith at this juncture to accept that the operation has been a success. Confidence in the surgeon and support from family and friends are a great help here.

For someone who has suffered from psychological stress as a result of a facial deformity, the long-term benefits of cosmetic surgery are legion and reach into all areas of life and work – the ability to make friends, professional performance, relationship with family and, most crucial of all, confidence in oneself. The cosmetic surgery may leave the patient more at ease with herself and more self-assured, as well as looking better. Taking all these things into account, it may really amount to starting a new life.

Face lift

This operation demands great precision, accuracy and attention to detail on the part of the surgeon. An unsuccessful face lift can leave the patient looking – and certainly feeling – far worse than she did beforehand.

The surgeon begins by trimming a few strands of hair back and making incisions on the scalp above the forehead, in front of (or just behind) the ears and underneath the earlobes. These cuts allow him to loosen the excess skin and pull what he judges to be an appropriate amount upwards and backwards. After the skin has been trimmed, the surgeon stitches the edges of the incisions back together again with meticulous care.

The effect of pulling the skin back and up is to tighten up sagging areas (round the cheeks and jawbone, for example) and to smoothe out to some extent frown lines on the forehead, crow's-feet round the eyes and wrinkles generally – none of these should be wholly eliminated, however, or the face can assume a look of mask-like artificiality. The scars left behind by the incisions are quick to blend with the surrounding skin and are normally hidden by hair and the natural fold in the area in front of the ear.

A face lift takes at least two hours to perform and it is always carried out in hospital and under a general anaesthetic. The usual length of stay in hospital is three days. As the surgeon generally treats the incised skin with a local anaesthetic, it is rare for there to be a lot of pain after the operation. The first 48 hours can, however, be depressing. The area of the operation is covered with a bulky dressing at this stage and even when this is removed, two days after the operation, the face looks red and swollen. Surgeons adopt different rules for timing the removal of stitches but generally stitches come out between five days and two weeks after the operation. The superficial swelling and bruising wear off gradually over the next few weeks.

Although the immediate after-effects of facial surgery take up to a month to disappear, there is no reason why they should prevent the patient from leading a fully active life within three days of the operation. A head scarf and dark glasses will camouflage the worst of the swelling and discolouration.

The full effect of the surgeon's work will not be plain until about three months after the face lift. During this period the swelling gradually subsides and healing of the deeper tissues takes place. Different people heal at different rates, so it may take a slightly longer or shorter time for the wounds to heal completely. It is even possible for the incisions on the different sides of the face to heal at different rates.

The results of a good face lift usually last roughly eight years. After about this long, the facial skin starts to sag again and the face begins to show signs of ageing. The most common age at which to have a face lift is in the early or middle forties. Furthermore, previous cosmetic surgery is no bar to further cosmetic operations and one person may have several face lifts, although most people are happy to stop after one.

Variations on the face lift

It is possible to carry out a partial face lift – for example, involving just the upper or lower face or even just the jawline and neck. Few good cosmetic surgeons would consider this, however, as the improvement in one part of the face only casts into relief the older appearance of the rest.

A fairly new approach advocated for older patients by some surgeons in the United States is 'total facial rejuvenation'. The term embraces a face lift, eyelid repair, dermabrasion of the deep wrinkles round the top lip (see pages 214–215) and neck rejuvenation (removal of loose folds of neck skin). If there is a nasal deformity, rhinoplasty is thrown in. (The nose is said to grow longer with advancing age and so shortening it is supposed to give a more youthful appearance.) All the operations may be done at one session or staggered over several months.

Some patients complain about a feeling of tightness round the neck or numbness round the ears for a few weeks or even months after this surgery, but the feeling almost always disappears eventually.

Another variation is to modify the muscle structure underlying the skin. This technique is said to help in eliminating frown lines, to give a more youthful contour to the cheek and mouth area and to leave less bruising and swelling after surgery. This kind of operation is even more delicate than an ordinary face lift and it takes longer to perform. It is likely to be available only in those parts of the world that treat cosmetic surgery as more or less a matter of course and where there is a high degree of sophistication in surgical techniques.

Blepharoplasty

This operation can be performed to remove sagging skin that makes the eyes look puffy, to raise a drooping eyelid or to reshape an eyebrow.

An incision is usually made in the natural fold of the upper lid, extending out into the smile lines around the eyes. For a lower lid the incision comes just below the eyelashes and also extends into the smile lines. After excess fat and tissue have been removed, the incision is stitched up.

The stitches come out 48 hours after the operation and within ten days the scars should have blended sufficiently so that they can be completely hidden by make-up. Immediately after a blepharoplasty dark glasses are useful to conceal the after-effects of the operation.

Blepharoplasty is always done in hospital under general anaesthetic. The normal stay is three days but some clinics allow a shorter stay.

Rhinoplasty

This operation aims to reshape the nose. Almost any shape of nose can be altered: a large one can be made smaller or a small one larger. The operation is tailored to suit the patient and she can usually have the shape or size of nose she wants.

The nose usually increases in growth at puberty and continues to grow until it reaches its mature size and shape at around the age of 15 or 16. Ideally, it should blend with the rest of the face harmoniously, looking feminine in a woman and masculine in a man. When the reverse happens, it can be very disturbing, especially during the traumas of adolescence. A teenager who is struggling with a sense of inadequacy and insecurity to begin with is likely to find it hard to summon up the courage to broach the topic of having cosmetic surgery to reshape her nose. Many people are in their early twenties before they are psychologically prepared for the operation. Rhinoplasty is possible at any age, although many surgeons set a minimum age of 18.

Before the operation, the patient decides with the surgeon on the shape and size of the new nose after surgery and goes into hospital the evening before the operation is due. The surgery is carried out either under a local anaesthetic while the patient is heavily sedated or under a general anaesthetic.

All the surgical work is carried out inside the nose so that after the operation no scars will be visible. Excess bone and cartilage are removed and the tissues inside the nose sculpted skilfully – to remove bumps, shorten the length, narrow the bridge and so on. If the nose is to be made larger, cartilage and silicone implants are inserted. The operation is not lengthy – most patients are back in their room within an hour.

After a brief stay in hospital (commonly three days) the patient goes home, wearing only a light dressing on the nose. The area round the nose is usually quite swollen and the skin round the eyes discoloured. The swelling inside the nose makes it feel stuffy and it is normally necessary to breathe through the mouth for two or three weeks after the operation. In addition there may be some numbness around the nose, rather like the after-effects of a local anaesthetic for dental treatment to an upper front tooth. These feelings wear off over the following month or two, but it takes about six months for the nose to assume its permanent shape, as bone and cartilage heal rather slowly.

Otoplasty

Protruding ears can cause a lot of anguish from an early age and so many cosmetic surgeons recommend dealing with them when a child is around five, before he or she starts being teased about them.

An incision is made behind the ear and the cartilage is stitched and then possibly bandaged back into a more normal position. Stitches are removed within five to seven days. The scars should fall into the groove behind the ear and the cosmetic results are usually excellent.

A child having otoplasty normally has the operation in hospital under a general anaesthetic, but an adult may be able to choose a local anaesthetic instead.

Cheekbone augmentation

Implants are used to augment cheekbones in much the same way as in chin augmentation (see below). The implants are inserted under local or general anaesthetic, either via the inside of the mouth or through an incision beneath the lower eyelashes. Straight after the operation the area will feel uncomfortable and the full results will not show until all swelling has subsided, several months later. Stitches are removed from beneath the eye five to seven days after the operation.

Double chin reduction

The sag of fat and loose skin that some people get under the chin can be dealt with during a face lift or as a separate operation. The Z- or T-shaped incision is made beneath the chin, so that any scar will be in shadow (see chart on pages 218–219 for further details). Sometimes chin augmentation (see below) is done at the same time, to enhance the effect of this operation.

Chin reduction

Bone and cartilage can be removed from the chin in much the same way as from the nose. The operation is performed from inside the mouth, so that it leaves no obvious scars.

The inside of the mouth feels sore for around ten days, so for this time it is sensible to eat only soft, pulpy food. Stitches are removed within a week of the operation and the immediate post-operative swelling subsides within a month.

If the chin is so large as to make a radical excision of bone necessary, the operation may have to be done from the outside. The incision is made beneath the chin, so that any scars are hidden in the shadow of the jaw.

Chin augmentation

This can produce virtually any size or shape of chin. Exact details of the desired contour are agreed between surgeon and patient beforehand.

The incision is usually made inside the mouth, along the lower gum. Then a previously moulded implant made from inert plastic is inserted to lie underneath the skin at the front of the chin to give the new shape. For the next ten days a tight bandage is worn round the chin to hold the implant exactly in position. During this period the patient should have a diet of soft food, to avoid dislodging the implant while chewing.

For further details of all pre-operative and post-operative conditions for facial surgery see the chart on pages 218–219. Virtually all scars can be camouflaged by skilfully applied make-up until they become less visible; for cover-up techniques see pages 205–207.

The Body

The recent upsurge of interest in keeping fit has underlined the fact that a slim, healthy body is a valuable asset. For those who are neither prepared to exercise and diet their bulges away, nor to resign themselves to a less than ideal figure, cosmetic body surgery provides a last resort.

Expense is one but not the only factor that should make body surgery a last resort in the search for beauty. Body contouring tends to be more serious from the medical standpoint than facial surgery. Some of the operations are lengthy, some involve a considerable spell of post-operative pain and immobility and all leave scars, albeit of varying degrees of conspicuousness. Perhaps as a result of this, some operations, such as hip and thigh reduction or a total body lift, are rare outside the main centres for cosmetic surgery on the American continent.

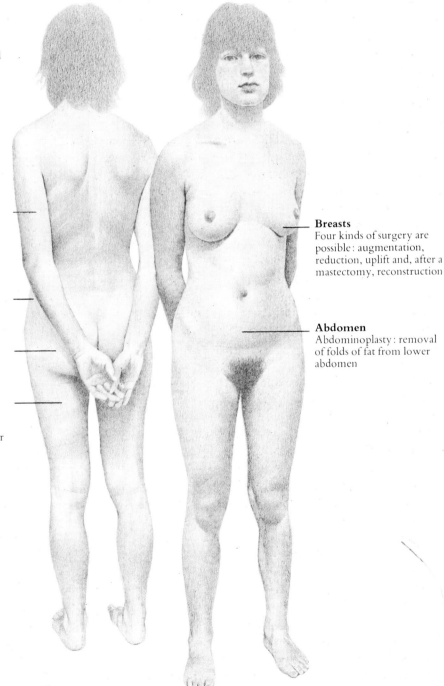

Total body lift
Removal of sagging skin from abdomen, buttocks, thighs, hips, arms, neck and face

Upper arms
Removal of loose folds of skin

Hips
Reduction : removal of excess fat and skin

Buttocks
Reduction : removal of excess fat and skin

Thighs
Reduction : removal of excess fat and skin, often known as jodphur thighs or riding breeches deformity

Breasts
Four kinds of surgery are possible : augmentation, reduction, uplift and, after a mastectomy, reconstruction

Abdomen
Abdominoplasty : removal of folds of fat from lower abdomen

Breasts

A woman's breasts are as individual as her fingerprint. Perhaps because of continual bombardment with information about what constitutes beautiful breasts, few of us are entirely satisfied with our own. Operations to change the size or shape of the breasts have been carried out for many years, although recent techniques have much improved the final result.

Breast augmentation

This is the most popular body operation in almost any cosmetic surgery clinic anywhere in the world. A typical candidate for it has already tried every other conceivable method to improve her bust: exercises, massage, bathing the breasts alternately in hot and cold water, so-called hormone creams. Sadly, the only successful way to enlarge the breasts is through surgery.

The first technique for breast augmentation was to inject liquid silicone directly into the breasts themselves. This was popular in the early 1960s but in 1965 the Food and Drugs Administration (the FDA) banned the practice in the United States until research should determine whether or not it was safe and effective. The research is still going on and so far the FDA has not received sufficient information about this substance for it to sanction the use of silicone injections. The operation is still illegal and no woman should contemplate it.

The second technique, introduced in 1962, was to implant silicone rubber devices to make the breasts bigger. These implants are legal, ethical, safe and widely used by cosmetic surgeons. In America more than half a million women have them permanently in their bodies.

The newest breast augmentation technique, which is not yet available in many parts of the world, uses an inflatable implant filled with physiological saline or salt water. These implants too are safe and effective and in consistency and feel they closely resemble normal breast tissue.

Before the operation patient and surgeon establish what size and shape the breasts are to be. It is not a good idea to be over ambitious: too large breasts may look unnatural or top-heavy. At this point you can ask to see a specimen of the implant material the surgeon intends to use.

Breast augmentation is rarely possible as an out-patient; most surgeons prefer the patient to be in hospital for at least three days. The operation is usually done under a general anaesthetic. The incision is made around the areola, the coloured area surrounding the nipple, where it will heal without leaving any obvious scar. The implant is then placed behind the normal breast tissue so that it lies against the pectoralis major, the largest muscle of the chest wall. The deeper layers of the wound are stitched together with soluble nylon that does not have to be removed and the stitches closing the incision round the areola come out a week after the operation.

The wound normally has only a light dressing, and it is kept clean and free of infection by the use of an antibiotic ointment. It is rare for there to be much discomfort, and any bruising usually disappears after a few weeks. Sometimes there may be some tingling or numbness round the nipple, but this usually wears off within a month. You should start wearing a bra in your new size as soon as it is comfortable to do so – buy one in advance and take it into hospital when you go for the operation.

It is better to avoid very active sports, such as swimming, tennis and volleyball, for about a month after breast augmentation. Movements that extend the arms high above the head and those that pull the elbows out at right angles at shoulder level should also be avoided, but otherwise the operation should not interfere with your mobility.

In the best hands this operation should have no complications, no leakage, no slipping, no infection and no rejection. The breast looks and feels natural. In this respect this new type of inflatable implant should not be confused with another type, made of silicone gel. Around a fifth of these become extremely hard after insertion, a complication that may call for further surgery. This is exceedingly rare with the new type of inflatable implant.

Breast reduction

Some women, rather than feeling inadequate about undeveloped breasts, are embarrassingly well endowed. Some breasts may be so pendulous that they may hang down to the thighs and so heavy that the bra straps ulcerate the skin of the shoulders. These breasts need to be reduced for medical – let alone psychological – reasons. In a less extreme case a woman may end up feeling like a freak and trying to camouflage her figure in shapeless clothes. Her problem may get even worse with age as the breast tissue grows thin and flabby and the nipples sag.

The first step is to have photographs taken of the breasts from every angle. On these photographs the new outline of the breasts can be sketched in during consultations between patient and surgeon before the operation.

For breast reduction an incision is made around the areola, just as for breast augmentation, and then all the way down the front underside of the breast, to where it meets the skin covering the chest wall. Skin, fat and breast tissue are removed, leaving enough to fashion a breast of normal shape and size. The nipples have to be moved upwards to an appropriate position on the re-shaped breasts but this should not affect their sensitivity and may not rule out breastfeeding later on provided the technique employed does not involve totally severing the milk ducts. Although the scars from this operation are nearly always more noticeable than those left by breast augmentation, they usually fade in time and can easily be hidden under make-up (see pages 205–207).

Breast reduction is a slightly more major operation than breast augmentation and generally involves a five-day stay in hospital and a general anaesthetic. There may be some bruising and discomfort immediately after the surgery but these effects should disappear after a few weeks. Provided that you avoid lifting heavy weights (anything over 13.5 kg or 30 lb) or stretching, normal activity can be resumed a month after the operation.

Be sure to take a bra in the new size into hospital with you so that you can start wearing it as soon as it is comfortable to do so.

Breast uplift (mastoplexy)

The breasts tend to droop as we get older. The suspensory ligaments, the skin and the breast tissue itself thin and become inelastic. Once this happens nothing will make the breast regain its former shape.

The operation uses virtually the same technique as breast reduction, but only skin, rather than skin, fat and breast tissue, is removed. Sometimes breast uplift is combined with breast augmentation or reduction, or the correction of a minor peculiarity like lopsidedness. A general anaesthetic is used. The normal length of stay in hospital is three days, but some clinics in the United States offer breast uplift operations to out-patients.

Breast reconstruction

In the United States, where breast reconstruction was pioneered, this operation is considered more or less the right of every woman who has had to have a breast removed. By far the commonest reason for breast removal (mastectomy) is breast cancer, but occasionally a breast may be removed in a very severe case of fibrocystic breast disease, which some doctors think is pre-cancerous.

A mastectomy operation can be either simple or radical. In simple mastectomy only the breast is removed; the muscles of the chest wall remain intact. In a radical mastectomy, the breast and the pectoral muscles are cleared from the chest wall and armpit. The technique of breast reconstruction depends on how complete the mastectomy has been.

After a simple mastectomy the breast can be reconstructed along the same basic lines as the breast augmentation operation described above. The operation can follow as soon as six weeks after the mastectomy (provided that there is no indication that the cancer may have spread to other areas of the body) and it involves only a three-day stay in hospital. Reconstruction after a radical mastectomy is more complicated, since the muscles of the chest wall have to be rebuilt first. Tissue from the arm muscles is often used for this purpose. The fatty tissue to form the bulk of the breast is very often taken from the abdomen and the whole is then covered by a skin graft. The second stage of the operation is carried out several months later, and involves putting in an implant, as in the breast augmentation operation. The inflatable type of implant gives the best results. Care is taken to fashion as natural looking nipple and areola tissue as possible – the most modern clinics reconstruct the nipple out of tissue taken from the patient's earlobe.

Post-operative care and restrictions for people who have had breast reconstruction are exactly the same as those for the other breast operations.

Breast reconstruction can rarely be completed without some residual scarring but the scars are not normally prominent. They are certainly not disfiguring, as those of mastectomy inevitably are. Because the operation is complex and done in stages, minor complications such as swelling and discolouration may occur but are normally temporary. Major complications are rare.

It is essential to approach this operation realistically. A reconstructed breast will hardly ever look as good as a natural one. Ask the surgeon to show you photographs of reconstructed breasts so that you avoid disappointment. Many women consider the psychological pay-off is more than sufficient.

Abdomen

The very obese are the obvious potential candidates for this type of cosmetic surgery but not the only ones. Even a slender woman may feel unhappy about wearing a revealing swimsuit on the beach if previous pregnancies have left her with a flabby tummy crisscrossed with indented stretch marks. Dieting and exercise may not resolve her problem. Cosmetic surgery offers people in this situation the only real hope of ever having a flat, attractive tummy again.

Abdominoplasty (apronectomy)

The abdomen can be lifted in much the same way as the face and this is the most popular of the body contouring operations. It is not a new idea: it was performed as long ago as 1899 by an American doctor on a 30-year-old woman with a massive pendulous abdomen. After the operation the patient should have a tight, flat tummy, a slimmer waistline and a natural looking navel. The scar should be scarcely noticeable.

Because abdominoplasty is a fairly major operation, it is always carried out in hospital under general anaesthetic. The stay in hospital is usually a week.

The surgeon begins by making a single incision across the lower part of the abdomen, across the groin. If any of the abdominal muscles have been split, they are repaired and then redundant fat and

skin are cut away. The remaining skin is pulled down taut and flat and joined to the skin at the groin. The navel nearly always has to be moved to a higher position, so that it will look normal.

After the operation a tube is usually inserted into either end of the incision to drain away any fluid that may collect in the wound – after this comes out on the fourth or fifth day the wound is dressed like any other abdominal surgery.

For the first three to five days after the operation the patient has to lie so that the body is slightly bent forward and then encouragement is given to her to straighten out gradually. No special support is necessary – any comfortable clothes may be worn. Stretching or lifting heavy weights should be avoided for around a month but bending does no harm straight away. Stitches are removed after about 14 days and after six weeks it is possible to undertake normal exercise. The scars will show up strongly at first but will fade to some extent over time. They should not show even when you wear a skimpy bikini.

Stretch marks

These may be treated as part of abdominoplasty, if the abdomen is flabby and pendulous, or by dermabrasion (see pages 214–215).

The most recent technique, used by some clinics in the United States, is very similar to facial dermabrasion and makes use of a high powered drill and a diamond burr under a general anaesthetic. The temporary biological dressing of pig skin used afterwards dries up and flakes off after about ten to 14 days, during which time the area should not be interfered with and must be kept clean. Most patients have to stay in hospital for about five days, the first two spent lying completely still on their back. Full mobility should be restored in a month and in six weeks it is possible to play active sports. Visible scars are rare.

Thighs, hips, buttocks

Very few women are without some degree of 'jodphur thighs', simply as a secondary sexual characteristic. Pads of fat laid down on the thighs and elsewhere from the time oestrogen begins to be secreted at puberty give the female body its distinctively curved contour. It may be difficult to lose fat from the thighs by dieting alone and even slim women may have a 'riding breeches' problem to some extent. The only solution for someone who is really determined to achieve slim thighs may be cosmetic surgery.

It was not until ten or 15 years ago that plastic surgeons developed techniques to correct top-heavy thighs. The longitudinal incisions made previously left unsightly scars and there was no efficient way of removing the fat. Cosmetic operations on the buttocks, hips and thighs are still available only in those parts of the world that make a speciality of cosmetic surgery.

Fat can be removed from all three sites in one operation – it is always carried out under general anaesthetic in a hospital. Crescent-shaped incisions are made beneath the buttocks and at the top of the inner and outer thigh. After excess skin and fat have been removed, the skin is pulled upwards, in rather the same way as one pulls on a stocking, and stitched into place.

Cosmetic surgical technique for this operation is so advanced that in certain clinics the patient may be able to get out of bed on the evening of the operation and sit on a chair with very little pain. On the other hand it is not uncommon to feel some discomfort on sitting down for two weeks. The only surgical dressing is one layer of gauze and the wound is treated with antibiotic ointment to prevent infection. Instructions are given on how to clean and dress the wound at home. The stitches are generally underneath the skin and can be left to dissolve on their own. Ordinary day-to-day activities can be resumed after two weeks and active exercise after a month. The scars will show when you wear nothing or only a very skimpy bikini, but not otherwise.

Upper arms

Sometimes flabby skin on the upper arms can produce a 'bat-wing' deformity between the elbows and shoulders, particularly as the skin sags with age. This can be corrected as part of a total body lift (see below) or on its own.

The surgeon makes an incision along the back of the upper arm from armpit to elbow, removes the excess fat and skin and stitches the edges of the cut back together. The scars can be hidden by sleeves or camouflaged with make-up (see pages 205–207 for cover-up techniques).

Total body lift

If the patient is fit and healthy, some surgeons will agree to treat several areas of the body during one operation – how many depends on the individual's ability to tolerate pain and immobility. As an alternative, several procedures can be staggered over a period of months.

A total body lift – including face lift, abdominoplasty, recontouring of hips, buttocks and thighs and removal of loose skin from the upper arms – is designed to take up the slackness and flabbiness that is common in ageing skin or may accompany drastic weight loss. If the excessive obesity was due to chronic bad eating habits, it is essential for the operation to be preceded by some form of counselling to warn the patient that she must never again put on too much weight.

Hair transplant

This is suitable only for treating conditions in which hair loss is permanent and complete over a circumscribed area and it is essential to consult a dermatologist beforehand to establish the suitability. The technique has changed little since it was first described in 1959. It still centres on transplanting full-thickness, hair-bearing skin in strips, plugs or combinations of both.

The skin to be grafted is normally taken from the back of the head, which is the last place to lose its hair. Up to 50 plugs, each around 5 mm ($\frac{1}{4}$ in) in diameter and containing ten or 12 hairs, may be implanted during one session. A local or general anaesthetic is used. After the operation a bulky dressing is applied to the scalp and kept in place for about a week. At the end of this period the dressing is removed and the grafted area may be gently shampooed and combed. The crusts that usually form round each of the plugs normally wash off in the first shampoo. Any that remain separate within a few days and the small swellings they leave subside over the next weeks.

After growing for a month, the hair in the transplants usually falls out – this is quite normal because the hair follicles in the grafted skin have entered the resting phase of their growth cycle (see page 31). They should start to grow again after around three months, but the full effect will not show for a year and it may be necessary to repeat the transplant to fill in spaces.

Cosmetic Dentistry

Starting good habits early

If you want to have a perfect white smile when you are 20, you (and your parents) will need to start working on it when you are five years old. It is no good thinking that primary or milk teeth are unimportant simply because children start to lose them around the age of six. Strong, well-positioned milk teeth guide the permanent teeth as they erupt and grow to take up their lifelong positions in the jawbones. If the baby teeth are overcrowded, the permanent ones may grow in crookedly. If a gap has been left by the removal of a decayed milk tooth, the permanent teeth on either side of the gap will not be encouraged to grow upright.

It is therefore worth while taking good care of baby teeth from the moment that they appear. Never offer a child a bottle filled with fruit juice as a pacifier – its sugar content rapidly decays the teeth and encourages a 'sweet tooth' in later life. It is helpful to give a baby hard foods to chew on as soon as he or she develops the liking for chomping, since chewing movements exercise the jaw muscles and help to make the teeth grow in straight. The chances of serious tooth decay can be minimized by attention to diet (avoiding a lot of sweet and starchy foods), careful tooth-brushing with the right kind of toothbrush (see page 57) and regular visits to the dentist. The use of fluoride either in tablet form or as toothpaste (see page 58) also helps stop decay.

Dentists hate taking out teeth, even baby ones, but occasionally an orthodontist will decide to take out a milk tooth to prevent overcrowding while the permanent teeth emerge. Most orthodontists feel that they have to 'educate' parents as well as treating the children, because parents often demand corrective treatment for malpositioned teeth long before it should be given. There is no point considering cosmetic dentistry for a child until it is eight, since it will not have the requisite number of teeth on which to fix a brace or wire. Most dentists would prefer to wait until a child is about 12 years old before undertaking orthodontic treatment because if this is given too early other faults may occur. In addition, many problems improve naturally if left to the correcting effects of chewing and the position of the tongue, cheeks and lips.

Whitening the teeth

According to the best dental opinion, no good 'cosmetics' for the teeth can be bought over the counter. Toothpastes that claim to whiten teeth usually do so by two methods. The first is really an optical illusion: the toothpaste contains a red pigment that turns the gums deep pink, so that the teeth look whiter in comparison. Toothpastes that use the second method, and claim to give a polished, gleaming smile, make the teeth shine by the use of abrasives (including one known as 'jeweller's rouge'). These substances are much too harsh to use on teeth – they work by scratching the surface enamel, which may be damaged or worn away through prolonged use of such toothpastes. Since there has been a move away from using abrasives on stainless steel kitchen sinks and ceramic baths and basins, it seems astonishing that we should continue to consider using them on our teeth.

The best and safest way to give your teeth a new look is to visit a dental hygienist. To keep your gums and teeth healthy you should go at least every six months – every three months is even better. The hygienist will remove from between the teeth calcareous deposits of plaque, which irritate the gums and make them bleed, and will descale your teeth and give them a good polish. This treatment makes everyone's teeth look several shades whiter, particularly smokers'.

What the cosmetic dentist can do

It is possible for a good, skilled cosmetic dentist to alter completely not just the look of your teeth or your smile, but also the set of your mouth and therefore, to some degree, your facial expression. If, for instance, your teeth have been ground away over the years either because you are a 'night grinder' or simply because you have especially strong masticating muscles, your jawbones will tend to come closer together. This accentuates the folds on either side of your mouth and may have an ageing appearance. A cosmetic dentist can open up the distance between the jawbones by repositioning the teeth, thereby stretching out the skin in your laughter lines. This procedure can also relieve pain and tenderness in the joints of the jaw, which become over-stressed when the teeth are ground away.

Virtually all forms of cosmetic dentistry will leave the area treated feeling tender and it is essential to ask your dentist what, and how, you may eat afterwards – it may be necessary to have soft, pulpy foods or to feed through a straw.

Repositioning teeth

In cosmetic dentistry much can be achieved by the use of simple methods and materials. It is quite possible to move the roots of teeth within the jawbone by perhaps a fraction of a millimetre, if they are pushed or pulled in one direction for any length of time. Even such a tiny adjustment makes a great difference to the overall effect. Very often sufficient force can be applied to a misaligned tooth simply by the expert use of elastic bands. For more severe deformities, wires and braces can be fitted to manipulate the teeth over a period of months into the desired position.

A tooth that is particularly badly out of line can be twisted or moved by cutting through the jawbone on either side of the roots. The tooth is then secured and the bone ends will heal in the new position exactly as a fracture does.

Caps, crowns and bridges

A broken, ugly or severely malpositioned tooth can be given a new appearance and a new lease of life by capping or crowning (the two terms are synonymous). This is usually done by filing the tooth away to form a 'peg' on to which the cap is cemented. Even a tooth that has snapped off or has had to be removed at the line of the gum margin can be capped. In such cases three or four 'posts' on to which the cap can be fixed are drilled into the remnants of the tooth.

Caps and crowns are made of a variety of materials. The most modern ones are composed of extremely strong porcelains and plastics, which come in a number of colours so that the finished cap will exactly match the rest of the teeth. The cap can be made in any shape to conform to the size and contour of the original tooth – indeed its shape may even be slightly imperfect in order to maintain a natural appearance.

A bridge consists of a clear plastic plate that has been moulded to fit over the hard palate. It may fill one gap or many – the requisite number of false teeth are secured in the appropriate places on the plate. The bridge slips easily into place and is held snugly in the mouth by wires that fit around existing teeth. It can be removed for cleaning, either with a sterilizing solution or a brush.

'Shortening' or 'lengthening' teeth

Almost any unsightly variation of bite (the way the top teeth sit on the bottom ones when the jaws are closed) or appearance can be corrected. In some cases the gums recede from the sides of the teeth, leaving a large part of them exposed; the same effect occurs if the teeth are genuinely too long. A good cosmetic dentist can correct this by exposing the roots of the teeth, to which the gum margins are attached, and cutting a thin flap from the surface of the gum. This is then swung down and applied over the exposed parts of the teeth. If after this the teeth are still too long, they can be filed away and given caps that will make them a little shorter than they were originally.

Some people have the reverse problem – the gums grow too far up the teeth so that they are, or appear to be, too short. In this instance the gum margins can be cut away (gingivectomy) and the teeth lengthened with caps that are slightly longer than the original teeth.

Buck teeth

Ideally buck teeth should be treated before the age of 14 by a paediatric orthodontist who will use braces and wires to pull the teeth into line with the rest. If you reach adulthood with buck teeth, cosmetic dentistry can correct the deformity by the use of caps. The malpositioned teeth are filed away and the caps fitted to follow the normal line.

Cosmetic dentistry at its best is highly creative and good practitioners will rise to almost any challenge to find an inventive way of correcting tooth deformity. One of the most beautiful and effective examples I have seen was the correction of malpositioned teeth in a person with a cleft palate. Because of the cleft, there were fewer teeth than is normal; in addition, they had moved round the jaw so that the front teeth were off-centre. The dentist transformed the appearance by using each of the existing teeth as the basis for a cap, but moving the position of every cap on its tooth a millimetre or so along in the direction that brought them all back to centre.

A–Z of Alternative Medicine

Any medicine that heals, cures or simply relieves discomfort without harmful side-effects is good medicine. It follows that any person who heals, cures or relieves a patient's discomfort without doing harm is practising good medicine. Good medicine therefore should have room for both orthodox and unorthodox therapy.

Orthodox medicine is based on allopathy, the doctrine of contraries, which originated in Asia Minor in the first century BC. It followed a principle so simple that it soon became accepted as common sense: when the working of the body goes wrong, counteract the symptoms. An example of this in practice would be to treat constipation with a laxative.

By contrast, the main branches of unorthodox medicine tend to preach that our bodies have a life force, which becomes disturbed in disease but which will reassert itself unaided to overcome the disease if the body is nourished only by the food that it needs and inessential or harmful ingredients are avoided.

Just like the best orthodox medicine, the best unorthodox medicine is holistic; it treats the patient as a whole rather than merely the symptoms. The true naturopath eschews symptomatic remedies because they fail to go to the root cause of the illness. For this reason the fashionable high-speed acupuncture therapist who treats a patient every ten minutes and deals with symptoms only is shunned by his holistic colleagues.

One of the reasons that unorthodox medicine is not readily accepted by mainstream doctors is that its techniques are not subjected to proper scientific scrutiny and objective analysis. Little account is taken of the natural variation that many illnesses exhibit or of spontaneous improvement. Until this changes, alternative medicine will remain on the fringe.

Acupressure
See Shiatzu, under **Massage**

Acupuncture
The word acupuncture comes from a Latin root meaning to pierce with a needle. The practice originated because it was noticed that Chinese soldiers wounded in battle by arrows not only recovered from the arrow wound but from other ailments as well. From these early observations the practice evolved of using a prick from a needle to activate certain parts of the body found to affect other parts.

The theory behind acupuncture is that a life force or energy flows through the body along lines or channels called meridians, quite distinct from the lines followed by nerves. The Chinese believe this life force must flow unimpeded if bodily health is to be maintained. When health breaks down, the energy flow in a particular meridian may be affected at a site considerably distant from the part of the body that is ailing.

The acupuncturist aims to restore the flow of energy in the affected meridian by the use of copper, silver or gold needles that are inserted into the flesh superficially at specific points on the meridian. If the therapist is good, this procedure should not hurt. The needle is thought to set up some kind of electrical current along the line of the meridian. It passes to the central nervous system and has an effect on the organ or area that is malfunctioning by re-establishing the flow of energy through the meridian in question.

Acupuncture is almost the only part of Eastern medicine that has come to be accepted in the West. It has been separated out from an entire system of oriental medicine, of which it is only a part. In Western countries therefore acupuncture tends to be practised in a way that would be disapproved of in the East.

However the uninformed or inexperienced may feel about acupuncture, it has undoubted success with many patients. Chinese films show patients having heart transplant surgery while the only alleged anaesthetic is acupuncture therapy. In the less pure form in which it is practised in the West it may be more difficult to prove the benefits of acupuncture.

Aromatherapy
This is a fairly recent addition to alternative medicine, although its roots go back through the millennia. For centuries pleasant smells have been associated with holiness – Buddha and the most holy Yogis supposedly gave off an aromatic smell. The burning of incense during religious ceremonies is another example of this link. In general sweet smells are supposed to appeal to our higher nature.

We have a highly developed sense of smell and can react to an odour within split seconds in an intensely personal and not always agreeable way. A small child who sniffs something offensive may vomit the next instant. There is no doubt that smells can and do affect our bodies, and aromatherapy is built upon this foundation.

According to aromatherapy, aromatic oil essences, such as musk, damask, sandalwood and so forth, are combined to suit the patient's personality. The aromas are smelled or inhaled to allow the essential ingredients to be absorbed through the lining of the air passages. The therapy is supposed to bring about mood changes according to the ingredients chosen: one mixture may tranquillize, another may excite, for instance. Through its tranquillizing effect aromatherapy is said to relieve tension and anxiety and improve relaxation. There are claims that it can help headaches and high blood pressure. With its mood-heightening effects it is said to increase efficiency and encourage a positive attitude to life and therefore greater enjoyment of it. In addition, aromatherapy is often used to boost the effect of other remedies – for example, aromatic oils may be used to intensify the benefits of massage.

Treatment centering on aromas ignores one of the basic physiological facts about the sense of smell, namely that it very quickly becomes exhausted. We can look at or hear something continuously over a long period, but a smell that is smelled for much longer than a minute can no longer be sensed. The olfactory organs speedily become saturated and cease to transmit data. Presumably the effects claimed for aromatherapy can last for only as long as it takes for the smell to exhaust our power to sense it.

Balneotherapy

Under this heading come all the variations on bath therapy stemming from the times of the Greeks and Romans – in fact even earlier civilizations made use of baths as centres of physical and mental rejuvenation. When the practice spread to Europe, areas where the water was believed to have special medicinal virtues became popular health spas. Different constituents in the water were supposed to help particular ailments. Sulphurous water, like that of the Dead Sea, was believed to benefit sufferers from psoriasis, and sulphur baths are still used to help people who suffer from this and many other skin complaints.

Other substances used in baths are Epsom salts and mud to draw out impurities from the skin; mustard to warm the skin, which is thought to be particularly useful for arthritics; oatmeal and peat to help hold heat in the skin; and pine to 'invigorate' the skin and to tranquillize the bather. Oxygen and ozone may be bubbled through the bath water for their allegedly energizing properties.

Some baths rely on particular procedures rather than special ingredients for their effects. Footbaths are recommended for sore or tired feet or to ward off a chill – a hot footbath containing mustard or a small amount of eucalyptus is a variation on this treatment. In Germany the scrubbing bath is still popular: this involves being scrubbed all over with a stiff brush, rubbed down with a dry towel and then resting in bed. The treatment is supposed to be good for people with poor circulation and for women going through the menopause, although it is hard to figure out how the procedure could help someone suffering from hot flushes. Another variant currently enjoying great popularity is the jet bath (jacusi) – see later entry under **Massage.**

Any of these baths might make you feel good but it is difficult to see how they could treat a specific disease. No form of balneotherapy should be taken by an eczema sufferer.

Biofeedback

This is the modern version of mind over matter. It includes a number of methods of relaying information to patients about what is going on in their bodies so that they can achieve some control over internal processes. An illustration is electroencephalography (EEG) to help the patient overcome anxiety and promote relaxation. The patient is connected to an EEG machine that relays on to a small screen the pattern of the brain waves being transmitted. The doctor points out a particular pattern that corresponds to 'tranquillity' and asks the patient to try to recreate it. By trial and error the patient gradually learns what she has to do and feel to produce the pattern and eventually she should be able to reproduce the same state of relaxation without the aid of the machine.

In some advanced medical centres biofeedback techniques may be used in the treatment of heart disease, high blood pressure and some psychiatric disorders. Simple portable biofeedback machines can be obtained for home or office use; they are claimed to help control blood pressure and tension.

Chiropractic

This term is derived from two Greek words: *cheir* meaning hand and *praktikos*, meaning practitioner. The system was founded by Daniel Palmer in the United States in the 1890s, in somewhat bizarre circumstances. Palmer overheard his janitor explaining how he had become instantaneously deaf some 17 years earlier when he had bent over and had felt something 'go' in his back. On examining the janitor's back, Palmer found that one of the vertebra was very slightly out of place, whereupon he proceeded to adjust it by manipulation and so managed to restore the janitor's hearing.

Chiropractic centres on the anatomy of the spinal cord and the nerves that branch out from it. Nerves run through each vertebra to particular segments of the body – a segment includes skin, bone, muscles, blood vessels and organs. The theory is that by manipulating a particular vertebra the health of the organ whose nerve supply runs through that vertebra can be influenced. For example, since the liver is supplied by nerves from the middle thoracic vertebrae (see page 64), manipulating these vertebrae can affect the way the liver works. Even minor derangements of the anatomy of the spinal cord, caused by bad posture or inflammation, can impair the working of a nerve and hence also the segment of the body it supplies.

The manipulation of the spinal vertebrae is done using rather short, sharp thrusts and movements intended to 'spring' a bone into place (such as a sudden downwards and upwards movement). The procedure demands great precision in terms of placing the adjusting hand, timing and the direction of the thrust itself. The movements are quite different from those used in osteopathy (see page 237).

Colour therapy

This adventurous theory takes off from fairly safe territory, the proposition that colour is a form of light and light a form of energy. It maintains that energy can be exploited to 'harmonize imbalances'. Restful colours are used to calm disturbed patients and violent colours for their stimulating effect.

The latest variation on this theme is colour 'breathing', where a patient imagines breathing a specific colour for therapeutic purposes.

Gerovital therapy

In 1956 Dr Ana Aslan, working in Rumania, reported the treatment of old and ageing people with a substance known as procaine hydrochloride or H_3, for which were claimed the following powers: to improve memory, concentration and perception, raise the levels of oestrogen circulating in the blood, make the skin plumper and stimulate hair growth, relieve angina, hypertension and the stiffness that accompanies Parkinson's disease, and help sufferers from arthritis and certain skin diseases. The conclusion Dr Aslan drew from her observations was that H_3 'reduces the biological age of the individual below its chronological age'.

Not surprisingly, this treatment (re-christened Gerovital H-3) became very popular and was widely used in Europe to attack the physical and mental symptoms of advancing age. When the first controlled research on Gerovital H-3 was made public six years later, the results scarcely supported the extravagant claims that had heralded its introduction.

The first study showed that the improvement in mood and activity that patients experienced on this treatment was only temporary. Most important of all, the death rate of Gerovital users was no different from the death rate among untreated patients of the same age nor from that of the geriatric hospital population as a whole. The obvious conclusion to be drawn was that Gerovital H-3 did not influence the most crucial biological characteristics of the ageing process.

A second study, carried out ten years later in the United States, produced equally disappointing findings – the only constant effect of the drug turned out to be to induce euphoria. This euphoric effect was later explained, however, by the discovery that H-3 inhibits the production of monoamine oxidase, high levels of which are normal in the elderly and the depressed. Later tests carried out in England could find no significant difference between patients on Gerovital H-3 and a control group receiving injections of sterile water or saline. The conclusion was drawn that there was no justification for using Gerovital H-3 in clinical practice as a rejuvenating agent.

Gravitonics

This theory, currently much in vogue on the West coast of America, originated in Hollywood. Patients are taught to exercise on a trapeze-like swing. A typical exercise might involve suspending oneself upside down while gripping the bar of the trapeze with the legs and feet. This is said to reduce tension in the lower back by removing the force of gravity and the weight of the body from the overworked back muscles.

One of the great advantages of this system is that one can use it at home – the swing is designed so that it can be fitted in an ordinary doorway.

Happiness cure

This theory has as its basis the truism that if you are happy you feel healthy. People who take the happiness cure try to think positively rather than negatively and to create happiness not just in themselves but in those around them. People are encouraged to do whatever they need to do to be happy and to express themselves in as many ways as possible. Teachers of this philosophy see themselves as helping people to find their true personalities and to express themselves in ways that foster self-esteem, self-confidence and the approval of the community in which they live. Another benefit claimed is that it frees its followers from frustration.

Herbalism

Some of the oldest methods of healing the sick were based on herbalism. Herbal lore was handed down largely through families, most of whom had their own family recipe book of favourite tonics and teas. The treatments matured through centuries of hit-or-miss practice until particular herbs could be definitely shown to have links with specific effects in particular diseases.

In ancient times a herb's effects and the individual's reaction to it could not be predicted with certainty. Most remedies were based on the theory that like cures like – hence yellow plants were used to cure jaundice and plants with heart-shaped leaves were thought to be good for the heart. Many plants take their name from their medical application: heartsease, liverwort, eyebright, spleenwort and bloodstone (the last is supposed to help stop bleeding).

Modern herbalism believes in correcting what is wrong with the body and strengthening its natural functions so that it may heal itself. Herbs – most of which should be fairly easy to get hold of over the counter – are classified according to the organs they may be used to treat. The list of disorders supposed to be amenable to herbal cures is impressive, ranging through anaemia, asthma, bladder trouble, 'female troubles', insomnia and so on.

Herbal remedies may well be worth a try. Most of them, even viewed sceptically, make up into an agreeable drink. And if you have faith in their power to cure, they may do just that. Bear in mind, however, the caveats on page 110.

Homeopathy

This theory of healing was known to Hippocrates and Paracelsus, but homeopathy as we know it now was founded in the eighteenth century by a German doctor named Samuel Hahnemann. Appalled at the medical practices of his time, which seemed to do more harm than good, Hahnemann sought a gentler, safer and more effective alternative.

According to Hahnemann, the human body has a great capacity to heal itself. The symptoms of a disease are simply a reflection of the body's struggle to overcome the forces threatening life. A doctor's work should be to discover and remove the cause of the trouble and then stimulate the vital self-healing force of nature. Hahnemann found his homeopathic remedies by himself taking doses of reputedly poisonous medicines and then noting the symptoms they produced. By treating patients suffering from similar symptoms with the substance that had provoked such symptoms in himself, he and his followers achieved encouraging results. Once having proved a substance to be effective, Hahnemann then went on to find the smallest effective dose, as the best possible way to avoid side-effects. Using a special method of dilution, he found that the greater the dilution, the greater the effect.

Homeopaths use medicinal substances of animal, vegetable and mineral origin: herbs and botanical medicines, drugs like morphine, cocaine and arsenic, substances like sand, charcoal, salt and pencil lead. However, the administration of medicines is only part of homeopathy. The emphasis is on treating the whole patient, not just the disease and for successful treatment, the homeopath must know about the patient's personality, past health, lifestyle and pattern of family health.

Homeopathy has many cures to its credit and is one branch of alternative medicine that lives quite happily alongside traditional practice.

Hydrotherapy

As its name suggests, this therapy relies on immersing the body, or part of it, in water. It aims to achieve both a surface effect – to increase blood flow to the skin, thereby eliminating 'toxins' from an area – and an internal effect – to draw blood to a specific area and then flush it out, thereby bringing nourishment and carrying away waste.

Most forms of hydrotherapy use hot and cold water alternately. The hot water is to make the blood vessels dilate, thus increasing the blood flow to the whole skin or that part of it that is immersed. This part of the treatment may last five, ten or 15 minutes, according to the severity of the condition and the patient's frailty. The second stage of the therapy involves douching, sluicing or showering in cold water. This causes the blood vessels to constrict down, reducing blood flow in the skin or the part of the body that is immersed, so driving blood back to the heart and the purifying organs such as the liver and kidneys.

This hot and cold water therapy should have two effects. First, it flushes blood through a diseased organ, nourishing it and, by carrying away waste material, encouraging healing. Second, it flushes blood through the skin to eliminate waste, and back through the liver and kidneys to cleanse the blood still further. Several

variations on this basic idea are listed below. No form of water therapy should be undertaken by eczema sufferers.

● Sauna

The early form of sauna was a succession of baths where one started off with immersion in warm water, followed by a cold bath or shower, then went back to the warm bath, and so on. The Finns, who developed modern saunas, substituted intense dry heat (from a stove) for the warm bath and they recommend staying in the heat for between eight and ten minutes, until the body is sweating profusely. After taking a cold shower, one returns to the sauna for a second, shorter period, to the point at which sweating begins again. A second cold shower is followed by a brisk rubdown with a towel, and then a rest.

The treatment improves circulation and is claimed to tone up the muscles, cleanse the skin and produce a feeling of well-being.

● Scotch douche

Hot and cold water are sprayed alternately up and down the spine. This is supposed to stimulate the spinal nerves by sluicing blood in and out of the spinal area. At the end of the therapy the spine tingles. This treatment is thought to help sufferers from migraine and various aches and pains in the back.

● Sitz bath

One sits rather than lies in a Sitz bath, the idea for which came from Germany. In fact two baths are used, one containing hot water and one cold.

The patient sits first in the hot bath for five to ten minutes with the feet immersed in cold water. This constricts the blood vessels in the feet and forces blood to the area where the skin is warm – the part in the hot bath. The patient then transfers to the cold Sitz bath and immerses the feet in hot water – this forces blood away from the pelvis and down into the legs. The combined effect of both stages is to flush blood into the pelvic area to nourish it and then out again to carry off waste material. Sitz baths are recommended for illnesses affecting the lower half of the body.

● Spanish mantle

The patient is first wrapped in a cold, wet sheet and then surrounded by hot water bottles and left to sweat for up to three hours. It is claimed that when the sheet is removed, the toxins eliminated through the skin may have turned the sheet yellow, grey or even black. The treatment's aim is to draw out impurities, or toxins, through the skin.

● Steam cabinet

This is another form of panthermal treatment, which works very much like the traditional Turkish bath, except that the head is left outside the steamy atmosphere, making the whole business rather more agreeable. Because the heat is wet rather than dry, it produces sweating faster and so is alleged to clear the skin more efficiently of waste materials. Again, because the sweat does not have the chance to evaporate off the skin, the body feels hotter than in a sauna and the process is fairly debilitating.

After about 15 minutes in the steam cabinet, the bather takes a cold shower to restore the skin temperature to normal. Like a sauna, the treatment should be followed by a rest.

Hypnosis

A classical description of the hypnotic state is 'a temporary condition of altered attention, the most striking feature of which is increased suggestibility'. Hypnosis has something in common with sleep, but the body tone is characteristic of waking rather than sleeping and the subject's mind is concentrated. In other words, hypnosis is a state in which people retain most of their faculties but – because they are deprived of full consciousness – may accept and act on suggestions made by the hypnotist.

Holistic practitioners hold that hypnosis should be used only as an adjunct to whole body therapy. They would disapprove of its use for symptomatic cures – for example, to help someone give up smoking, conquer drug addiction or cure obsessive eating. Their view that this would be treating the condition superficially and not reaching the root cause is absolutely right. Used properly, however, hypnosis is a method of disciplining mind and body that can help people to control anxiety and cope better with stress.

The power of suggestion during a hypnotic trance shows in the following experiment. The person under hypnosis is told that a burning match is about to be placed on one hand. When the hand is then touched with a pencil, the subject draws back quickly and the hand becomes red and swollen. When the subject comes round, the hand still feels as if it had been burned.

If patients could learn to exert this kind of power over their own ailments, hypnosis could be a very promising aid to medical treatment.

Inhalation therapy

This is supposed to help people with chest complaints – bronchitis, emphysema or asthma, for example. Steam containing various natural ingredients is directed at the patient's face. The patient sits a few feet away from the source of the steam and breathes in the warm, moist air. Rosemary may be added to the water to produce an energizing effect, camomile to tranquillize. Olbas, camphor, menthol or eucalyptus may also be added to soothe inflammation and clear bronchial passages. Steam that has been subject to ultra-violet radiation (rather misleadingly called 'dry steam') is said to be especially useful for relaxing the constricted bronchii in asthma and so making breathing easier.

A holistic therapist would never prescribe inhalation therapy on its own – it would be combined with relaxation and breathing exercises. Biofeedback systems (see page 233) added to inhalation therapy help patients to improve their breathing considerably.

Jacusi
See **Massage**

Massage
The various types of massage described here are said to improve circulation, disperse tension and promote healing of the body or particular parts of it. For Swedish massage and the use of massage in health spas see pages 239–240.

● Jacusi

Taken in a special bath, this is a deep, forceful type of massage. The body is bombarded with jets of water from all directions. Because the body can move and float freely in the bath while this is going on, it is a safe and very relaxing form of massage, especially recommended for people with arthritis, muscular and rheumatic complaints. It is not, however, suitable for eczema sufferers.

● Neuromuscular

This is a fingertip massage, adapted from an Indian technique in the 1930s by Stanley Lief, an osteopath who wanted to find a way of relaxing patients' muscles before osteopathic manipulation (see page 237 for details of osteopathic techniques).

During this massage, specific motor points of muscles are massaged deeply with the fingertips. The effect seems to be to damp down the output to the sensory nerves in the area, thus breaking the vicious circle of pain/tense muscle/muscle spasm/ pain/muscle over-tenseness. Once muscular tension has been relieved by this technique, the muscle should not spring back into its previous tense position and osteopathic manipulation can be carried out more effectively.

● Shiatzu

This type of massage is similar in many respects to neuromuscular massage, but the pressure is applied to points on energy meridians (see **Acupuncture**, page 232) rather than to muscles.

The massage – performed with the thumb, force-fully and occasionally even painfully – is intended to restore interrupted energy flow along the meridians by stimulating specific points. Pressure is applied very precisely, in the hope of stimulating some nerves and damping down others, to the benefit of the distant organ that is supplied by the stimulated nerve.

This technique is claimed to improve overall health and also to help specific organs by bringing about the release of blocked energy.

Megavitamin therapy
The principle underlying this treatment is that illnesses may be prevented or cured by massive intake of certain vitamins – hence it clashes with homeopathic practice from the outset. Different vitamins are prescribed for various conditions, for example, vitamin C for infections and vitamin E for cardiovascular disorders. Many eminent men have carried out research in this

field, including Dr Linus Pauling, and extensive experiments have shown that vitamins given in about 100 times the usual recommended dose can have an effect, although not necessarily a specific one, as the patients might not previously have been vitamin deficient.

Naturopathy

Most systems of alternative medicine are based on naturopathy. Its principles – some of which have been outlined earlier – are worth summarizing again.

- The patient is treated, not the disease.
- The whole patient is treated, not merely a part.
- The factors causing the disease must be removed.
- Disease is a disturbance of the life force, demonstrated by tension, rigidity or congestion somewhere in the body – the muscles, for example.
- The patient's own life force is the true healer – it is the healing power of nature itself that cures.
- The body has to go through a healing crisis, in which the life force cleanses the body by eliminating accumulated 'toxins'. The potent drugs of orthodox medicine, while superficially curing the disease, drive it deeper within the body and leave behind a chronic condition for the future.

Naturopaths consider nutrition to be the sheet anchor of health and advocate fasts and other dietary constraints. Water should be pure and food organically grown, unprocessed and (as much as possible) uncooked. Animal protein, while not altogether ruled out, should not make up more than 25 per cent of the diet and should be taken in its purest form (such as simply cooked meat or fish).

Apart from adhering to this kind of diet, naturopaths believe that health depends on the patient adopting the right attitude of mind. Relaxation exercises, yoga, meditation and even psychotherapy may be used to help achieve this. Other ingredients in the naturopathic recipe for good health are proper breathing and sufficient exercise to keep the muscles toned up and the body supple.

Osteopathy

Manipulation was one of the earliest forms of medical practice: its benefits are listed in the *Kung Fu*, written 5,000 years ago. Osteopathy as it is practised today was founded by an American doctor, Andrew Still, in 1874 after the death of three daughters from spinal meningitis. Dr Still's original thesis remains the basis of osteopathic practice: the body has the ability to regulate and heal itself provided that its structure is sound and that blood and nerve impulses can move freely.

Harmful structural changes to the body may arise as a consequence of poor posture, trauma, a sudden movement or sleeping on too soft a bed. Osteopathic manipulation tries to rectify these changes by manipulating the vertebrae and it is claimed that by allowing the nervous system to resume its healthy functioning, far-reaching improvements to health may be achieved. Osteopaths also believe that relief of muscle spasm cures illnesses stemming from stress and strain on these tissues. Such illnesses are said to be caused by venous congestion and impaired nutrition.

The two basic techniques of osteopathy are massage of muscles in spasm and manipulative correction of disaligned bones in the spine. The technique is different from that used in chiropractic and usually involves gentle leverage of one part of the body against another – for example, the chin against the neck to adjust the position of a vertebra at the base of the skull. A new cranial technique aims to make minute adjustments to the bones of the skull by manipulating the spine, sacrum and pelvis. This is claimed to help not only muscle, bone and joint illnesses but also disorders of organs such as the liver, heart and kidneys, by relieving pressure on the nerves that supply these organs.

Osteopathy can claim many well-documented cures and is gaining acceptance by the medical profession.

Radionics and radiesthesia

The basis of these closely allied systems is the belief that illness is due to a disorder of energy flow – in this respect they relate closely to acupuncture and homeopathy.

Both systems employ specific diagnostic tools, the best known of which is the pendulum swung by the therapist. From its movements he deduces information about the state of the patient's health. This system is supposedly almost mathematically precise in assessing the function of organs and the severity of a disease.

Treatment can be prescribed from many different branches of alternative medicine: a specific homeopathic remedy, an acupuncture point for treatment, a vitamin supplement or the exact location of an osteopathic lesion for manipulation.

Reflexology

According to this theory the sole of the foot is like a map of the body, with nerve endings and 'reflexes' that correspond to different organs. These were charted and used for healing hundreds of years ago in China and Tibet.

Disorders are said to show up on the foot as tiny crystalline deposits in the area of skin corresponding to the organ. By breaking down these deposits, reflexology restores the circulation of blood and vital energy to the organ, promoting healing. A special 'reflex roller' can be used in various different ways to assist the massage process.

Sauna
See **Hydrotherapy**

Shiatzu
See **Massage**

Health Clinics

Most health clinics or spas adhere to one or more of the forms of alternative medicine – naturopathy, osteopathy, homeopathy and so forth (see pages 232–237). Many spas were first founded by leading practitioners in one of these fields. They vary a great deal, however, in the seriousness with which they approach health and apply their regimes, so there is quite a wide range for the would-be slimmer, health seeker or sick person to choose from.

In some health spas, all the staff right down to the maids take the treatment very seriously. They pay assiduous attention to the exact details of diet and do everything possible to make the patient feel better. Such clinics run their timetables and routines along much the same lines as a hospital, but their impact tends to be very different. Because of the friendly, informal atmosphere, the luxurious surroundings and the freedom in the last resort to take it or leave it, the routine is not in any way irksome but is welcome to most patients. Many health spas are set deep in the country, in spacious elegant buildings and beautiful grounds. A stay in one of these places can add up to a spell in the hospital of your dreams.

At the other end of the spectrum are clinics that place the accent on beauty rather than health. Patients tend to treat their stay here like a luxurious holiday. They pay a little attention to diet, a little attention to exercise and a great deal of attention to pampering themselves with beauty routines. In the evening they can go out to enjoy a drink or dinner with friends. It is essentially up to you to choose how industrious and abstemious or how self-indulgent and lazy you want to be.

One aspect of life in a health clinic that is sometimes overlooked is its quietness. Patients can enjoy prolonged solitude if this is what they want. Rest is considered an important part of the treatment and the medical staff usually do not mind anyone missing out a treatment session if the reason is to catch up on sleep. The emphasis on peace and quiet is an important factor to bear in mind when weighing up the claims clinics make for their treatment. It may be that simply by making an effort to spend more time resting in quiet surroundings you can give your health all the boost it needs without incurring the expense of going to a health spa.

A stay in a health clinic can last as long as the money to pay for it does, but many clinics have a minimum stay of four or even seven days. This is particularly true of the more serious places, because the medical staff there would say that four days is the shortest period that allows a patient to rest and enjoy the effects of a proper diet and appropriate treatments for several consecutive days. Other health spas take a less strict view of their role and some advertise 'bargain break' stays of three or even two days. These stays may be billed as 'slimming sessions' or just as a relaxing weekend. An astonishing variety of different treatments may be crammed into this short stay: body massage, Slendertone, saunas, yoga, facial massage and jogging, to mention just a few. It would be unreasonable to expect an individually tailored programme in a place that operates on this basis and short-stay clinics concentrate heavily on beauty rather than health care.

On arrival

On the first day at a serious health clinic, usually in the afternoon, it is customary to have a consultation with one of the medical staff. This is a rather leisurely version of an orthodox medical interview. The consultant asks about the reasons for coming to the clinic and past medical history, including details of any current medical complaints, previous illnesses and the treatment received for these in the past. Weight and blood pressure are generally measured, although a full medical is rare. At an osteopathic clinic the examination includes a general osteopathic assessment and any abnormal findings are noted. When these preliminaries are complete, the consultant goes on to discuss at some length what the patient hopes to gain from the stay and how this can be achieved. Details of diet, exercise and particular treatments are explained and the patient's questions answered. At the best clinics it should be clear from the outset that the aim is to examine and treat all aspects of the patient's health rather than just a few symptoms – this is what is known as the holistic approach.

Diet

Most naturopaths believe that sound nutrition is a key factor in maintaining health, just as faulty nutrition is an important cause of disease. For this reason diet is stressed as an integral part of any health cure.

As a general rule patients at a health clinic begin by spending two or three days fasting or semi-fasting. On a fast you have only hot water and lemon juice three or four times a day, plus as much water as you want. On a semi-fast fruit is allowed as well – an apple and a peach, or a pear and grapes, or a plum and a slice of melon – and a glass of hot water three or four times a day. The theory behind this sort of diet is that abstaining from food allows the body to divert to other uses the energy it normally spends on digesting and assimilating food and eliminating waste. One effect of fasting is supposed to be the elimination of 'toxins' from the body. These toxic substances are extremely difficult to give a scientific label to but they feature prominently in naturopathic literature. Ridding the body of them is considered to be the first step towards restoring health. Most people experience some unpleasant symptoms during a fast, including headaches, slight sickness and possibly dizziness too. These symptoms can be discussed with the medical consultant if they cause uneasiness, but they are quite normal effects of going without food.

How long you spend fasting or semi-fasting is really up to you. Most of us find two or three days on this kind of regime enough, but convinced naturopaths may continue on water and lemon juice for up to three weeks. This does no harm – in fact general health and specific illnesses often improve while the fasting goes on.

After the fasting phase is over, a gentle diet of fresh, virtually uncooked food is introduced. Typical menus for the first three days after the fast are shown below.

Day 1

Breakfast	Lightly stewed fruit, yogurt, bran and honey. Hot water and lemon.
Lunch	Vegetable soup (potassium broth, yeast extract and tomato juice), fresh fruit. Hot water and lemon.
Tea	Tea with skimmed milk or lemon.
Supper	Fresh fruit, yogurt. Wheatgerm and honey. Hot water and lemon.

Day 2

Breakfast	As Day 1.
Lunch	Salad of mixed vegetables. Fresh fruit, stewed fruit or yogurt. Wheatgerm and honey.
Tea	As Day 1.
Supper	Vegetable soup. Fresh fruit or yogurt. Wheatgerm and honey.

Day 3

Breakfast	As Day 1.
Lunch	As Day 1, plus a baked potato, crispbread and butter.
Tea	As Day 1.
Supper	A portion of lean meat, chicken or fish. Lightly cooked vegetables and a baked potato. Stewed or fresh fruit or yogurt.

Of course, this fairly restrictive diet is not compulsory and patients can depart from it if they wish, provided they choose food that is available at the health spa. One can ask to have tea and toast for breakfast and one can have the kind of food listed on Day 3 right from the beginning. However, refined or processed foods are not likely to be served at all and the only cooked or baked foods on offer are those made on the premises. Most spas grow their own vegetables according to organic gardening methods, that is, with no chemical fertilizers.

Massage

Massage plays an essential part in most treatment programmes. It is advocated for releasing tensions, stimulating circulation and for assisting in the elimination of toxins (discussed above) through the skin. One thing massage does not do is help you lose weight: it is rather like having your muscles exercised for you and uses up none of your energy. The masseur or masseuse works extremely hard, but the person having the massage loses no more fat than she would lying in bed.

Many claims are made about the virtues of massage or a particular type of massage technique. Some claims are false, others are plausible and some indisputable. Massage helps break down fat (false). Massage releases emotional tension when it breaks down muscular tension (plausible). Massage stimulates circulation locally and generally and by improving nourishment of the tissues speeds up the healing process (true). It may or may not be an agreeable process, depending on the type of massage, the expertise of the masseur and the response of the individual body. Until you get used to it, it may be uncomfortable for the first day or two of the treatment.

During a massage session the parts of the body are treated in a specific order. The direction of massage is always towards the heart, thereby helping the return of blood through the veins to the heart. First the patient lies on her back and the masseur massages the front of one leg, the ankle and the sole of the foot and then does the same with the other leg. The abdomen is massaged next if this is indicated (as in cases of hepatitis or colonic complaints) and then each arm, wrist, hand and finger. When this has been done, the patient rolls over on to her front and the masseur massages the backs of the legs, the back, the shoulders and the neck. These movements are carried out with energy and some force in Swedish massage. There are long, heavy stroking movements over the large muscle masses such as the calves, thighs and back, slapping movements, used mainly on the back, and beating movements with the side of the hand, going, for example, from the bottom of the back up to the top and then back down again. Sometimes the masseur may give a slap extra force by shaping her hand into a cup before hitting the skin, so that extra air is trapped inside it. The whole process is far from gentle, but may be surprisingly relaxing once you have become accustomed to it.

Swedish massage is far from the only technique likely to be found in a health spa. Shiatzu, jacusi and neuromuscular massage are the most popular variations (for more information on all these techniques, turn to page 236).

Heat
Heat features in the treatment regimes of most health spas. In some cases the heat is panthermal (applied to the whole body), in others it is specific to a particular area.
- Moor, oatmeal, peat or seaweed bath
The ingredients of these four baths (a moor bath, as the name suggests, contains a mixture of moorland ingredients such as heather and bracken) promote relaxation when the body is tired and tense but not sufficiently strong to respond to the greater heat of the hot blanket, steam bath or sauna (see below). For the use of baths in alternative medicine see Balneotherapy, page 233.
- Poultices
These are used primarily in cases of arthritis, sprains, strains or muscle injury and they may be applied to a specific joint or to a small area of the body. The purpose of using poultices is to heat up the area treated and to keep it hot for as long as possible. This improves circulation to that part of the body and hence its nourishment. The effect is to alleviate discomfort, if not remove pain. The good effects of a single poulticing may wear off after a few hours, but applying poultices repeatedly on successive days can speed up the healing process.
- Sauna, steam cabinet, hot blanket
These procedures are used to increase body temperature so as to induce the body to get rid of 'toxins' through the skin by stimulating the sweat and sebaceous glands. Because they improve circulation, they may also relieve fatigue. Hot blanket treatment consists simply of lying wrapped in a specially designed electric blanket; see pages 235–236 for further details of sauna and steam cabinet.
- Sitz bath
This is a special treatment to tone up the muscles and organs in the abdominal and pelvic cavities. It improves circulation to these parts of the body and is supposed to strengthen the supporting tissues. For more details see page 235.

Physiotherapy
The facilities available in some modern clinics are as good as those in a hospital physiotherapy department. The kind of treatment selected will depend on the individual patient's complaint.
- Exercise
As well as exercises and sporting activities to help tone up patients who are basically healthy but out of condition, there may also be specially designed programmes to strengthen damaged muscles, weakened joints or make breathing more efficient. People whose movements are limited (for example, by arthritis) may have exercises to be carried out in warm water or a heated pool, to improve the mobility of the body. Exercises may be performed on machines (see pages 166–167).

● Heat

Heat therapy is used primarily to treat small joints, such as those in the hands and feet, after an injury or damage by arthritis. Wax baths, where the hands are immersed and then exercised in melted wax, can be beneficial. The hands may be wrapped in warm wax after the exercises to prolong the benefits of this heat treatment.

● Light

Ultra-violet radiation is used in various forms. One method is to use a short burst (no more than a minute) of narrow spectrum ultra-violet radiation to kill off bacteria on the surface of the skin. Although ultra-violet therapy may be used to imitate the effect of sunshine and to promote a suntan, this treatment always damages the collagen within the skin (see pages 18–19).

The infra-red part of the light spectrum is warm and produces radiant heat that can be used to treat the deeper layers of injured muscles and joints and so promote healing.

● Inhalation exercises

Physiotherapists take patients with chest complaints through a daily exercise programme to improve their breathing. Steam inhalations, possibly combined with aromatic oils (see Inhalation therapy, page 236), can be used to soothe and open up the air passages.

● Electrical stimulation

The standard methods of using electricity to treat inflamed or swollen muscles and joints include:
Microwave – This makes use of the same basic principles as a microwave oven and works in exactly the same way. It promotes healing by heating the affected part from within as a result of stimulation of the cells by microwave energy.
Slendertone – This is a method of making the muscles contract and relax alternately without taking exercise. It is used to tone up flaccid muscles and is claimed to help break down deposits of fat. There is no evidence that it actually does the latter. It does not help anyone to lose weight, since it uses up no energy. During a treatment session the patient lies on a couch and pads are strapped singly or in groups over areas where fat has accumulated, such as the upper thighs or abdomen. When the current is switched on a tingling sensation may be felt under the pads and the muscles beneath them alternately contract and relax due to the electrical stimulation. A session usually lasts less than half an hour.

● Ultrasound

This technique uses sound waves of very short wavelength. These penetrate to the deep layers of muscles and joints and create a vibration, which in turn creates heat. This helps some obstinate conditions, notably frozen shoulder, tennis elbow and strains and sprains.

Enemas and colonic irrigation

These still feature in some health clinic programmes because fasting is supposed to stimulate the gastro-intestinal tract to eliminate toxins that have to be washed out by the introduction of warm water through the rectum (an enema). The old theory of auto-intoxication, long disproved, looms behind these practices. Contrary to what it states, faeces not immediately eliminated from the body do no harm.

Relaxation and yoga

Most clinics hold optional daily classes in relaxation and yoga, to promote loss of tension and stress and improve the suppleness of the body (see pages 162–165 for yoga postures to try and pages 168–171 for relaxation techniques).

A typical day at a health clinic

7.00 A.M.	Breakfast brought to your room
7.30–8.00	Consultant or sister visits your room to check on progress, answer your queries and adjust treatments
8.15–11.15	Treatments:
	Massage
	Steam cabinet
	Sitz bath
	Cold shower
	Rest
11.30	Meeting with your consultant for review or osteopathic treatment
12.15 P.M.	Lunch
1.30	Treatment with ultrasonics in physiotherapy department
3.00	Relaxation exercises
4.00	Tea
4.30	Yoga classes
6.15	Supper
7.30	Lecture by outside speaker

Beauty Clinics

Few young women who have clear complexions and unlined faces are found among beauty clinic clients. In general beauty clinics serve older women who are beginning to show the signs of age: wrinkles, sagging skin, puffy eyes, crow's-feet. Part of the motivation to go to a beauty clinic stems from the desire to slow down the ageing process or to control its effects. Unfortunately there is no treatment on offer in any beauty clinic anywhere that will achieve either of these two aims.

No substance or process yet known to science can restore permanently the proteins, fats and moisture that provide the supple support for the skin, or do anything to repair the fractures that develop in the collagen within the dermis as the body grows older.

Cosmetic creams certainly cannot hold lines or wrinkles at bay, no matter what exotic ingredients they lay claim to. A cream that contains collagen can do nothing more for the skin than any simple moisturizer; there is no route by which the substances it contains can penetrate deeply enough to have any impact on the natural collagen and protein within the skin.

Another claim frequently made is that a cream containing the hormones oestrogen and pro-gestogen 'rejuvenates' the skin, but these creams have never been proved effective. It is worth noting here that hormones are powerful drugs and that any cream with a sufficiently high hormone content to produce a change in the skin when applied externally would never be available for sale over the counter. No doctor, moreover, would consider prescribing hormones on other than clear medical grounds – certainly not for cosmetic reasons. The 'hormone' creams used in skin beauty treatments contain only a tiny amount of oestrogen or progestogen, and only a tiny fraction of this amount ever penetrates even the outer layers of the skin. There is no evidence that the hormones that do enter the outer layers of skin improve it in any way.

There is equally little point in using a cream that contains vitamins: none of the vitamins it incorporates can be absorbed by the skin to the extent that they have any lasting effect. This applies to the much-publicized vitamin E creams no less than to others. There is no medical evidence to support the claim that this type of cream smoothes out wrinkles or improves the skin's texture. Finally, there is no evidence that extracts from vegetables, fruits or herbs, placental extracts or royal jelly from queen bees – to mention just a few of the bizarre possibilities – have any beneficial effects at all upon the skin.

The very most that can be said in favour of creams is that they help the skin to retain water, making its surface look fresh and feel less dry. This effect wears off within hours, so the cream has to be applied frequently. They do not bring about any permanent or even long-lasting change.

Another of the fundamental laws preached by beauty clinics is that the skin must be kept clean. Cleanliness tends to be not merely advocated but obsessively pursued. No routine is performed in a beauty clinic until the skin has been viciously cleansed. From a dermatological point of view there is neither physiological evidence nor logic to support this fanaticism. As pointed out on page 20, skin does not need to be clean to be healthy. Of all the reasons put forward by beauticians and cosmetologists in favour of cleansing, only social ones have any force. No others are valid.

Certain types of vigorous cleansing, such as brushing (see page 245), can actually harm the skin. This has been demonstrated by an experiment on surgeons who were 'scrubbing up' before performing surgery. The surgeons were checked periodically during scrubbing up to find out when their skin became surgically clean – that is, at what point the surface bacteria had been removed by the action of brushing and rubbing with soap. It transpired that the optimum time for scrubbing up was 45 seconds; at this point the bacterial count on the skin surface was lowest. If the scrubbing went on for longer than this, the bacterial count began to climb again. The reason for this somewhat surprising discovery is that continued scrubbing liberates bacteria from the deeper layers of the skin, where they live peacefully, doing no harm at all, and brings them up to the surface, where they may be harmful. Hence long scrubbing up routines make the skin surface dirtier rather than cleaner. In the light of this, the brushing routines of up to 15 minutes advocated for facial cleansing do not even have the rationale that they are cleaning the face.

Many techniques used in beauty clinics rely on electrical therapy in one form or another – perhaps the need to maintain client interest explains the number of gadgets employed. One favourite electrical treatment is iontophoresis (see page 245), a technique whereby substances are electrically driven into the skin, the favourite one being water to moisturize it. This practice too has no sound physiological basis. The skin loses water continually into the air that surrounds us. The drier the air, the more and the faster water is lost from the skin. The only way to slow down this inevitable evaporation of water for any length of time is by surrounding the skin with air that contains more water than the skin, which is hardly practicable for the majority of us. Hence the effects of iontophoresis can last no more than a couple of hours.

Electrical stimulation of body muscles – another technique that is very popular in beauty clinics – produces contractions of muscle groups that are sometimes alleged to help people lose weight. This claim is false: an exercise that burns up no calories will never help you slim. Electrical stimulation may also be used to tone up the muscles of the face, on the grounds that this tightens the skin and gives a more youthful appearance. This claim is transparently false: what could be better exercise for the facial muscles than talking, chewing and smiling? Why should a few minutes of electrical stimulation do more than the actions that are part of our everyday lives? The answer is that they do not.

A dermatologist is forced to conclude that most treatments offered by beauty clinics and advocated by cosmetologists and beauty therapists have at best a transient effect. They can in no way slow down the rate at which a person's skin naturally ages.

It is important to remember here that any treatment capable of altering the skin's appearance semi-permanently, that is, for up to a year, should be delivered only by a medically qualified person such as a dermatologist or a plastic surgeon. The reason for stating this so categorically is that treatments that have radical effects have side-effects too and can damage the skin if used improperly. No person without medical qualifications has sufficient knowledge to make the fine judgement about when and how much of this treatment can be safely given without entering the danger zone. The fact that treatments given by non-medically qualified personnel do not have sufficient effect on the skin to bring about a substantial change is simply the other side of the same coin.

One further aspect of beauty treatment and cosmetology that raises suspicions in a scientist's mind is the type of language used to describe the effects of treatment. In a standard textbook on beauty therapy, the action of a cucumber face pack is set down as 'to stimulate the skin, increase cellular function and refine skin texture'. As a trained dermatologist, I have no idea what any of these claims means. No scientist knows in what way the skin can be stimulated, which of the millions of cells in the skin are to have their function increased, or how skin texture can be refined. The phrases are meaningless.

While occasionally it may be justified in orthodox medical practice to use a substance for its placebo effect – indeed doctors agree that there is a recognized place in medicine for placebos – placebo beauty techniques are quite another matter. Beauty clinics charge high prices, claim quite specific effects for each and every treatment they offer and often wrap their claims up in quasi-scientific language. Hence it comes as quite a shock to find a sentence in the same standard text on beauty therapy referred to above advocating the use of electrical brush cleansing as an alternative to manual methods simply to vary the facial routine and maintain client interest. I hope this will make people think twice before making their next trip to a beauty salon and having the treatments described below.

Facial massage

According to beauticians, the main purpose of facial massage is to 'increase the skin's capacity to function more efficiently'. Facial massage certainly stimulates blood circulation within the skin and this is supposed to increase natural cellular regeneration and help to keep the skin's oil and fluid content well balanced. However, a normal, healthy skin does all this efficiently on its own without the aid of facial massage. By all means use this technique if you find it soothing and relaxing, as many people do. See the step-by-step guide on pages 176–177 for instructions on how to carry out a facial massage yourself. The belief that the procedure will improve the skin as well as make you feel more relaxed, however, is unjustified.

Sometimes a variation on the standard massage called 'continental facial treatment' is recommended for ageing skin. This procedure comprises cleansing, vacuum massage (see page 245), manual massage of the face, neck and shoulders, a non-setting facial mask, skin toning treatment and make-up. A Viennese facial treatment – involving cleansing, massage with high-frequency current (see below), a non-setting facial mask, skin toning and make-up – is another variation that may be recommended. Although any of these procedures may be agreeable to experience and give one a pampered feeling, none of them has any sound physiological rationale.

Face masks

The face mask is a well-tried weapon in the beauty-therapist's arsenal. It is claimed to perform many tasks: to stimulate, to refine, to cleanse by removing dead skin, to soothe and nourish the skin, to unblock the pores and to control blackheads.

Whatever exotic ingredients the mask contains (such as wheatgerm, honey, egg yolk, peach, avocado or glycerine) it achieves very much the same modest effect: to increase blood flow to the skin and to cleanse its surface. This in no way enlivens ageing skin or restores the collagen that gives it its elasticity. Pores cannot permanently shrink and the feeling of tightness that follows the removal of a face mask wears off quickly.

Time spent wearing a facial mask may add up to a pleasant, relaxing interval, but it has no other special justification. If you enjoy the ritual of facial masks, it would make sense to give yourself one occasionally (following the guide on page 25 for instructions) rather than go to the expense of having essentially the same process carried out at a beauty clinic.

Electrical treatments

- Audiosonic vibration

This sort of apparatus comes with a sponge head, which is used to give gentle face and neck massage, plus a flat disc head, which has a more intense action and is generally used on muscles or joints. Audiosonic vibrators are designed to increase the circulation of blood in the locality being treated. Sometimes the additional claim is made that electrical treatment, used as an adjunct to manual methods, can 'increase cellular activity' and so delay or arrest the development of wrinkles, crepey skin and the other symptoms of advancing age. There is absolutely no scientific evidence to support this claim.

- Diathermy

This involves coagulating tissues by heating them, usually done by applying a fine wire or metal point, which becomes red hot when an electrical current is passed through it. The technique is used by dermatologists, as described on page 215.

Beauty clinics make use of diathermy to treat unwanted facial hair by killing the hair root (see page 47). In the hands of an expert this is safe, fairly painless, effective and should leave no scars. Diathermy is sometimes used to coagulate broken veins on the cheeks and face. Because it is essential that the person carrying out this delicate task should have full medical training, it makes sense to consult a dermatologist rather than go to a beauty clinic for this type of treatment. A dermatologist can assess the overall condition of the skin and decide whether or not it would be safe to treat the broken veins by coagulation (electrical or chemical). He will refer patients on to a suitable practitioner if he cannot carry out the treatment personally. No beauty therapist without medical training is in such a strong position to give sound advice.

- High frequency treatment

During this treatment, a direct high frequency alternating current is applied to the skin to dry, 'refine' and heal it and to produce a germicidal layer of ozone on the skin surface.

High frequency electrical treatment of the skin generates a transient feeling of warmth and may also have a relaxing effect. The claim that it has a germicidal effect too by limiting sebum secretion runs counter to a basic physiological truth, namely that sebum itself is the skin's own natural antiseptic (see page 14).

If this form of treatment is used incorrectly on the skin, it can leave permanent scars.

- Vibrator treatment

A facial vibrator can be used to produce a series of mechanical vibrations that simulate the effects of massage with the hands. This treatment claims exactly the same benefits as manual massage, namely those of stimulating circulation and having a general relaxing effect. These claims may be true (see also pages 172, 239–240) but massage has no particular virtues so far as skin care is concerned.

Brush cleansing and massage

The aim of brush cleansing is to improve skin texture by desquammation (peeling off the dead cutaneous cells from the rough skin surface). By replacing the brush cleansing head with a pumice block a more abrasive effect can be achieved. As pointed out on page 242, carrying out this type of vigorous cleansing routine for longer than 45 seconds leaves the surface of the skin with more bacteria on it than a milder treatment does.

Pressure spray toning (vaporizers)

These can be used to direct a fine spray of water under pressure on to the face or to help remove a facial mask. It is claimed that the water the vaporizer produces forms a fine, penetrating film that is readily absorbed into the skin. While it is true that water can be made to enter the skin, it is lost very quickly into the surrounding air, unless this is extremely humid. Hence any good that vaporizing does literally evaporates within a few hours. It cannot permanently hydrate the skin.

Facial vacuum treatment

This may be used to reinforce the cleansing or massaging technique after initial cleansing has been done manually or by steaming. As well as helping remove blackheads and oily secretions, vacuum cleansing is supposed to improve the drainage of lymph and the nutritional state of the tissues. The treatment lasts from three to five minutes for cleansing and from ten to 12 minutes for massage and drainage of the lymph vessels.

All the lymph vessels in the face, head and neck drain downwards quite efficiently under the influence of gravity alone and any improvement in lymph drainage brought about by applying a vacuum cup will be infinitesimal.

Ozone therapy

Under this heading falls a group of treatments that are said to dry, heal and stimulate seborrhoeic skin and areas of acne by applying ozone, which is chemically related to pure oxygen but with one more oxygen atom in the molecule. Beauticians claim that ozone is beneficial to a 'disturbed and blemished' skin and that ozone steaming is a useful adjunct to direct high frequency electrical treatment (see page 244) and ultra-violet radiation (see page 241).

Many years ago there used to be speculation that ozone might turn out to have medicinal properties, but these have never been clearly defined, let alone proved.

Galvanic skin treatments

- Iontophoresis

This is a process that uses a galvanic current to introduce water-soluble chemicals into the upper layers of the skin. It works as follows. When an electrical current is passed through a solution, particles become positively or negatively charged. Positive ions are attracted to the cathode and negative ones repelled from the anode, so when the anode is used positive ions are driven into the skin through a pad and the reverse happens if the cathode is used.

It is said that the acidic substances that form around the anode have an astringent effect on the skin, whereas those at the cathode open up the pores. Applying a galvanic current is supposed to make the cells of the skin expand and increase their blood supply. There are various substances available in ampoule form that beauticians use for three to 12 minutes to moisturize or 'normalize' the skin.

Any substance that enters the skin by iontophoresis can penetrate only the outermost layers. Positively or negatively charged particles and water are rapidly lost once the electrical current is removed. The claim that frequent, regular and prolonged courses of this treatment have a lasting effect upon the skin are quite without foundation.

- Disencrustation

This is not a medical word but in beauty terms it means removing blockages in the skin, removing surface oiliness and regulating secretions. Disencrustation fluid is contained in ampoules for use with the galvanic electrical apparatus, although it is claimed (by beauticians) that simple saline solution (salt in water) is just as effective. See the preceding entry on iontophoresis for why this kind of treatment has no lasting effect.

Skin peeling

Beauty clinics carry out skin peeling by biological (fruit and vegetable extracts), chemical (various aids) and abrasive (abrasive brushes or stone pads) methods. The aim of skin peeling is to improve the quality of the complexion by removing dead cells from its surface and to increase the rate at which the skin naturally loses dead cells (desquammation). After skin peeling the skin is supposed to look fresh and clean. Skin peeling methods are used not only for general cleansing purposes but also for problem skins with blocked pores and oiliness, for 'sallow complexions' and for post-acne scarring.

One of the aspects of a beautician's credo that a doctor takes greatest issue with on purely physiological grounds is the belief that removing the surface layer of dead cells (keratin) from the skin is necessarily a good thing. It is not. In the first place keratin is one of the skin's natural barriers (see page 12). Second, the skin has a perfectly good mechanism of its own for getting rid of dead cells; it is desquammating all the time. We naturally lose millions of dead cells from the skin's surface every day and there is no reason why we should need to lose them any faster. Third, the rate at which the skin produces new cells is controlled from within the body and there is nothing we can do with beauty treatments to increase it. Indeed we would not want to do so. When the production of cells in the basal layer (see page 12) is increased, the dead cells reaching the surface of the skin cannot be desquammated fast enough. The result is piles of scales such as you see in psoriasis. Much of the practice of dermatology is in fact aimed at slowing the speed at which the skin replaces itself, or as the beautician would claim, quite wrongly, rejuvenates itself.

Many applications prescribed by dermatologists have the sole aim of preventing over-rapid replacement of skin cells. In other words, their aim is to tranquillize the skin and damp down its sensitivity rather than to heighten it. It is only when the skin is irritated that it is stimulated to increase the production of new cells. It is therefore wrong to try to improve the appearance of the skin by making use of a process or a product that irritates it; the effect will be exactly the opposite of that desired. For this reason most dermatologists would be against any of the treatments that beauticians claim 'stimulate' the skin.

Regenerative cell therapy

Occasionally extravagant claims are made about new methods of 'rejuvenating' or 'revitalizing' the skin and the body. Such is the demand from an insecure public for these treatments that they often become widely used in the absence of any proof that they are effective. A currently popular treatment is one that was proposed in the 1930s by Dr Paul Niehans, known as regenerative cell therapy. This involves injecting patients with a mixture of cells from the glands of freshly slaughtered animals. It is claimed that a study using a geiger counter confirmed Dr Niehans' theory that cells from a particular animal organ find their way directly to the same organ in the patient. So when liver cells from animals were injected into a patient, they were supposedly traced to the liver by the use of a geiger counter. Similarly, pancreas cells from animals made their way to the patient's pancreas. Dr Niehans treats each affected human organ with injections of a corresponding animal organ and this is alleged to have helped many eminent people.

Of course, not all patients in Dr Niehans' Geneva clinic get well, but in his opinion the failures are not due to failures of treatment but to improper administration of his cell therapy. In other words, the failures do not damn his method but the technique by which the method is used.

The treatment is extremely expensive. The cost of a single injection is rarely less than $1,000 and many injections may be prescribed.

Beside the fact that Dr Niehans' therapy has never been put to scientific test and therefore its efficacy has never been proved, there are basic physiological questions one must ask about it. If its efficacy is thought to be connected with the effect of *live* animal cells, then the whole theory is shaky. The body has several in-built mechanisms to protect it from invasion by live foreign cells.

Any such alien material, especially if it is animal in origin, is immediately attacked and speedily rendered inactive. Second, it is highly unlikely that a substance that is injected can reach a specific organ in any concentration. It mixes with 4.8–6 l (8–10 pt) of blood, which greatly dilute it, and as the heart is not specific about which artery it directs the blood into, the substance will be pumped to all parts of the body.

In purely mechanical terms, it is impossible for the injected material to settle in only one organ. The fact that Dr Niehans was able to trace radioactive cells to the liver means nothing. The liver is the major purifying organ of the body and it automatically sifts, sieves and strains any foreign material out of the blood. This happens the first time the blood circulates through the liver. As the circulation time of blood round the body is about 12 seconds, the vast proportion of an injected foreign substance is cleaned out of the blood and into the liver during its first pass through the organ – that is, in 12 seconds. What the study was recording was a normal physiological event, not proof of an organ-specific treatment.

Slimming treatments

Most beauty clinics offer several seductive methods for losing weight. They are seductive because they require no effort, physical or mental, on the part of the would-be slimmer. For exactly the same reason they are ineffective. There are only two ways to lose weight.

1 Take in fewer calories: eat less food or less fattening food.
2 Use up more calories: lead a more active life or take up an active exercise programme.

You may of course lose weight as the result of beauty clinic treatments but it is 'artificial' weight loss. In the first place it involves the use of and adherence to regimes to which you yourself have no access in the course of your everyday life. To maintain weight loss by beauty clinic methods therefore you must continue to attend beauty clinics. This is not what correct weight maintenance is about.

Second, the weight loss is temporary. Very often it is due to 'forced' fluid loss. The body is self-correcting and once the force, such as sweating or wrapping, is removed it will compensate by retaining fluid until it has re-equilibrated. So while some beauty clinic methods (by no means all) leave the body a few pounds lighter the effect is transient. It is up to you and you alone to attain your ideal weight and maintain it (see pages 112–117).

• Electrical muscle stimulation (Slendertone) (see page 241)

The claim made for this form of weight reducing treatment is that it takes all the hard work and monotony out of exercise. Unfortunately it does not consume any calories at all. It will therefore not help anyone to lose weight, not even from difficult areas such as the thighs and upper arms.

• Massage

Massage will not in any circumstances cause you to shed weight, unless you are the masseuse.

• Suction cupping

By the application to the skin of a rubber cup connected to an air-pump a vacuum can be created that sucks the skin and subcutaneous fat into the cup. Several cups may be applied over a pad of fat such as the outer thigh. Fat loss is claimed by improving lymphatic drainage. This is fallacious: lymphatic drainage, be it good, bad or indifferent, does not help true weight loss. ·

• Sweating

Saunas and steam cabinets (see pages 235–236) make the body sweat and you can lose up to 1.25 kg (3 lb) or 1.8 l (3 pt) of sweat at one session. When you climb on to the weighing machine immediately afterwards, the loss is impressive. However, unless you drink no fluid over the next 36 hours your body will compensate by retaining the same amount of fluid as was lost.

• Wrapping

This form of treatment involves wrapping the body in cloths, which may be impregnated with lotions, gels and extracts (usually vegetable or herbal) claimed to make the treatment more efficient. The client may be 'wrapped' for several hours, during which time sweat is secreted with resultant weight loss. Various claims for the treatment include improving congestion (blood flow), improving lymphatic drainage, breaking down fat (this cannot be done through the skin by any means known to science) and water loss through sweat. Even if any of these claims are true, none will lead to a lasting weight loss.

Psychotherapy

Psychotherapy has its origins in primitive medicine. Hippocrates taught that the mind and body were inseparable and should be treated together. Babylonian priests attempting to cure a sick person would recite the names of various devils until one of these evoked a visible response; that devil was then blamed for the disease.

It was Freud, however, who attempted to develop a scientific theory of psychotherapy (called psychoanalysis) that would have the same status as modern medicine. He found that if he encouraged a patient with a hysterical or nervous disorder to talk freely, it was possible to trace from what the patient said, from pauses and from changes of mood or subject what his or her emotional disturbances were, even though these had been suppressed in the unconscious mind years before. Moreover, Freud discovered that if he could make the patient recall and describe the traumatic incident, whether real or imaginary, the repressed feelings were released and the illness often disappeared. Although the term psychotherapy has several meanings, to Freudians it meant (and still does) the use of psychoanalysis as a therapeutic method, rather than simply as a scientific exploration of the mind.

Mental disease can be divided into two broad types: psychosis, which is a true disease of the mind, is quite abnormal and includes episodes of complete breaks with reality, and neurosis, which is an emotional disturbance that many doctors feel is simply an exaggeration of the norm. Neurotic symptoms are very common and only in rare instances is the neurosis severe enough to warrant hospital admission. It is therefore a public problem, one that in affluent societies may affect as much as 30 per cent of the population. Psychotherapy was taken up very quickly for the treatment of neurosis because it claimed to be able to treat neurotic patients who were not amenable to, or whose symptoms were not severe enough to require, in-patient hospital treatment.

Mind and body

The classification of mental illness into psychotic and neurotic led to a differentiation between physical symptoms as 'organic' and 'functional'. Organic diseases are regarded as real and objective, with a traceable cause that can be removed or healed, while functional symptoms are held to be invented or imaginary, with no observable cause.

The followers of Freud went a little further in their examination of functional and organic disorders. They established the hypothesis of psychosomatic medicine, which reverted to the primitive idea that mind and body are inextricably linked in the causation of illness. But because the medical profession as a whole emphasized the physical aspects of disease, psychosomatic illness came to imply illness of an emotional origin; the fairly commonly held view was that psychosomatic conditions were not deemed worthy of serious consideration by scientific medicine.

Medical orthodoxy, in an attempt to circumscribe psychosomatic illness, linked it to specific disorders such as asthma, skin diseases and peptic ulcers. Subsequent research widened the range of physical symptoms that could be connected with emotional disturbances – for instance, the level of sugar in the blood of a diabetic. Studies also showed that the blood pressure of heart patients could be increased by anxiety and stress and in 1958 the results of a ten-year study of 100 heart patients in New York suggested that 'undue emotional strain associated with job responsibility is far more significant than heredity or a prodigiously high fat diet'.

Most doctors would now agree that in order to treat patients properly the physical symptoms, personality, emotional disturbances and social and domestic background should all be considered together. They would also concede that conditions that are attributed to a definite cause such as bacteria may occur because stress has weakened the patient's defence mechanisms. It follows that people become ill because of inadequacies of the mind as well as of the body. Doctors cannot afford to neglect some of the greatest health problems facing society now, problems resulting from insufficient adjustment to a myriad of social and psychological stresses.

Psychotherapy today

Much psychiatric medicine as it is currently practised precludes the relating of treatment to the patient's home and what is happening there. Yet mental illness should never be considered in isolation, since it involves relationships between people, and unless the disturbance of these relationships is understood, the treatment will have little chance of success. Psychotherapy can provide an alternative answer, avoiding as it generally does attendance at a psychiatric clinic or admission to a mental hospital entailing the removal of the patient from family and job.

Whatever the method employed, psychotherapy aims to help a patient to acquire insight into herself and her behaviour so that she can learn to deal with her own difficulties. It does not concentrate only on her symptoms or seek to 'cure' them, but to explain the underlying reasons for them.

Psychotherapists often find that the patient who requests their help feels that there is a great disparity between what she actually is and what she ought to be. The therapy will be designed to change the patient's concept of herself so that she comes to feel not just acceptable, but self-determinate and worthy of her own respect. Once this change of perception has occurred, it is found that all anxiety and tensions are reduced.

Critics of psychotherapy claim, however, that achieving insight into oneself is not always useful or necessary. Indeed for some it may be an intolerable strain. If it leads a patient to realize the truth about herself – that she is not in love with her husband, or that she is homosexual – she may conclude that she cannot bear to go on living. In this way a psychotherapist could be responsible for releasing powerful feelings that might, for instance, lead to the break-up of a marriage; although this may be to the long-term good, it will obviously be painful in the short term.

Where psychotherapy can help

In its widest sense psychotherapy can be used for the treatment of almost any condition whose background is at least partly psychological, or due to an inability to adjust to stress. Such conditions might include overeating leading to obesity, depression, anorexia nervosa, frigidity, nymphomania, etc. The form of therapy used varies according to the illness, the patient's personality and the psychotherapist's method of treatment.

Before undertaking any form of psychotherapy, there are certain basic conditions that the patient must be prepared to fulfil. These are:

• that she is willing and able to explore her feelings.

• that she is capable of working in a close and intimate way with a psychotherapist who will interpret her personality, inadequacies, motivation and symptoms.

• that she will accept some kind of therapeutic plan as part of her treatment regime.

Psychoanalysis

As described above, this is the best-known form of psychotherapy. It does, however, have certain disadvantages. It is expensive and it takes a very long time – the patient may be required to undergo analysis five days a week for four or five years. Moreover, while it has its zealots in those whom it has helped, the patients' friends and relatives may not always be as enthusiastic about the results, finding the patients changed – and not always for the better.

Whereas psychoanalysis requires a large number of regular sessions, anything less frequent is often referred to as intensive psychotherapy or psychoanalytically orientated psychotherapy. This usually involves regular treatment, say, two or three times a week over one year, or even several years. A less intensive regime would mean attendance once a week for six months or so – this is called brief psychotherapy, or focal therapy.

Interpretive psychotherapy

This attempts to help the patient understand the cause of her difficulties and the symptoms that they give rise to. The psychotherapist cannot do this without understanding what has happened in every aspect of the patient's life, including childhood, adolescence, family and personal relationships. He may interpret the significance of the patient's symptoms as they relate to her present life, but quite often a special technique is employed involving the transference of relationships between patient and therapist.

'Transference' is the process by which the patient displaces on to the therapist feelings and ideas that she has had in the past. She therefore begins to relate to the therapist as if he were a person with whom she has formerly had a relationship, so that he takes on the emotional significance of that other person. In this way, the disturbing aspect of that relationship can be worked through in detail with the therapist during the treatment.

Short-term therapy

This recently developed form of therapy claims that neurotic symptoms can be successfully treated without recourse to the personality problems of the patient. It is said that there are three conditions necessary for this kind of therapy. First, there has to be 'congruence' in the therapist's experience of the patient's thoughts and behaviour – in other words, he must be sincere in his desire to help. Second, there must be 'empathy' so that the therapist is able to understand what the patient tells him and can convey this understanding back to her. Third, there has to be 'unconditional positive regard'. This is a warm appreciative feeling for the patient and the ability to convey a sense of valuing her whatever she may say. The aim of this joint endeavour is that the patient should become free of mental symptoms, especially excess anxiety, and able to direct her energies towards personal growth and maturation, without feelings of jealousy, envy or greed. She should be able to give and accept love and tenderness and to form lasting relationships of emotional and physical intimacy.

In the short-term treatment process, the therapist has to work quickly to establish with the patient a rapport and a feeling of equality and warmth, while at the same time he must assess her psychological condition and get an idea of what she is like and what she wants to be. Indeed, to be successful, the therapist's work depends entirely on a good interaction with the patient.

Suggestive psychotherapy

Here, reliance is placed on resolving the patient's difficulties by making direct suggestions. One of the most intense and dramatic of suggestive therapies is hypnosis, in which the patient's state of consciousness is altered and active directions are given. Although hypnotherapy is often used to change patterns of behaviour, it can also be used to encourage the patient to release repressed memories. This use is based on the theory that it is possible to make closer contact with the sub-conscious mind when the patient is hypnotized.

Supportive psychotherapy

The essence of this form of therapy is that the therapist listens to the patient in an understanding and concerned way. The patient is encouraged to explore her own thoughts and to express problems, conflicts and anxieties. The therapist may help with advice and may give reassurance by offering his own experiences so the patient can identify with or reject them as appropriate.

Group therapy

After the Second World War group psychotherapy spread rapidly. In 'small group' therapy seven or eight strangers meet together with a therapist under strictly defined conditions. Their common denominator is their inability to deal with stress in their lives. Within the group framework the interactions between them can be studied easily and specific therapy worked out. Often the group is set the task of observing and understanding its own behaviour and tensions.

When such groups were studied initially, three main patterns emerged. The first was characterized by dependency – an attempt to make the therapist omnipotent and to give him all responsibility. The second was the fight and flight pattern, in which solutions were sought by conflict or escape. The third was pairing – the establishment of a relationship between two members, in the interaction between whom the rest of the group would look for a solution.

The objective is that, with the help of others as well as the therapist, a patient will first discover, then rationalize, then adjust to and finally cope with her problems. The presence of others with similar difficulties gives her an insight into her own. With the realization that others are acting irrationally she may rapidly conclude that her own behaviour is equally unreasonable, which can then help her to correct it. Thus, what happens in group therapy should follow a logical and purposeful development with, as its end product, a patient who no longer depends on the group to feel at one with herself and society.

Phobias and behavioural therapy

There is no doubt that certain psychological illnesses benefit greatly from therapy. Among these are phobias. A phobia is an overwhelming though unreasonable fear about a certain situation. Most of the people who suffer from one are aware that they are behaving irrationally, but are quite unable to control their fear. Very often a phobia can be the result of an earlier distressing event that has been forgotten. Phobic patients can be helped particularly by the different forms of behavioural therapy, the main ones of which are described below.

• Aversion therapy

This is often used for the treatment of addictions – for instance to alcohol, smoking, drugs or gambling – and some fetishes and perversions. Its aim is to teach the patient that indulging in the behaviour under treatment leads to unpleasant consequences.

The original aversion techniques were used for the treatment of alcoholism. Patients were administered a nausea-inducing drug. Just before they started to be sick, they were allowed to pour themselves a glass of their favourite drink. The intention was to build an association between the sight and taste of alcohol and the overwhelming feeling of nausea. In other forms of aversion therapy, electric shocks are used.

• Cognitive manipulation

The essence of this form of therapy is that the patient tells herself again and again that she is not afraid, in the hope that the feeling of fear will eventually be dissipated. The therapy is usually accompanied by the recording of a body function, say the pulse, or breathing rate. One example would be a person who is afraid of snakes and whose heartbeat increases on seeing one. She will be told over and over, and encouraged to repeat herself, that her heart rate will not quicken when she sees a snake. At the same time the soundtrack of a heart beating normally will be played to her. If the treatment is successful she will stop avoiding snakes. Furthermore, if she sees one, she should experience no increase in her heart rate.

• Desensitization

One of the most successful of the behavioural therapies, desensitization combines the phobic situation with a pleasurable experience. Thus, someone who suffers from claustrophobia could be placed in an enclosed space, but listening all the while to her favourite music. The therapy is accompanied by exercises in relaxation, and when complete relaxation is achieved, the patient is asked to imagine increasingly unpleasant situations. An important aspect of this therapy is the encouragement of the patient to persevere by reporting progress, by charting improvements and by rewarding effort with praise and giving constant support. During desensitization therapy, the presence of a relation or trusted friend can be very helpful.

• Flooding

The patient is encouraged to visualize the phobic situation as vividly as she can for as long as possible, with the aim that eventually it should no longer arouse fear. This method has been used successfully to treat students who suffer from examination phobias.

• Logo therapy

Here the situation and symptoms of the phobia are exaggerated and the patient is asked to try to discipline her terror rather than run away from the situation. After repeated disciplining the patient should no longer be haunted by her fears.

• Modelling

This involves exposing the phobic person to other people who are untroubled in what is for her a phobic situation. If this kind of group therapy is repeated, the fear will gradually diminish because the patient will try to imitate the fearless behaviour of the other people in the group.

Encounter group therapy

A form of therapy that gained prevalence in the early 1960s, encounter group therapy centres round the potent pressure of the group to remove the members' constraints against what is normally felt to be 'forbidden'. The group demands complete openness to any impulse – whether it be to touch, to be caressed, to undress or to curse – and such is the variety of groups available that anything promoting this openness – nudity, marathons, screaming, bathing, etc. – will be used by one or other of them. Although they may vary in methods, encounter groups all function by imposing a liberating imperative.

The members usually recognize that the kind of openness and intimacy achieved in the group setting should not be carried into everyday life, and it is therefore better that contacts within the group are brief and impersonal.

Index

Index prepared by Ann C.
Hall, registered indexer of
The Society of Indexers

A

abdomen, 17, 76-9, 131, 240;
    exercises for, 77, 135-7,
    147-9, 164-6
abdominoplasty, 218-19, 225,
    228
abrasion, 47, 246
abscess, 26, 58
aches *see* complaints
acidity, of skin, 14, 16; of
    urine, 178
acne, 14, 26, 29, 245; cover-
    up techniques for, 205,
    207; and sun, 18, 63;
    surgical and chemical
    treatments for, 213-15
acupressure, 232; *see* shiatzu
acupuncture, 117, 232, 237
addiction, treatment for, 251;
    see also drugs
adrenalin, 168
aerobic exercise, 128
ageing, 13, 208-9, 216, 220,
    242, 244; *see also* cosmetic
    surgery; wrinkles
alcohol, 109, 119, 121, 179;
    see also wine
Alexander principle, 132-3
allergies, 26, 45, 61, 108-9,
    180, 213
allopathy, 232
alopecia, 32
amino acids, 98, 102, 122
anaemia, 82, 100, 102, 234;
    see also blood system
androgen, 14
ankles, 91; *see also* legs
anorexia nervosa, 127, 249
ante-natal exercises, 77, 147-
    9; *see also* pregnancy
antihistamines, 26, 28
anti-perspirant, 14
antiseptic, 14, 33
anxiety, 14, 112, 132, 233,
    248, 250; *see also*
    psychotherapy; stress
appetite suppressants, 116
apronectomy, 117, 228
archery, 151
arms, 80-1; cosmetic surgery
    for, 218-19, 225, 229;
    exercises for, 132, 142-3,
    151, 154-61 *passim*, 164
aromatherapy, 232-3
arthritis, 67, 81-2; treatment
    for, 163, 233-4, 236, 240-1
ascorbic acid, 102
Aslan, Dr Ana, 234
asthma, 108, 134, 234, 236
astringent, 21-2
atherosclerosis, 109
athlete's foot, 91

athletics, 151; *see also*
    exercises
audiosonic vibration, 244
aversion therapy, 251

B

back, 17, 62-5; exercises for,
    137, 140-1, 148-9, 152-3,
    163-5, 167; and posture,
    130-1, 133; *see also* spinal
    column
backache, 64-5, 68, 113, 162
bacteria, as food, 107;
    infections, 26, 29; and skin,
    25, 241-2, 246; and sweat,
    14
badminton, 152
balance, and posture, 130-1;
    yoga exercise for, 163
balneotherapy, 233, 240; *see
    also* hydrotherapy
bangs, 36, 39, 41, 61
barbiturates, 179
barrier, skin as, 12, 15
basal metabolic rate, 96-7,
    104
baths, 16-17, 179, 233, 235,
    240; *see also* hydrotherapy
beauty clinics, 213, 242-7
behavioural therapy, 250-1
Benson, Dr Herbert, 168-9
Berenson, Marisa, 178
beverages *see* alcohol; drinks
biofeedback, 14, 233, 236
birthmarks, 205, 207, 214-15
blackheads, 14, 22, 26, 59, 63,
    245; *see also* spots
bleaching hair, 45, 47
blemishes, covering, 205-7
blepharitis, 51
blepharoplasty, 218-19, 221,
    223
blisters, 26-7
blood pressure, high, 101,
    109, 113, 168, 232-3, 248
blood system, 13, 15, 92, 96,
    100, 178, 233, 235, 237,
    244, 247; and massage,
    172-3, 176-7, 244
blow drying, 39; *see also* hair
blushers, 188-9, 191, 203, 205,
    208
BMR *see* basal metabolic rate
body and mind, 132-3, 160-2,
    248
body hair, 15, 31, 46-7, 127
body size, 97
body surgery, 218-19, 225;
    see also cosmetic surgery
boil *see* abscess
bottom, 13, 66, 69; cosmetic
    surgery for, 218-19, 225,
    228-9; exercises for, 135,
    138-40
bowling, tenpin, 160
bra, 73, 226-7

bran, 109, 120
bread, 98-102, 105, 111, 120
breastfeeding, 73, 218, 227
breasts, 13, 17, 70-5; exercises
    for, 142-3; operations on,
    74-5, 217-19, 225-8; self-
    examination, 74-5
breath, bad, 58
breathing, 96, 147, 162, 169,
    171, 234, 236-7, 241
bruising, 13
brushes, make-up, 182-3, 187,
    200-1
brushing, hair, 34; skin, 242,
    245; teeth, 57-8, 230
buck teeth, 231
bunion, 90-1
bust *see* breasts
butter, 99, 101, 105, 120
butterfly machine, 167
buttocks *see* bottom

C

calamine lotion, 19, 28
calcium, 100, 103-4, 111
calluses, 17, 92
calories, 96-7, 114, 118, 120-1,
    151-61; *see also* slimming
calves, 144-5; *see also* legs
camouflage, 15, 205-7
cancer, 18, 32, 45, 58, 74-5,
    218, 227
canoeing, 152
capping teeth, 231
carbohydrates, 96, 98-102,
    104-5, 119-21
carotene, 101
cellulite, 69, 89, 117
cellulose, 98, 100
cereals, 99-102, 105, 107, 109,
    111, 120, 126
cervix, 79
cetrimide, 26, 29
chapping, 27, 59
cheekbones, 187; cosmetic
    surgery for, 218-21, 224;
    see also cheeks, make-up
cheeks, make-up, 188-91,
    202-4
cheese, 98-102, 105, 109, 111,
    118-20
chemical skin treatment, 213-
    14, 246
chignon, 36, 42
chilblains, 27
chin, 17, 59, 187; cosmetic
    surgery for, 218-21, 224;
    make-up, 188-91
chiropractic, 65, 233, 237
chloasma, 18, 27
chloride, 101
chocolate, 99, 108-9, 121
cholecalciferol, 103
cholesterol, 99, 109
Citizens' Advice Bureau, 212
Clarke, Linda, 212

cleanliness *see* hygiene
cleansing skin, 15, 20-3, 193,
    199, 205, 242-5
climbing, 152
clinics *see* beauty; health
clips, hair, 35
clothes, 61, 69, 72, 78, 89
club cut, 36
club hair, 31
clubs, slimming, 117
coeliac disease, 108
coffee, 77, 109; *see also*
    drinks
cognitive manipulation, 251
cold, common, 55, 102
cold feet, 92
cold sores, 59
collagen, 12-13, 18, 29, 209,
    242
colostrum, 72
colour, hair, 31-2, 44-6, 208-
    9; make-up, 184, 186-200,
    202-9; skin, 14-15;
    therapy, 233-4
combination hair, 38
combination skin, 22, 25
combs, 34-5
comfort, 168
complaints: back, 64-5, 68,
    113; bacterial, 26, 29;
    chest, 236; deficiency, 101-
    3; diabetic, 113, 248;
    digestive, 108-9; eye, 51;
    hand, 81-2; heart, 109, 113,
    168, 233; leg, 89-92;
    mouth, 58-9; nose, 26, 55;
    organic, 248; rheumatic,
    164; sciatic, 64, 163, 165;
    urinary, 165; *see also*
    allergies; arthritis; asthma;
    blood pressure; damage;
    medicine; migraine; skin
conditioning hair, 33, 38
conjunctivitis, 51
contact lenses, 51, 193
contour colour, 187-91, 202-
    4, 208
convalescence, 126
cooking, 102-3, 106-7
corns, 17, 92
cortisol, 15, 178
cosmetic dentistry, 230-1
cosmetic surgery, 13, 54-5,
    59, 117, 205, 212-13, 216-
    29; *see also* dental surgery;
    medicine
cosmetics *see* make-up
cover-ups, 205-7
crash diets, 124-5
cricket, 152
croquet, 152-3
crowning teeth, 231
crow's-feet, 23, 27, 193, 222;
    see also wrinkles
cryotherapy, 214
curettage, 214
cuticle, hair, 38; nail, 82-5
cutting hair, 36
cycling, 153; machine, 166-7
cysts, 213-14

D

daily minimum exercises, 128, 134-5
damage, to hair, 32, 38, 41; to skin, 18, 47, 242; see also complaints
dance, 153
dandruff, 33
deafness, 53-4
deficiency diseases, 101-3
deformity, 216, 221-4, 231
dehydration, 14, 16-17, 20-1, 34, 97, 215
dental, floss, 57, 59; splinting, 116; surgery, 230-1; see also teeth
deodorant, 14
depilatory cream, 47
depression, 113, 179, 222; see also stress
dermabrasion, 29, 214-15, 218-19, 221, 223, 228
dermatitis, 18, 27-8; seborrhoeic, 33, 51; see also skin
desensitization, 251
desquammation, 245-6
detergent, 16, 81
diabetes, 113, 248
diarrhoea, 108
diathermy, short-wave, 46-7, 244; see also electrocoagulation
diet, 56, 96-111, 238-9
dieting see slimming; weight, loss
digestion, 96, 98, 100, 106, 108-9, 164, 178
disc, slipped, 64-5; see also back
disclosing tablets, 57
disease see complaints; medicine
disencrustation, 245-6
disfigurement, 205-7
dislocation of shoulder, 63
distraction, 169
diuretics, 54, 77
dizziness, 54
douche, Scotch, 235
dreaming, 178
drinks, 99, 109, 119, 121; see also alcohol; coffee; water
drugs, 109, 127, 179, 212, 235, 237
dry hair, 34, 37-8
dry skin, 22, 24-5, 61
dryers, hair, 34, 39
dye, hair, 31-2, 44-5

E

ears, 52-4, 217; cosmetic surgery for, 218-19, 224
eczema, 27-8, 108, 215, 233, 235-6; see also skin

EFA see essential fatty acids
effleurage, 172-3, 176
eggs, 98, 101-3, 105, 107-8, 111, 118, 120
elbows, 17, 81, 170; see also arms
electrical therapy, 241, 243-5, 247, 251
electrocoagulation, 215
electrodesiccation, 27, 215
electroencephalography, 233
electrolysis, 20, 46-7
emotional problems, 212; see also anxiety; stress
encounter group therapy, 251
end-gaining theory, 133
energy, 96-7, 104, 112, 114, 126
enzymes, 109
epidermis, 12, 15, 16
erogenous zones, 13
essential fatty acids, 100; see also fats
evening make-up, 202-4
excision, 28, 215
excretion, 96
exercises, 128-67; abdomen, 77, 135-7, 147-9, 164-6; ante-natal, 147-8; back, 137, 140-1, 148-9, 152-3, 163-5, 167; facial, 59, 146, 177, 243; heart, 151-60, 165, 167; limbs, 81, 89-91, 138-9, 142-3, 148, 151-61, 164; machines for, 116, 166-7, 240; neck, 61, 146; in physiotherapy, 240; post-natal, 148-9; posture, 130-1; and pregnancy, 77, 147-9, 159; reasons for, 128; as relaxation, 169; and sport, 150-61; see also yoga
eyebrows, 31, 183, 190, 194-5, 197-8, 202-4, 209, 221, 223
eyelashes, 31, 182-3, 193, 196-8, 204, 207, 209
eyelids, cosmetic surgery for, 217-19, 233
eyes, 48-51, 101; exercises for, 146, 177; make-up, 21, 183, 192-9, 202-4, 209; skin round, 21-4, 50; and sun, 49; see also blepharoplasty

F

face, cosmetic surgery for, 216-24; exercises for, 59, 146, 177, 243; hair on, 46-7, 244; mask, 25, 244; massage, 176-7, 179, 243-5; nerves of, 13; relaxation of, 171; shape, 187-8; skin care of, 20-5
fallen arches, 92
false nails, 83

fasting, 124-5, 237, 239
fat, body, 12-13, 69, 81, 89, 97, 112, 114, 122, 126, 172, 174; see also obesity; weight
fats in food, 96, 99-101, 105, 107, 109, 119-23, 125
FDA see United States Food and Drugs Administration
feet, 17, 86-7, 90-2; exercises for, 144-5, 148, 153, 164; massage, 93, 175, 240; relaxation, 171; see also pedicure
fencing, 153-4
fibre, 100, 109-10, 123
finger kneading, 173, 175-6
fish, 98-100, 102-3, 105, 107, 111, 118, 120
fitness, 128
flooding therapy, 251
floss, dental, 57, 59
fluid balance, 97, 114-15, 117, 122, 124-5; retention, 77, 115; see also water
fluoride, 58, 101
focal therapy, 249
folic acid, 102
follicles, hair, 13-15, 20, 31-2; nail, 82
folliculitis, 26
food, 56, 96-111, 120-1, 237, 239; see also slimming
forehead, 22, 187-8, 190
foundation, 20, 22, 184-7, 203-9
freckles, 28, 206-7
freezing food, 107-8
freezing skin, 214
French pleat, 36, 43
Freud, 248
fringe, 36, 39, 41, 61
frozen shoulder, 63, 241
fructose, 99
fruit, 99-101, 103, 105, 119, 121
fungal infection, 28, 91

G

galvanic treatment, 245-6
genitals, 13, 68
Gerovital therapy, 234
gingivitis, 59
ginseng, 110-11
glasses see spectacles
glaucoma, 51
glitter, 203-4
glucose, 99
gluten, 108
glycerides, 99
glycerol, 99
glycogen, 114-15, 124-5
gold powder, 203-4
golf, 154
gravitonics, 234
greasy hair, 34, 37-8

Grenz rays, 215
grips, hair, 35, 182
group therapy, 250-1
groups see clubs
groups, food, 105
gums, 56-9; see also teeth
gymnastics, 154

H

hack squat machine, 167
Hahnemann, Dr Samuel, 234-5
hair, 30-47; body, 15, 31, 46-7, 89, 127; care, 33-5, 38; colour, 31-2, 44-6, 208-9; cut, 36; damaged, 32-3, 38, 41, 44; drying, 34, 39; equipment, 34-5, 182; facial, 46-7, 244; follicles, 13-15, 20, 31-2; growth, 31-3; and hormones, 31, 33, 46; keratin in, 33, 44; leg, 46-7, 89; lice in, 28; loss, 32-3, 125; perming, 31-2, 44-5; removal, 46-7; setting, 40-1; styles, 36, 40-3; types, 38; washing, 33, 37-8; wigs and hairpieces, 46
halibut liver oil, 101
halitosis, 58
hands, 80-5; care of, 16-17, 81-2, 84-5, 171; exercises for, 142-3
hang-gliding, 154
hangnails, 82-3
happiness cure, 234
hay fever, 26, 193
health clinics, farms, 116-17, 212-13, 238-41
healthfoods, 110-11
heart, disease, 109, 113, 168, 233; exercises for, 151-60, 165, 167; slowed rate, 178
heat therapy, 240-1
heels, 17; see also feet
henna, 46
herbal remedies, 110, 234-6; see also vegetables
herbalism, 234
high frequency treatment, 244
highlighting, 45, 189-92, 202-4
high protein diet, 122
hips, 66-7; exercises for, 138-9, 141, 148-9, 163-4, 167; operations on, 67, 218-19, 225, 228-9
hirsutism, 33, 46-7; see also hair
hockey, 154-5
hollows, facial, 188, 208
home exercise, 134-49
homeopathy, 213, 234-8
honey, 99, 110-11, 121

hormones, 101-2; and breasts, 72-3; in cosmetics, 20, 242; and fat, 228; and hair, 31, 46; and menopause, 78; and menstruation, 77; and muscles, 155, 157, 166; in pregnancy, 78; and skin, 14-15, 27, 29, 61; and sleep, 178-9
hydrocortisone, 63, 81
hydrotherapy, 213, 235-6, 247
hygiene, 17, 33-4, 37, 57-8, 73; dental, 230; food, 108
hypnosis, 117, 169, 236, 250
hypo-allergenic make-up, 180, 184, 187, 192

I

ice skating, 155
ideal weight, 112-13, 247
illness see complaints
impetigo, 28; see also skin
implants, breast, 218-19, 226
infections see complaints
infra-red light, 241
ingredients of make-up, 184, 186-7, 192-3, 200
ingrowing toe nails, 92
inhalation therapy, 236, 241; see also breathing
injections, desensitizing, 26; rejuvenating, 246-7
insomnia, 162, 168-9, 178-9, 213, 234
intestinal bypass, 117
'invisible' fat, 99, 123
iodine, 101
iontophoresis, 243, 245
iron, 100-1, 104
isometrics, 155
isotonics, 155
itching, 28
Iyengar, B.K.S., 162

J

Jacobson, Dr Edmund, 169
jacusi massage, 233, 236, 240
jawline, 177, 189, 208, 223
jogging, 155-6
judo, 156

K

karate, 156
keratin, in hair, 33, 44; in skin, 12, 25-6, 246
ketosis, 119, 122, 125

kidneys, human, 15, 77, 97, 235, 237
kilocalories, 96-7; see also calories
kneading, 172-3, 176
knees, 17, 88-9, 148, 164, 171; see also legs

L

lacrosse, 156
lactose, 99
lanolin, 23, 50, 184
lanugo, 127
lecithin, 99
legs, 16-17, 86-93; exercises for, 135, 138-41, 144-64 passim, 167; hair on, 46-7, 89; massage, 90; relaxation of, 171; see also knees
lice, 28
Lief, Stanley, 236
light treatment, 241
lignin, 100
lipids, 99
lips, 13, 56, 59; make-up for, 182-3, 200-4, 208-9
liver, as food, 101-2, 105, 107, 111, 120
liver, human, 79, 101, 103, 114, 164, 233, 235, 237, 246-7
logo therapy, 251
loss of hair, 32-3, 125
loss of nutrients, 106-7
loss of weight see slimming; weight, loss
low calorie diet, 118-22, 125
low carbohydrate diet, 117, 119-23
low fat diet, 123
low protein diet, 122-3
lumps, breast, 74-5
lungs, 15, 100, 151-60, 167
lymph glands, 75
lymphatic drainage, 245, 247

M

machines, exercise, 116, 166-7, 240
magnesium, 101
make-up, 16, 20-2, 59, 180-209, 212-13; allergies to, 180, 184, 192, 200, 204; attitudes to, 180; for camouflage, 205-7; ingredients of, 184, 186-7, 192-3, 200; for older skin, 208-9; party, 202-4; see also moisturizer
manicure, 17, 84-5; see also hands; nails
manipulation, 172, 233, 237

margarine, 99, 101, 103, 105, 111, 120; see also fats
mascara see eyes
massage, 172-7, 213, 232, 236-7, 247; facial, 24, 176-7, 179, 243-5; feet, 93, 175; in health clinic, 239-40; leg, 90; mechanical, 245; neck, 61, 177, 179; for relaxation, 169, 173-7
mastectomy, 75, 218, 227-8
mastoplexy, 227
meal pattern, 106
meat, 98-9, 101-2, 105, 107, 111, 118-20
medicine, alternative, 212-13, 232-7; orthodox, 213, 232; see also complaints; cosmetic surgery; psychotherapy
meditation, 159, 162, 169, 213, 237
megavitamin therapy, 236-7; see also vitamins
melanin, 14-15, 18, 28, 31, 103
melanocytes, 14-15, 28-9, 31
membrane, skin, 12
Ménière's syndrome, 54
menopause, 73, 78, 233
menstruation, and anorexia, 127; and breasts, 72, 74; and fluid retention, 77, 114-15; and iron, 100; pain, exercise for, 141; and perfume, 61; regulation of, 165; and spots, 29
metabolism, 96-8, 101, 104, 106, 112
methylcellulose, 116
microwave energy, 241
migraine, 108-9, 235
milia, 29
milk, 96-103, 105, 107-8, 111, 118, 120
milk glands, 72-3
mind and body, 132-3, 160-2, 248
minerals, 100-1
Mitchell method of relaxation, 170-1
mites, 28
mobility see exercise
modelling therapy, 251
moisture loss, 14, 16-17, 20-1, 34
moisturized foundation, 184
moisturizer, 14, 16-17, 20-4, 61, 89, 176-7, 209; see also make-up
moles, 28, 215
monoamine oxidases, 109, 234
monosaccharides, 99
moodiness, 77
mouth, 52, 56-9, 102
muscles, and hormones, 155, 157, 166; modification of, 223; stimulation of, 172-3, 241, 247; see also exercise

N

nails, 13-14, 17, 81-5, 91-3; see also hands
naturopathy, 213, 232, 237-9
neck, care of, 59-61; cosmetic surgery, 218-19, 221, 223, 225; exercises for, 59, 146, 163, massage, 172-3, 177, 179; and posture, 61, 130-3
nerves, 12-13, 49, 53, 56, 64, 72, 132, 162, 170, 232-3, 237
netball, 156
nettlerash, 26
neuromuscular massage, 236, 240
neuroses, 248-51
niacin, 102; see also vitamins
nicotinic acid, 101-2, 105, 107; see also vitamins
Niehans, Dr Paul, 246-7
nitrogen, liquid, 214
nits, 28
nose, 22, 49, 52-3, 55, 58, 176-7, 189-90; cosmetic surgery, 216, 218-21, 223-4
nosebleeds, 55
nutrients, nutrition see food
nuts, 98-100, 102, 105, 111, 121

O

obesity, 112-13, 117, 122, 125, 228, 249; see also fat; slimming; weight
oedema, 125
oestrogen, 27, 31, 46, 72, 78, 228, 234, 242; see also hormones
oil: bath, 16; in moisturizer, 21-2; see also aromatherapy; make-up, ingredients of
oil, olive, 38
oil, vegetable, 25, 38, 99, 109, 120
oily hair see greasy hair
oily skin, 21-2, 24-6, 61, 184, 186, 245-6
older face, make-up for, 208-9; see also ageing; cosmetic surgery; wrinkles
operations see cosmetic surgery; dental surgery
organic diseases, 248; see also complaints
organic food, 237, 239; see also healthfoods; wholefoods
orthodontists, 230-1
orthopaedic mattress, 65
osteoarthritis, 67
osteomalacia, 103
osteopathy, 65, 213, 233, 236-8

otoplasty, 54, 218-19, 221, 224
ovaries, 165
overweight, 59; see also obesity; slimming
ozone therapy, 233, 245

P

Palmer, Daniel, 233
'palming', 50
parachuting, 156-7
party make-up, 202-4
patting, in massage, 177
Pauling, Dr Linus, 237
pectins, 100
pectoral muscles, 72, 142-3, 167, 226-7
pedicure, 17, 93; see also feet
peeling, chemical skin, 213-14, 246
pelvis, 66-9, 88, 130-1, 147-9, 235, 237, 240
perfume, 61, 184, 186, 200; see also aromatherapy
periods see menstruation
perms, 31-2, 38-40, 44-6
phenol, 213-14
phobias, 250-1
phospholipids, 99
phosphorus, 101, 103
physiological relaxation, 170-1
physiotherapy, 240-1
piercing, ear, 53
pigmentation, skin, 15, 18, 27-9, 205, 207, 215
pimples, 29, 63, 205; see also acne; blackheads; spots
pincurls, 40
pins, hair, 35
placebos, 102, 110, 116, 243; see also medicine
plaque, 56-7, 59, 230
plucking eyebrows, 194
poisoning, food, 108
polyneuritis, 125
polysaccharides, 99
polyunsaturated fats, 100, 109
pores see sebaceous glands; sweat glands
post-natal exercises, 147-9, 159
posture, 61, 63-5, 72, 77, 128, 130-3, 147-9, 152, 155-6, 160; see also yoga
potassium, 101, 125
poultices, 26, 240
powder, 180, 182-3, 186-7, 202-8
pre-eclampsia, 78, 91
pregnancy, 32-3, 57, 67-8, 72-3, 77-9, 81, 91-2, 147-9, 179; and exercises, 77, 147-9, 159; food in, 100, 102, 104, 106, 111
pre-menstrual tension, 77

pre-ski trainer, 167
procaine hydrochloride, 234
progesterone, 27, 29, 78; see also hormones
progestogen, 27, 77, 242; see also hormones
progressive relaxation, 169
prolactin, 72
prostheses, 75
protection factor, in sunscreens, 19
protein, 37, 96, 98, 104-7, 111, 122-5, 237
psoriasis, 18, 233, 246
psychoanalysis, 248-9
psychosomatic illness, 248
psychotherapy, 116, 127, 212-13, 221, 248-51; see also medicine
puberty, 13-14, 17, 22, 26, 29, 31, 72
pubic hair, 31
pubic lice, 28
pulses, 98, 100, 105, 111
pyorrhoea, 59
pyridoxin, 102

R

radiesthesia, 237
radionics, 237
radiotherapy, 75
reflexology, 237
regenerative cell therapy, 246-7
rejuvenation, 223, 233-4, 242, 246-7; see also cosmetic surgery
relaxation, 147, 168-77, 179, 213, 232-3, 237, 240-1, 251; exercises for, 134, 146, 160-6; facial treatments for, 243-5; see also Alexander principle
replacement meals, 117
resorcinol, 213
retinol, 101
rheumatism, 164, 236
rhinoplasty, 216, 218-19, 221, 223-4
riboflavin, 102
rickets, 67
riding, 157
ringworm, 28
rollers, hair, 34-5, 40-2, 44
roller-skating, 157
roughage see fibre
rowing, 157
running, 151, 157-8

S

sailing, 158
salt, 49, 101

saturated fat, 100, 109, 120; see also fats
sauces, 121
sauna, 117, 235-6, 240, 247; facial, 25
scabies, 28-9
scalp, 33, 37-8, 44-5, 229
scars, 13, 205, 207, 213-15, 217, 219, 222-9, 244, 246; see also cosmetic surgery
sciatica, 64, 163, 165
Scotch douche, 235
sebaceous glands, 12-15, 17-18, 20, 22, 25-6, 38, 59, 72, 214, 240
seborrhoeic dermatitis, 33, 51
sebum, 14, 16, 21-2, 25, 34, 38, 44, 59, 72, 244
setting hair, 40-2
sexual intercourse, 89
shampoo, 16, 33, 37-8, 229; see also hair
shaving, 46-7
shiatzu massage, 236, 240
shoes, 78, 89-92; in sports, 151-161
shoulders, 62-3, 130-2, 146, 151-2, 163-5, 170, 204, 240
shower, 16-17
Shuster, Prof. Sam, 18
side-effects, drug, 109
silicone, 226
silver powder, 204
sinuses, sinusitis, 55
sit-up board, 166
Sitz bath, 235, 240-1
skating, 155, 157
skiing, 158, 161
skin, 10-29; acidity, 14, 16; bacteria, 25, 241-2, 245; care of, 16-25; colour, 14-15; complaints, 16, 18, 26-9, 59, 108, 205, 207; round eyes, 21-4, 50, 209; and hormones, 13, 15, 26-7, 29, 242; keratin in, 12, 25-6, 246; and pregnancy, 77-8; structure, 12-15; and sun, 18-19, 26, 63, 103, 241; treatments, 213-15, 233-4, 242-6; type, 22, 25, 184; see also allergies; cleansing; cosmetic surgery; make-up; massage; moisturizer; wrinkles
skin rolling, in massage, 174
skipping, 158
sleep, 96, 178-9
Slendertone, 241, 247
slimming, 112-25, 218, 247; see also weight, loss
smell, sense of, 55, 58, 61, 232-3
smoking, 58, 82, 128, 162, 236, 251
soap, 16, 20-2
social eating, 118-19
sodium, 101
soya bean products, 111
Spanish mantle, 235

spas see hydrotherapy
spectacles, 49, 51, 193, 209
spinal column, 63-4, 130-1, 233, 235, 237; see also back
split ends, 38
sponges, 182, 184-5, 205-6
sports, 150-61
spots, 22, 29, 59, 205, 213; see also acne; pimples; scars; warts
starches, 98-9
starter's kit, make-up, 193, 195, 197
starvation, 125
steam cabinets, 235-6, 247
steroids, 26
Still, Dr Andrew, 237
stockings, 89-91
stomach, 135-7, 160; see also abdomen
streaking hair, 45
stress, 59, 168-170; see also anxiety; depression; psychotherapy
stretch marks, 17, 77-8, 214, 228
stroking, in massage, 172, 174-5
stye, 51
styling, hair, 34-6, 40-3
sucrose, 99
suction cupping, 247
sugar, 56, 98-9, 105, 107, 110, 121, 230
suggestive psychotherapy, 250
sulphur, 233
sun, effects of, 15, 18-19, 49, 63, 103, 215; see also light treatment; tan
sunglasses, 49
sunscreen index, 19
suppleness see exercise
support stockings, 17, 90, 92
supportive psychotherapy, 250
surfing, 159
surgery see cosmetic surgery; dental surgery; mastectomy; medicine
sweat glands, 13-15, 17, 20, 97
sweating, 117, 235, 240, 247
sweaty feet, 92
Swedish massage, 239-40; see also massage
swimming, 159
swollen ankles, 91

T

table tennis, 159
T'ai Chi, 159-60
talcum powder, 172, 186, 203-5
tan, fake, 19, 202, 204; see also sun
tapôtement, 172

taste, 58
tattoos, 215
tears, 49-50
teeth, 56-9, 230-1
temperature, body, 178
temperature control, 15
tennis, 160
tennis elbow, 81, 241
tenpin bowling, 160
tension *see* anxiety;
    relaxation; stress
testosterone, 31, 155, 157,
    166; *see also* hormones
tests, allergy, 108
textured vegetable protein,
    107, 111
thermic effect, 126
thiamin, 102; *see also* vitamins
thighs, 13, 17; cosmetic
    surgery for, 218-19, 225,
    228-9; exercises for, 135,
    138-41, 167; *see also* legs
throat, 16-17, 25, 60-1
thrombosis, 92
thyroid gland, 101, 165
thyroxine, 101
tights, 89-91
tinnitus, 54
tinting *see* colouring
tocopherols, 103
toners, 20-3
tongs, curling, 34
tongue, 58
toothbrush, 57, 230
toothpaste, 57-8
toxins, elimination of, 235,
    237, 239-40
trampolining, 154
tranquillizers, 169, 179, 212
treatment *see* medicine
trichlorocetic acid, 213-14
triglycerides, 99
Turkish bath, 117, 235
TVP *see* textured vegetable
    protein
tweezers, 182-3, 196
twist machine, 167

urinary disorders, 165
urine, 97, 178
uterus, 77, 79; *see also*
    pregnancy

vacuum, facial, 245
vagina, 14, 17, 68, 79
vaporizers, 245
Vaseline, 59
vegans, 111
vegetable protein, 98, 111,
    123
vegetables, 96, 98-103, 105-7,
    111, 118-21, 123
vegetarians, 102, 111
veins, broken, 16, 20, 22, 25,
    27, 89, 215, 244; cover-up
    techniques for, 206-7;
    knee, 17; varicose, 92
vellus hair *see* hair, body
verruca, 92, 214; *see also*
    warts
vertigo, 54
vibration treatment, 244-5
vibrations, in massage, 174
virus infections, 29, 59
visualization, 169
vitamin A, 101-2, 105-6
vitamin B, 101-2, 104-5, 107,
    111
vitamin C, 96, 102-7, 236
vitamin creams, 242
vitamin D, 15, 18, 67, 103,
    105-6, 111
vitamin E, 103, 236, 242
vitamin K, 103
vitamin pills, 110, 124
vitiligo, 18, 29
volleyball, 160

also fat; obesity; slimming
weight-training, 151, 166
whiteheads, 29
whitlow, 29
wholefoods, 110-11; *see also*
    healthfoods
wigs, 46
windsurfing, 161
wine, 99, 119, 121
wrapping, 247
wrinkles, 13, 18, 20, 29, 50,
    61, 193, 205, 207-9, 213,
    218; *see also* ageing;
    cosmetic surgery

yeasts, 107
yoga, 161-5, 179, 213, 237, 241
yogurt, 98, 100, 105, 110,
    120, 239

X-rays, soft, 215

Acknowledgments

The Publishers would like to thank the following
individuals and organizations for their assistance:
Dr Wilfred Barlow, author of *The Alexander Principle*
and Medical Director of the Alexander Institute;
Body Designs Ltd; Boots the Chemists; Louise
Callan; Sylvia Caplin; Debbie Churchill; the Clinical
Cosmetic Centre; Concept Public Relations; Sarah
Culshaw; Dance Centre Ltd; Johanna Donat; Julie
Hazelwood; Health Education Council; Roger
Hillier; Anne-Marie Hughes; Debbie Jeacock; John
Jeffs; Leslie Kenton; Dr Annabella Marks; Maria
Mosby; Ravelle's London Lady Health and Beauty
Clinic; John Ringshall; Amy Roberts; Scholl; Naomi
Simons-Schroter; Starcross School; Donna Sturm;
Dr A.J. Tyler; Sue Wason; Davina Waterhouse;
Ray and Joyce Wyatt; Leigh Young; Barbara Yung.

Roller styles, p. 41, by Pin-Up
Classic Hairstyles, pp. 42–43, by Karin at John
Olofson
Party Tricks Make-up, pp. 202–203, by Anne-Marie
MacKay
Leotards by Flexatard and Dance Centre Ltd.

Photographs
Fausto Dorelli: all colour photographs
Chris Harvey: 129 134–149 158–159 163–165
John Smallwood: 150–157 160–161
Roger Walton: 4–5

Artwork
Giovanni Caselli: 12 32 50 54 56 64 68 73 79 82 88 131
133
Pat Doyle: 9 95 181 211
Howard Pemberton: 17 23–25 34–43 51 57 61 65
74–75 83–85 91 93 130 166–167 170–177 221 225
Malcolm Smythe: 96–97 114 124
Kathy Wyatt: 183–201 206–208

ulcer, mouth, 59
ultrasound therapy, 81, 241
ultra-violet rays, 18, 241, 245;
    see also sun
underarms, cleanliness, 17;
    hair, 31, 46-7
underweight, 126-7; *see also*
    weight
United States, 112, 123, 159,
    192-3, 216, 223, 226-8, 234
United States Food, Drug
    and Cosmetics Act, 192-3
United States Food and
    Drugs Administration, 32,
    226
unsaturated fat, 100, 109; *see*
    also fats

waist, 76-8, 136-7, 163, 167
walking, 91, 96, 154, 160-1,
    179
warts, 29, 214-15; *see also*
    spots
washing, hair, 33, 37-8; *see*
    also hygiene
waste elimination, 15
water, in diet, 96-7, 109, 237,
    239; *see also* fluid;
    hydrotherapy
water skiing, 161
wax baths, 241
wax, ear, 53-4
waxing hair, 47
weight, control, 97, 114-17;
    gain, 78, 81, 126-7; ideal,
    112-13, 247; loss, 69, 104,
    111-25, 127-8, 153, 158,
    160-1, 166, 243, 247; *see*